THE
C·O·M·P·L·E·T·E
BOOK OF
VITAMINS
ALL NEW EDITION

by the editors of *Prevention*® magazine

Rodale Press Emmaus, Pa.

Library of Congress Cataloging in Publication Data
Main entry under title:

The Complete book of vitamins.

    Includes index.
    1. Vitamin therapy. 2. Vitamins. I. Prevention
(Emmaus, Pa.)
RM259.C65 1984   615.8'54   83-24583
ISBN 0-87857-495-6 hardcover
ISBN 0-87857-503-0 hardcover deluxe

    6 8 10 9 7 5   hardcover
        8 10 9   hardcover deluxe

Editors: William Gottlieb, Carl Lowe, Mark Bricklin, Susan Zarrow
Contributions by: Stefan Bechtel, Dominick Bosco, Mark Bricklin,
    Randolph Byrd, Colin Covert, Bruce Fellman, John Feltman,
    Alan R. Gaby, M.D., Emil Ginter, Ph.D., William Gottlieb, John
    Kalantari, Jane Kinderlehrer, Jody Kolodzey, Laurie Lucas, Eileen
    Mazer, Emrika Padus, Kerry Pechter, Linda Shaw, Carl Sherman,
    Larry Stains, Debora Tkac, Jonathan Uhlaner, Lewis Vaughn, Tom
    Voss, John Yates
Research Chief: Carol Baldwin
Assistant Research Chief, Prevention Health Books: Christy Kohler
Research Project Coordinator: Carol Sitler Pribulka
Research Associates: Martha Capwell, Tawna Clelan, Christy Kohler,
    Christine Konopelski, Joseph Kosch, Pam Mohr, David Palmer,
    Carole Rapp, Janice Saad, Nancy Smerkanich, Pamela Uhl,
    Diana Witte, Susan Zarrow
Design Project Assistant: John Pepper
Copy Editor: Louise Doucette
Supervisor of Publication Recipe Testing: Anita Hirsch
Office Personnel: Diana Gottshall, Susan Lagler, Carol Petrakovich,
    Cindy Harig, Marge Kressley, Donna Strubeck, Cindy Christman

Notice

THE
C·O·M·P·L·E·T·E
BOOK OF
VITAMINS
ALL NEW EDITION

CONTENTS

List of Tables

BOOK I

Vitamins in Your Daily Life

INTRODUCTION

"A questionable and potentially harmful practice."

That's a quote from researchers at the government's Food and Drug Administration (FDA). The "practice" they're talking about isn't voodoo or child beating. It's taking vitamins.

In a phone survey, the FDA found out that 43 percent of the thousands of people they talked to used supplements. When they asked them *why*, "the most frequently cited benefits of taking supplements were that they made the person feel better and prevented illness."

What's questionable and harmful about that?

Nothing. At least not to you and me. But some experts in the government and the medical establishment seem to have a fixation about vitamins. They don't believe you need to take them. If you do take them, they don't believe they work. (And if *you* say vitamins work, as those folks on the phone did, they think you're deluding yourself.) And so TV and magazines are blitzed with programs and articles telling you that, if you eat a "balanced diet," there's no reason to take a vitamin supplement. And that if you do take one, you'll probably overdose on it and kill yourself. Well, book 1—Vitamins in Your Daily Life—is out to debunk those official myths.

We'll tell you right off the bat why you probably *do* need food supplements. We'll investigate the government's Recommended Dietary Allowances (RDAs) of vitamins and show why they're not set at levels that keep you really healthy. We'll look into the possibility of overdosing on vitamins and show you why a sensible supplement program is virtually risk free. (And we'll give you a program suited to your individual needs.) We'll also describe studies which show that older people could use more vitamins in their diets. And so could people who live where it's polluted. And people who take prescription drugs. And people who diet. And people who have surgery. In short, just about everybody.

So keep up that "practice." It could make your health perfect.

CHAPTER

1

WHY WE NEED
VITAMIN SUPPLEMENTS

The evidence that many people feel better and do better when they take vitamin supplements (along with a good diet) is so overwhelming that few who have investigated the subject with an open mind doubt it. Besides all that's been published, millions of people believe it as a result of personal experience.

Yet, even those of us who are convinced of the wisdom of supplements must stop and wonder every once in a while why so many people seem to need them. Surely nature didn't design human beings to gulp down a handful of pills every day in order to be healthy and strong. Nor is there any famine upon the land: What we see sticking out is not ribs, but bellies. So why should it be that so many people do so much better with supplements? *What's wrong with plain old food?*

Plenty. Probably more than you ever imagined. For instance, you may have asked yourself why so many people seem to need supplements of vitamin C in order to keep their resistance at peak levels. Isn't there enough vitamin C in fresh fruits and vegetables to keep them healthy?

Sure there is, as long as you eat all your fruits and vegetables right in the orchard or garden. If you eat them as most of us do,

4

at home or in a restaurant, you can run into some unexpected problems.

Take oranges, for instance. The orange peel is nature's nutrition preservative. As soon as you take it off and begin to fool around with the orange, the vitamin C begins disappearing.

If you take a fresh orange and juice it yourself, you might think you're getting all the vitamin C that was in the orange, but you aren't. You're leaving about 30 percent of it behind in the residue of the section membranes.

Even if you eat the residue, you've still lost nutrition. The simple act of *juicing* an orange reduces the vitamin C because vitamin C is very sensitive to oxygen. When you break the orange segments and let the juice splash around, you start to destroy vitamin C. When you process oranges (or other C-rich fruits) in a blender, every whirl of the blades encourages vitamin C destruction.

If you buy your orange juice in a waxed cardboard container, pasteurized, and take it to a laboratory, they will probably tell you that the juice has lost something on the order of 20 percent of its original vitamin C. But what they probably won't tell you, because they didn't test it, is that half or more of the vitamin C which is there is biologically inactive—of no apparent use in maintaining or building health.

One of the most surprising examples of unexpected vitamin C loss was reported by Israeli scientists who found that, when oranges are blended with bananas (often to make a fruit mixture for infants), fully 75 to 80 percent of the vitamin C content vanishes—apparently through a reaction between vitamin C and a factor in the bananas *(International Journal for Vitamin and Nutrition Research).*

Vitamin C is so sensitive to human manipulation that, as soon as you put a knife to a fruit or vegetable, the bruise causes vitamin loss. The finer you chop or shred your food, the more vitamin C is lost. And the longer you keep it before eating it, the more is lost. Generally speaking, fruits and vegetables which are processed in the home and kept a day or two before they're eaten have lost anywhere from 30 to 70 percent of their vitamin C.

One final example: Potatoes are not that high in vitamin C but, because many people eat potatoes on a regular basis, they are an extremely important source of that vitamin in the diet. But today, many people eat potatoes reconstituted from instant mixes or eat potato chips which have been made by reassembling dehydrated potatoes. How many consumers realize these products contain no vitamin C whatsoever? According to Richard H. Barnes, Ph.D., former dean of the graduate school of nutrition at Cornell University, "We wonder if anyone knows of any values that are realistic in terms of the ascorbic acid [vitamin C] intake of the American public. It would appear to be something very, very much less than the values that have been calculated from food consumption surveys" *(Nutrients in Processed Foods).*

Government Food Tables May Be Inaccurate

Other people are wondering, too. When Mary K. Head, Ph.D., formerly of the department of food science at North Carolina State University in Raleigh, investigated the nutritional content of foods which were actually being served to students at a cafeteria, she found that the way the food was prepared and served caused considerable nutrient loss *(Journal of the American Dietetic Association).* When we compare some of her figures to those in official government food tables, we find some big differences. Take thiamine, for instance—needed for emotional health, among other things. Government tables say that a 3½-ounce serving of green beans, even when cooked the worst possible way—in lots of water and for a long time—contains 0.06 milligram of thiamine. But the average value found by Dr. Head was only one-third that much! Government tables also say that about 7 ounces of spaghetti with sauce contain 8 milligrams of vitamin C (from the tomato sauce), but Dr. Head's figures show that what the students were eating contained a mere 1.2 milligrams. Eighty-five percent of the vitamin C had dropped out.

The examples of how nutrients are missing or lost in unexpected ways are practically endless. Some of them are no big secret. A good example is that milling whole grain products to produce white flour reduces valuable vitamins, minerals and fiber by an average of 70 to 80 percent. Many also know that boiling vegetables in water for extended periods of time is nutritional murder. Folate (folic acid) is vital to healthy blood, energy and a smoothly functioning nervous system. Boil most vegetables in water until they're done, and you wind up with more folate in the water than you have in the vegetables! Boil cabbage until it's done, and you have only 25 percent of the vitamin C you had when you dropped it into the pot.

Canning is another killer. One recent study showed that 44 percent of the vitamin C originally present in raw peas is lost in the canning process. There was no big surprise in that, scientists reported. Food composition tables will tell you the same. The surprise, they said, is that 42 percent of the vitamin C which is left is actually found in the liquid in which the peas are canned, rather than the peas themselves. So if you want to get the amount of vitamic C the food tables tell you you're supposed to get, you'll have to eat your peas with a spoon instead of a fork!

Many people believe that organ meats are rich sources of the B vitamins—and rightly so. The problem, again, is the difference between theory and practice. When you brown various organ meats on top of your stove, for instance, you are losing from one-third to two-thirds of the thiamine (B_1) and about one-third of the riboflavin (vitamin B_2). Just the thaw drip from frozen meats that you are preparing to cook can seriously deplete B vitamins. Fully one-third of all pantothenate (pantothenic acid) in beefsteak, for example, literally drips out of your meat before you even cook it—which will, of course, destroy still more. Vitamin B_6 is another nutrient, particularly important to women and older people, which is destroyed in cooking. While meat is generally a good source of vitamin B_6, if you eat your meat well done, you may lose up to 70 percent of the B_6 in the cooking process.

Cooking methods aside, what's in the water you cook with can also make a difference. Baking soda added to vegetables causes considerable destruction to thiamine. Japanese scientists recently demonstrated that, when rice is cooked in water which has been chlorinated, there is considerably more destruction of thiamine than when it's cooked in distilled water because chlorine reacts chemically with thiamine (*Journal of Nutritional Science and Vitaminology*, vol. 25, no. 4, 1979). And speaking of rice, be aware that, if you wash your rice before boiling it, you are destroying anywhere from 10 to 25 percent of the thiamine before you even cook it!

Remember, we aren't even talking about people who need extra nutrients because of special stress or illness or dieting. We're only talking about how reasonably healthy people, eating a normal, typical diet, are being shortchanged of nutrition. But even without special problems, getting the proper nutrition from your food isn't as easy as it's cracked up to be. The often-heard statement that you can get all the nutrition you need from a well-balanced diet of "ordinary food" is totally out of touch with reality. Food may be good enough on paper, but not in real life. It's like getting a salary that's adequate—until you pay all your taxes and deductions!

Our food is being taxed the very same way. Only many of the taxes are invisible. We think the food value is there, but it isn't.

And that, in a nutshell, is why so many people who use vitamin supplements as one method of improving nutrition so often find themselves feeling more alert, energetic and less bothered by a host of ailments, minor and major. When combined with smarter food selections and better food preparation, supplements can make a big difference. It's like giving your health a "raise"!

2

SUPPLEMENTS FOR OPTIMAL HEALTH: WHY THE RDAs AREN'T HIGH ENOUGH

Vitamins are powerful substances. We need only microscopic amounts of them in our diets to stay healthy, but take away those teeny quantities and our bodies soon run into deep metabolic trouble.

Scientists originally discovered vitamins while examining deficiency diseases—the devastating medical problems that occur when your diet lacks a particular vitamin. First, they pinpointed what foods could cure these diseases, and then they isolated the chemicals in the foods that were the sources of the cure.

The chemicals they discovered function in our bodies as coenzymes. That means they combine with the body's enzymes to promote the intimate processes that take place in each of the cells. They act as catalysts. They help vital chemical reactions take place that could not occur without their presence.

All vitamins are organic. In their natural state, they're all produced by plants or animals and they find their way into your body when you eat a plant or animal that contains them. But even though plants and some animals can make vitamins, human bodies generally can't. If you don't take in a vitamin in the food you eat or in a vitamin supplement, then you don't get it.

RDAs—Health Designed by Committee

Most of us are familiar with the phrase "Recommended Dietary Allowance (RDA)." You often see the RDAs referred to as part of the nutrition information on food labels. Or else they may be used in an advertising campaign: "One ounce of our cereal contains 75 percent of the Recommended Dietary Allowances of these seven important vitamins." The RDA is the amount of each nutrient which, according to a panel of nutrition authorities, is enough to keep the average person healthy.

Most orthodox nutritionists believe that, if your diet contains the RDA for all nutrients, there is nothing to be gained by taking additional supplements. A growing group of scientists, doctors and informed laymen disagree. They contend that many people can benefit from taking some nutrients in amounts greater than the RDAs.

This controversy, which has been brewing for many years, will not be resolved anytime soon. It is therefore important that anyone interested in nutrition understand what the RDAs actually mean. How are they determined? To whom do they apply? How should they be used? What are their limitations?

The Recommended Dietary Allowances are discussed in a book with the same title. This book is revised about every five years to keep up with new research. It is written by a panel of scientists considered to be experts in the field of nutrition. None of the well-known dissenters in the field, however, such as Linus Pauling, Ph.D., Roger Williams, Ph.D., Carlton Fredericks, Ph.D., or Emanuel Cheraskin, M.D., are members of this panel.

The RDAs are defined as "the levels of intake of essential nutrients considered, in the judgment of the Committee on Dietary Allowances of the Food and Nutrition Board on the basis of available scientific knowledge, to be adequate to meet the known nutritional needs of practically all healthy persons." This definition seems easy enough to understand, but it is not as straightforward as it looks. It is a very carefully worded statement which must be just as carefully interpreted.

What, for example, is meant by the phrase "practically all"? Researchers know that nutrient requirements vary widely from person to person—some need considerably more than others. Because of this variation, a small group of research subjects cannot be reliably used to predict the needs of an entire population. Since it is not possible to guarantee that everyone will be protected, a level of intake is chosen which the statistician predicts will cover the needs of 97 percent. In other words, about 3 percent of the people need more than the RDA for any particular nutrient. There is, unfortunately, no way of knowing whether you are among the unlucky few who will develop a deficiency by consuming what the committee has recommended.

You might argue that a 3-percent risk is not great enough to justify taking a bunch of supplements. That, of course, is an individual choice. But your chances of having a deficiency are actually much greater than 3 percent. That is because you are taking the same risk with each of the 40 or so essential nutrients. When you have to take the same 3-percent risk 40 times, your odds do not look very good. A mathematician would tell you that, if you take in exactly the RDA for each essential nutrient, you will have at least a 50-50 chance of becoming deficient in one or more nutrients. With those odds, it is not unreasonable to take out an insurance policy of sorts by consuming more than the RDAs. While that may or may not improve your health, it is quite unlikely to do any harm.

Another phrase in the RDA definition that requires explanation is "healthy persons." The committee clearly points out that the RDAs apply only to those in good health. "Special needs for nutrients arising from such problems as . . . inherited metabolic disorders, infections, chronic disease and the use of medications require special dietary and therapeutic measures. These conditions are not covered by the RDA.''

So if you find that increasing your intake of vitamins and minerals relieves the symptoms of your arthritis (a chronic disease), you should get no argument from believers in the RDA. Likewise, the vitamin C requirement for the common cold (an infection) is not included in these nutritional guidelines. If you have developed unexplained depression after using an oral contraceptive, that drug has probably caused an unusually large need for vitamin B_6. If you have heart disease, diabetes, cancer, recurrent infections, chronic diarrhea, anemia or other disorders, your nutritional needs are likely to be increased.

What if you do not have any of these diseases? Does that mean you are healthy? Does the RDA apply to you? Actually, a case could be made that very few of us are truly healthy—that we are a nation of chronically ill people. One out of three of us will develop heart disease; one out of five will die of cancer. Three of ten women will develop severe thinning of their bones after the reproductive years. Millions of men will suffer from prostate troubles as they get older. While our bodies are slowly developing these problems, we should not be considered healthy even though we may feel well. For if we were better nourished, the degeneration would probably proceed at a slower pace. It might even be prevented entirely. The millions who require medication for anxiety, depression or pain are also chronically ill. Perhaps better nutrition could help these people, too.

Another large group of people for whom the RDAs may not apply are the elderly. As people get older, they lose the ability to absorb nutrients efficiently. As a result, nutrient needs become greater. The committee is aware of these increased needs. But since few experiments have been done with the elderly, no one is sure how much to recommend.

So there are quite a few people who are not covered by the standards set forth in the RDAs. But what about those to whom the guidelines do apply? What do the RDAs mean? How are they determined? The committee answers these questions as follows: ''For certain nutrients the requirements may be assessed as the amount that will just prevent failure of a specific function or the development of specific deficiency signs—an amount that may differ greatly from that required to maintain maximum body stores. Thus, there are differences of opinion about the criteria that should be used to establish requirements.''

In other words, the committee is setting minimal requirements for minimal health. It is clear they are not interested in the question of whether larger amounts can promote metabolic excellence or optimal health. But accumulating evidence suggests that better nutrition can do just that.

Nutritional supplements can help detoxify environmental poisons. They may decrease the adverse physical and emotional effects of stress, minimize the risk of infections and promote more healthy skin. The list of possible benefits from optimal nutrition is long. The goal of promoting excellent health obviously demands different nutritional standards than the mere desire to avoid serious illness.

We might, therefore, wish to use other criteria than the committee has decided upon. For example, those with elevated levels of serum cholesterol may need more of the nutrients that can lower cholesterol, such as niacin, calcium and vitamin C. Another criterion that could be used is the activity of our blood platelets. Many people have overactive platelets, which might increase their risk of developing a dangerous blood clot in an artery or vein. These people may have a greater need for vitamin E, vitamin B_6 and essential fatty acids, all of which can reduce platelet activity (if you are taking an anticoagulant medication, consult your doctor before acting on this information).

The requirement for the antioxidant nutrients (selenium, vitamin E, vitamin C and zinc) might depend on the number of pollutants and cancer-causing agents that are working at oxidizing your cells. The need for calcium and chromium should vary with the amount of sugar you consume, since these nutrients are known to be depleted by excess sugar.

When you use criteria such as these to establish nutrient needs, a comprehensive nutrition program beings to look more sensible than the traditionalists would have you believe.

Some Misleading Statements from the Food Industry

One additional point to keep in mind is that the RDAs can be used by industry to make a product appear more nutritious than it really is. For example, a manufacturer might create a "fruit drink" from sugar, artificial color, artificial flavor, preservatives and vitamin C. Advertisements for this product would focus on the fact that it contains 100 percent of the RDA for vitamin C. It might not occur to the consumer that this drink has little else to offer and could even be harmful. Or else consider a cereal made from grain which has been refined to the point where dozens of different nutrients have been lost. If a few of these nutrients are added back in the "enriching" process, claims can be made that the cereal contains 100 percent of the RDA for various vitamins. Do not let these advertisements persuade you that everything lost in the refining process has been replaced.

Minimal or Optimal Nutrition?

The RDAs were originally designed to ensure that large segments of the population would not develop serious nutritional deficiencies. They were first published during World War II, when there was concern about the adequacy of the K rations being fed to our troops. For these purposes, the RDAs have provided valuable information. But if you are trying to do more with nutrition, if you are interested in relieving the suffering of disease, preventing chronic illness, warding off the effects of stress, increasing your energy level, relieving anxiety or depression or getting rid of the cramps in your legs or the numbness and tingling in your fingers, then the RDAs have little to offer.

We are, of course, grateful to the hard-working experts who have spent much time in producing the Recommended Dietary

Allowances. But we must recognize, as they do, the three major limitations of these guidelines:

1. They apply only to healthy people, a group that is rapidly becoming extinct in our polluted and stressful environment.
2. Their purpose is to guarantee a minimal, rather than optimal, level of nutrition.
3. There is a high probability that even a totally healthy person looking only for the minimum will need more than the RDA for some nutrients.

So, when planning your nutrition program, be sure to keep the RDAs in mind. That way you will not forget to include at least the bare minimum for all the known essential nutrients. But remember that the ultimate in good health requires more than just the bare minimum.

3

HOW MUCH? A GUIDE TO PERSONAL VITAMIN SUPPLEMENTATION

No one can say what level of supplementation is exactly right for you. With changes occurring almost continuously in our bodies, our diets and our environments—not to mention changes in nutritional science itself—it is just not possible to be terribly precise.

Still, we need some general guidelines that will put us in the right church, if not the exact pew, so far as supplements are concerned. That's what we're trying to provide here.

Please keep in mind the following:

1. These guidelines are not specific recommendations, but rather general, informational statements which inevitably reflect a certain degree of personal opinion as well as current research.

2. For each nutrient, read the paragraph of descriptive statements accompanying the various amounts. *Find the paragraph which most sounds like you.* It is not necessary, or in some cases even possible, for each sentence in the paragraph to describe you spe-

cifically. Go with the one that, *overall,* seems most applicable.
3. Don't try to use the information here to pin-point nutritional causes of symptoms. Analyzing serious symptoms is your doctor's job.

Vitamin A

5,000 international units: Your diet regularly includes liver, carrots, broccoli, apricots, sweet potatoes and spinach. You are generally in excellent health, your resistance is very high and the environment in which you live is low in pollutants. Naturally, you are not a smoker and never have been. Nor are there any smokers in your household. There is nothing in your family history that makes you particularly concerned about cancer.

10,000 international units: You eat vitamin A–rich foods such as liver, carrots and sweet potatoes occasionally, but they're not on your menu every day. Your health is better than average, but you are not invulnerable, and you know that when your resistance gets low you tend to become ill, perhaps with upper respiratory symptoms. Skin problems are not unknown to you. You are exposed to an average amount of pollution from various sources.

25,000 international units: Occasionally, you notice patches of dry, bumpy skin on your legs or arms. Not dry and flaky, but dry and *bumpy.* Recently, you may have been involved in a serious health crisis such as surgery, an injury, a burn or another problem that had you out of circulation for more than just a few days. Your vision, especially at dusk, is not what it could be. Foods such as liver, spinach and carrots have been known to appear on your dining room table, but they are hardly fixtures.

(Normally, supplements of vitamin A should not exceed about 40,000 international units per day. Very large amounts— usually well over 100,000 international units per day—can cause symptoms of toxicity, such as dry skin and loss of appetite. The amounts mentioned in this guide, however, are perfectly safe for adults.)

Thiamine (Vitamin B$_1$)

5 milligrams: You're practically famous for your perpetual good mood and unflagging energy. Your diet regularly includes brewer's yeast, wheat germ, whole grain products, nuts, liver and sunflower seeds.

10 milligrams: You're generally a frisky sort, even though you aren't necessarily ready to conquer the world at the dawn of each and every day. There are times when you wish your nerves were better behaved, and you sometimes think you drink too much coffee or tea for your own good. Your diet is average.

25 milligrams: Your nerves are definitely in a state, and you may be suffering from depression, loss of appetite or similar emotional and neurological problems. Your energy levels are at best undependable, as is your memory. Possibly, you are in your retirement years, when absorption of thiamine—as well as other B vitamins—is very much reduced.

Riboflavin (Vitamin B$_2$)

5 milligrams: You're a great one for dairy foods like milk, cheese and eggs. Almonds, asparagus, broccoli, liver, wheat germ and other riboflavin-rich foods appear in your daily fare. Your eyes are clear and bright and the skin around your mouth is perfectly smooth—except when you smile, which you do frequently.

10 milligrams: Milk and liver you don't care for, cheese and eggs have too much cholesterol for you, and wild rice and asparagus are too expensive. So you don't get that much riboflavin in your diet except from your whole grain bread. You are also getting up there in years.

25 milligrams: If you look in the mirror carefully, you will see small cracks around your mouth, or your tongue may be smooth and purplish. Your eyes may burn, itch, be abnormally sensitive to bright light or simply feel worn out. You may feel depressed. You are no spring chicken.

Niacin

10 milligrams: Your diet regularly includes fish, beans, organ meats, peanuts, poultry, whole wheat products and brewer's yeast—or at least half of those foods. Your disposition is strictly blue sky. The only time you are irritable is when enemy tanks invade your neighborhood.

25 milligrams: Your diet is nothing to brag about, particularly, and occasionally you wonder if there is some reason why it's becoming so difficult for you to fall asleep or if your headaches have some peculiar origin.

50 milligrams: Your nerves and your personality are definitely not what they used to be and not what your friends or family would like them to be. You may have thought about visiting a psychologist or psychiatrist, and you would be grateful if something could be done about your insomnia.

Vitamin B$_6$ (Pyridoxine)

5 milligrams: You practically radiate good health, and your positive, energetic attitude is reflected in your intelligently varied diet, which includes wheat germ, brown rice, salmon, peanuts, liver, bananas and, of course, whole grains.

10 milligrams: You certainly aren't sick, but you sometimes wonder why your skin isn't better or why your nerves aren't calmer. You may tend to retain a lot of fluid before your menstrual periods.

50 milligrams: Your monthly periods cause you considerable distress, not only because of fluid retention, but because of emotional problems at that time—or perhaps *all* the time. Possibly, you are on birth control pills. Life is looking more and more like an ordeal.

Vitamin B₁₂

5 micrograms: You are healthy, energetic, haven't yet reached retirement age, and you regularly eat animal foods such as meat, fish or chicken.

10 micrograms: You've passed your 60th birthday, and your ability to absorb this vitamin in a useful form may be on the wane.

25 micrograms: Lately, your energy level, and possibly your nerves, just haven't been up to snuff. Possibly, you've been ill or had surgery. You may be a strict vegan, one who avoids all animal-source foods. These symptoms may well be serious enough to suggest a thorough medical evaluation.

Folate (Folic Acid)

400 micrograms: You eat a lot of raw green vegetables such as broccoli, asparagus and spinach. You're a liver lover from way back, and you eat it with onions. You are full of energy, and retirement is something that's far in the future.

400 to 800 micrograms: You must remind yourself that y⸱u should eat raw green vegetables more frequently, and you wish you were able to work out a way to eat beans, broccoli, asparagus, wheat germ, tempeh and whole wheat products more often than you do. Your health is about average.

800 to 2,000 micrograms: Lately, you feel as though you've been under considerable emotional stress, and you haven't been able to handle it as well as you should. Your nerves in general have been in such a state that you have given serious consideration to seeking some kind of help, whether medical, psychological or even nutritional. You are over 70 years of age and your absorption of folate, therefore, is likely to be impaired. Possibly, you have recently undergone surgery. Your doctor may have reason to believe you have folate deficiency anemia, which causes, among other things, inflammation of the tongue, digestive problems and diarrhea. (When taking folate supplements, always take vitamin B_{12} with them.)

Vitamin C

100 milligrams: You can hardly remember the last time you were ill. Your health is excellent, and your gums are clear, firm and never bleed. Your daily diet includes generous measures of such vitamin C–rich foods as broccoli, cabbage, melons, citrus fruits and green peppers.

500 milligrams: You feel that your resistance must be maintained at a high level in order to keep you feeling your best. There may be some chronic health problem or stress in your life, such as a bad back, allergies or exposure to cigarette smoke. Your diet is not bad by a long shot, but it does not supply the amount of vitamin C you feel you should get.

2,000 milligrams: You are definitely susceptible to stresses such as infection, pain or skin problems. Possibly, you are recovering from surgery, an injury or any other serious bout with illness. In the past, you have noticed that injury or surgical incisions seem to heal very slowly. Your diet could be better, but it is difficult for you to eat raw foods, high in vitamin C, because they tend to make your gums bleed. You may want to step down to a lower level of vitamin C supplementation when the health problem or crisis you are now undergoing disappears.

Vitamin D

0 to 200 international units: You live in an area where the sun shines strong and bright, such as Florida or southern California. What's more, you move around quite a bit outdoors, so sunlight strikes your body, causing your system to manufacture its own vitamin D. If you have a year-round tan, you probably don't need any supplemental vitamin D at all.

400 international units: You live in an area such as Pennsylvania or Washington state, where a beautiful sunshiny day is a real event. You are not a big drinker of milk, which is fortified with vitamin D, usually at the rate of about 400 international units per quart. Occasionally, however, you do eat fish containing vitamin D, such as herring, mackerel, salmon, sardines and tuna.

800 international units: You probably live in the northern United States, Canada or England, where, except for a few weeks in the middle of summer, intense sunshine may be as rare as rainbows. What's more, for one reason or another, you do not get very much exercise outdoors. Possibly you have had a problem with your bones, suffering a fracture or pain. Although a physician may recommend considerably higher supplements, you should not ordinarily take more than this amount on your own each day, as vitamin D tends to accumulate in the body, and very large amounts (usually many thousands of international units) can become toxic.

Vitamin E

100 international units: You are relatively young, in fine health, and you live in an exceptionally clean area, where there is remarkably little pollution.

400 international units: You may have a health condition which may be prevented or improved with vitamin E, such as intermittent claudication (cramping of the calf on walking) or any one of a number of skin problems. The air you breathe, the water you drink and, possibly, the food you eat contain the usual amount of pollutants found in our modern world. Your diet contains a substantial amount of polyunsaturated fats such as corn oil.

600 international units: You may be concerned about a circulation problem and feel that the beneficial effect of vitamin E on blood elements is something that you want to take advantage of in full measure.

CHAPTER

4

GETTING THE MOST FROM YOUR VITAMINS: A PLAN FOR MAXIMAL ABSORPTION

Even if you're taking all the right vitamin supplements, you may be getting less out of them than you think you are! But don't despair—nutritional "fuel efficiency" is easy to achieve if you keep a few simple concepts in mind.

"Generally, vitamins are absorbed best when they are taken with other foods and minerals," counsels Harold Rosenberg, M.D., past president of the International Academy of Preventive Medicine, in *The Doctor's Book of Vitamin Therapy* (G. P. Putnam's Sons, 1974). "The best time is after meals and as evenly throughout the day as possible."

This matter of good timing can't be overemphasized either, for taken at the wrong time—on an empty stomach, in particular—even the most beneficial supplement can pass through your body with less than optimal results. After all, it's only the nutrients actually *absorbed* by your digestive system—this takes place primarily in your small intestine—that can work their metabolic magic.

Combining supplements with meals, then, is the best way to give nature a helping hand.

"The nutrients were in your food in the first place," Dr. Rosenberg says. "And when you're eating, tastes and odors—

the entire range of gustatory and sensual factors—stimulate and excite the digestive enzymes. Primed by even something as simple as a piece of fruit or a slice of whole wheat bread, these enzymes are ready for the vitamins and minerals.''

So you needn't fear your supplements will get lost in a crowd.

"Though everything goes in the kettle at the same time, the body has a fairly broad tolerance level for unscrambling what we put in in scrambled form,'' explains Rebecca Riales, Ph.D., a clinical nutritionist from Parkersburg, West Virginia.

And once unscrambled, many nutrients must form partnerships with other substances found in food in order to be absorbed fully.

Vitamins That Need Fat

Fat in your meal acts like a chauffeur service for vitamins A, D, E and K, the fat-soluble vitamins.

"For example, if you take vitamin E on an empty stomach, there's almost no absorption,'' Dr. Riales notes. "And you'll have the same trouble if you take a multivitamin with, say, a breakfast of skim milk and cold cereal—there's almost no fat in the meal and you'll wind up absorbing very little of the fat-soluble vitamins.''

But drink a glass of whole milk, add a pat of butter to your oatmeal or some vinegar and oil to your salad, and the increase in nutrient absorption can be "tremendous,'' according to Hugo Gallo-Torres, M.D., Ph.D., senior research physician of the department of gastroenterology, medical research, at Hoffmann-La Roche, Inc.

"Fat-containing foods may also prolong absorption,'' he explains, citing a wealth of recent research from Japan.

But what about the water-soluble vitamins—the B complex and C?

"These are well absorbed with or without food, but taking them with a meal can slow the *rate* of absorption (although it won't decrease the total amount absorbed),'' says Dr. Riales.

And that can be beneficial.

Initially, you might absorb more of a B or C supplement on an empty stomach than you would with a meal. But doses absorbed too quickly are excreted too quickly to have long-term effects on body concentrations. On the other hand, stretching out the absorption time as you digest your food will result in increased levels of the nutrient in your blood over a longer period of time.

It's a case of "slow and steady" winning the race, and it has inspired the suggestion that you take your supplements in divided doses throughout the day, rather than all at once.

Michael Mayersohn, Ph.D., and his colleagues at the University of Arizona tested this idea with vitamin C. Working with three people, they gave each a gram (1,000 milligrams) of vitamin C daily for two weeks. One person took the vitamin in a single dose, the second received the gram in eight small doses and the third also took the entire dose of the supplement at once, but after eating a high-fat meal.

"The divided dose and after-meal treatments produced a significant increase in AA [ascorbic acid, i.e., vitamin C] absorption compared to the corresponding control experiment, 72 percent and 69 percent increase, respectively," they wrote (*Life Sciences,* vol. 28, no. 22, 1981).

"From a practical point of view, efficiency of AA absorption may be improved by either dividing up a daily dose into several smaller doses taken during the day or by ingesting the vitamin after a meal."

Dr. Rosenberg mentions that the B vitamins are also best taken throughout the day.

"Every requirement of the human body operates on a twenty-four-hour cycle. Your cells do not go to sleep when you do, nor can they survive without continuous oxygen and nutrients."

Nutrient Interactions

Some nutrients just naturally go together, practicing a kind of vitamin-and-mineral teamwork when it comes to maximizing absorption.

Take calcium, for example.

Divided doses of the mineral teamed with vitamin C can increase the percentage of calcium absorbed, notes Dr. Riales. And combining vitamin C with calcium is "worthwhile—especially if you're older. Vitamin C's acidity seems to help calcium remain soluble and hence available for absorption."

And, of course, there's the team of vitamin D—the "sunshine vitamin"—and calcium. This vitamin regulates how much of the bone-building mineral is absorbed through your intestine, so you'll want both on your team.

There are many other examples of nutrient teamwork, but most of them take place *after* absorption.

But that's not so with vitamin C and iron.

If you're a woman eating less red meat and gaining more of your protein from plant sources, this vitamin-mineral pair's teamwork is especially important.

The iron in plants plays "hard to get," but vitamin C can overcome that and make a sizable portion of the mineral ready, willing and able when it comes to intestinal absorption, according to Sean Lynch, M.D., of the department of medicine at the University of Kansas.

"But you have to take the vitamin with your meals," he emphasizes.

And again, taking the C in divided doses—say, with each meal—makes that much more iron available from your food.

Zinc Helps Folate Absorption

If you want maximum folate (folic acid) absorption from your food or vitamin supplements, it's a good idea to take zinc along with it.

Researchers at the University of California at Berkeley found that, when healthy volunteers were put on a diet that depleted their reserves of zinc, the absorption of folate dropped sharply. Why? The folate-containing compounds in foods, polyglutamyl folates, must be split by an enzyme before folate can be absorbed. And this enzyme, they suggested, requires zinc *(FASEB Proceedings)*.

While you're making sure your diet has all the nutrients essential for healthy absorption, you might also consider the negative effect of nonessentials like additives. According to one study, the common preservative EDTA can reduce the absorption of iron.

Nutrient Absorption Declines with Age

In general, the older you are, the greater the chance you'll run into absorption problems. A decline of secretions of stomach acid and digestive enzymes means poorer absorption of iron and protein.

Less and less of the B vitamins and such minerals as calcium, too, make it out of your digestive tract and into your bloodstream. This is one reason why older people are so often beset with nutritional ills. Poor absorption means poor nutrition, which will impair absorption further—starting a cycle that is difficult to stop. Is this inevitable?

"There are widespread differences in the ability to absorb nutrients," says Mark Tager, M.D., who practices wellness-oriented medicine in Oregon. "At least part is rooted in individual history—how a person has used or abused his digestive tract during his lifetime." The continual use of stimulants, like caffeine, may take its toll over time. So can years of neglected stomach and bowel problems.

By the same token, attention to those things that promote healthy digestion and absorption pays a double bonus: now and in the future. Making mealtime (and the hours afterward) relaxed and pleasant is more than just a civilized idea for this reason. "I'd suggest a quiet period surrounding digestion," says Dr. Tager. "It does little good to throw in good food and then damage digestion by stress."

Exercise will give your digestive system the same benefits it gives the rest of your body. "Individuals who don't exercise, who don't get enough oxygen to the cells, tend to have poor absorption patterns," Dr. Tager says. "Yoga exercises that aim at using stomach and intestinal muscles can do particular good."

But where digestion and absorption are concerned, the main thing, appropriately enough, is food. Dr. Tager emphasizes the virtues of raw foods, whole grains and vegetables. Many people may want to add vitamin and mineral supplements to sound diets based on whole, natural foods, to ensure an adequate supply of all the nutrients necessary for efficient absorption. What it comes down to is this: A high-quality diet will help your body get from your food all the good things that nature put into it.

And that logic is hard to question.

CHAPTER
5

DO YOU HAVE "HIDDEN HUNGER"?

Suppose for a moment that you were usually so dog tired you couldn't even get out of your chair to do your household chores. Or suppose you couldn't sleep at night. Or you were so cranky most of the time that you felt like snapping everyone's head off. Or you were just getting sick much too often.

If this sounds like you, then your body may be telling you it has a "hidden hunger" for the proper levels of vitamins.

Technically, such hidden hunger is called subclinical, or marginal, malnutrition. "If a person has a subclinical nutritional deficiency, he or she might appear perfectly normal," says Frank Beaudet, an instructor at the Leonard Davis School of Gerontology, University of Southern California. "There will be no obvious symptoms that anything is wrong nutritionally. But when the person is under physical or emotional stress, then we will see the full impact of marginal levels of nutrition."

A person with hidden hunger sounds like an accident waiting to happen. "In many ways that's true," Beaudet says. "Subclinical malnutrition can lead to, among other things, an increased susceptibility to disease and a longer recovery time from surgery. It could even lead to an adverse reaction to a flu vaccination due to lowered immune response."

Is subclinical malnutrition something new? "Not really," says Beaudet. "But it has only been recognized within about the past five years. Our knowledge of, and ability to recognize, subclinical malnutrition have developed along with the renaissance in nutrition, in general, and, geriatric nutrition, in particular."

Is the problem very widespread? "Malnutrition itself is not an epidemic among older adults," Beaudet says. "But countless numbers suffer from subclinical malnutrition—and may not even be aware of it."

Your body may have a hidden hunger for one or more vitamins. "In the United States today, we rarely see cases of classical vitamin deficiency, such as scurvy and pellagra," says Richard Rivlin, M.D., of the Memorial Sloan-Kettering Cancer Center and New York Hospital–Cornell Medical Center, New York City. "But we are now beginning to recognize a vast new series of marginal deficiencies related to disease and therapy. . . . Marginal deficiency, it now appears, may be a surprisingly common phenomenon."

In a paper presented to the Vitamin Nutrition Issues Symposium in Boca Raton, Florida, in October, 1979, Dr. Rivlin used riboflavin (vitamin B_2) to illustrate his point. He noted that animal studies have shown that, when your body is low in riboflavin, the production of an enzyme that the body needs to use the riboflavin in the first place is inhibited. "The less [riboflavin] you have," said Dr. Rivlin, "the less you are able to utilize; once the body gets sick, it gets sicker, because it lacks the enzyme and therefore cannot utilize what little vitamin there is in the diet. . . . The important concept is that deficiency itself produces changes in the ability to utilize that same vitamin.

"Riboflavin is important in blood formation, in the brain, in fat metabolism, in degrading drugs and foreign substances and in maintaining the skin. And because one vitamin is involved in the metabolism of another, the effects of one deficiency are compounded by effects upon others."

Several other factors also can create a hidden hunger for riboflavin. "Boric acid, for example, which is present in some 400 home products such as mouth washes, suppositories and imported foods, claws onto the sugar portion of the riboflavin, binds it and takes it out in the urine. The amount of boric acid ingested by the population is obviously variable; but if individuals are taking boric acid over a long period of time in low amounts, they may be at risk for gradually getting a degree of vitamin depletion."

Dr. Rivlin pointed out that drugs such as the tranquilizer chlorpromazine, if taken over a long period of time, can also cause a riboflavin deficiency. "The same principle is true for other nutrients," he said. "Drugs and hormones may act as antagonists or enhancers, and one should really look at nutrition not only from the standpoint of diet, but also from the standpoint of metabolism.

"While there are many challenging problems that lie ahead in nutrition, we are very much concerned with the fact that marginal deficiencies due to drugs or hormones may be a very common problem. We are actively pursuing these problems, and I think this is the type of thing that one will be hearing much more about in future years."

Guarding against Hidden Hunger

Subclinical malnutrition is a complex problem and one whose seriousness is only now being fully recognized. Although the answers aren't all in, health professionals do recommend various steps you can take to make sure you don't have hidden hunger.

Arnold Schaefer, Ph.D., executive director of the Swanson Center for Nutrition in Omaha, Nebraska, says that drug-induced vitamin and mineral deficiencies can be avoided if you take high-potency nutritional supplements.

Frank Beaudet points out that, since our taste perception decreases with age, many older people do not eat properly because their food seems relatively tasteless. "We should increase the amount of seasoning in our food as we grow older," says Beaudet. "That means using more of such green herbs as basil and tarragon and using more garlic or onion for a more flavorful diet.

"The best recommendation I can make for older people is to try to eat a diet with foods as high in nutrient density as possible." Beaudet says, "That means foods with high nutrition per calorie. Foods with low nutrient density, like pastry, should be avoided.

"Older people are regularly under emotional and physical stresses, and proper nutrition can cushion the effects of those stresses. No older person should have to suffer from the effects of subclinical malnutrition."

CHAPTER
6

NUTRIENTS FOR
THE CRITICAL YEARS

We all know there are often health problems and pain involved in aging. We know that drugs can relieve pain and sometimes correct the causes of it. But drugs very seldom act on the body in one single, beneficial way. There is generally a mixed bag of effects, and the bag gets larger the more drugs you take.

The really disturbing thing about this situation is that the medications the elderly take can often deplete nutritional stores that are already dangerously low. A host of prescription and nonprescription drugs, everything from aspirin to glucocorticoids, have been shown to rob the body of essential nutrients. Many of those drugs are routinely taken by older people for years, to counter the effects of chronic illnesses.

At the same time, as people get older, their bodies change. They make changes in the way they live, including their meal patterns. Often the result is a system denied the nutrients it needs to handle the stresses of old age, including the stress of increased medication.

Large segments of the elderly population of the United States are suffering from multiple nutritional deficiencies. A survey of older Missouri residents found that half of the women and one-fifth of the men were getting less than 67 percent of the Recommended Dietary Allowance for one or more nutrients *(American Journal of Clinical Nutrition)*.

A government survey of low-income districts in ten states discovered that at least half of the elderly women and a third of the elderly men were getting inadequate amounts of niacin in their diets. Thirty percent of the elderly people in that survey had unacceptably low levels of protein in their blood.

Nearly all of the subjects of a survey of older people in Montgomery County, Virginia, reported that they took in less than the recommended allowance for vitamin B_6 *(Nutrition Reports International)*.

Drugs That Destroy Vitamins

And the elderly are the people who consume more prescription drugs than any other group in the country. People 65 or over, although just one-tenth of the U.S. population, consume nearly a quarter of all drugs prescribed. The average elderly American takes 13 different drugs in the course of a single year. *That means that the people nutritionally least equipped to cope with the stress of medication receive the most of it.*

For example, there is evidence that barbiturates, prescribed as tranquilizers and sleeping aids, may lower the amount of calcium in the blood by disrupting the metabolism of vitamin D. Vitamin D is necessary for the proper absorption and utilization of calcium. Phenobarbital, a barbiturate that in high doses is used to prevent epileptic seizures, has been linked to altered vitamin D metabolism and resulting cases of osteomalacia, a softening of the bone caused by a lack of calcium.

In other research, scientists have found that barbiturates increase the excretion of vitamin C from the body, as well.

Glucocorticoids—the family of anti-inflammatory drugs used to relieve the symptoms of arthritis—can also play havoc with the body's nutritional balance. Glucocorticoid treatment can cause a form of osteoporosis, a classic deficiency disease in which bone density drops as a result of a lack of calcium. Children receiving long-term glucocorticoid therapy for kidney disease have been shown to have low blood levels of the most active metabolic product of vitamin D *(Lancet)*. Scientists believe the action of the glucocortocoids against vitamin D produces low levels of calcium in the blood, which, in turn, can cause bone-weakening osteoporosis. Treatment with the same drugs may also lead to potassium deficiency and can have a similar effect on vitamin C levels.

Older people receiving treatment for heart ailments are up against an array of drugs which can undermine their nutritional defenses.

Digitalis, for example, can increase the body's requirements for thiamine. Hydralazine, a drug used to treat hypertension, can cause vitamin B_6 deficiency.

Diuretics administered to counter high blood pressure can flush enough potassium out of the system to cause a deficiency. The diuretic triamterene works without depleting the body's potassium, but, unfortunately, it interferes with the utilization of folate (folic acid), an essential member of the B vitamin group. Like other diuretics, it can also produce excessive excretion of calcium.

The Problem with Mineral Oil

Nutritional problems may crop up even in the course of treatment of minor ailments like headaches and constipation. Mineral oil and phenolphthalein, used as laxatives, can block normal absorption in the digestive tract. Mineral oil dissolves the naturally occurring source of vitamin A, carotene, and it slips untouched through the stomach and intestine. Mineral oil interferes with the absorption of all the fat-soluble vitamins—A, D, E and K—and chronic use, the kind that older people with chronic constipation would practice, may cause deficiencies in all those vitamins.

Headache relief can be just as costly in nutritional terms. Aspirin depletes body tissues of vitamin C; even a small dose can cause the excretion of C from the body to increase threefold. Aspirin also disrupts the body's utilization of folate.

The more you look at this situation, the more you are struck by the way the problem acts to make itself worse. You keep finding vicious circles in which problems turn back in on themselves or pile up on top of each other in ways that can be very discouraging.

For instance, several drugs, including barbiturates, glucocorticoids and aspirin, act to deplete vitamin C. Vitamin C, in turn, is important for the proper metabolism of drugs in the body. If drugs are not metabolized at the correct rate, their effects can be prolonged or their possible toxic side effects increased. And so you have one drug side effect, the depletion of vitamin C, making the dangers of other side effects even worse.

That puts older people, who are often being treated for a number of conditions at once, in a scary position. "Multiple pathology often leads to multiple pharmacy with the increased risk of interactions between drugs and increased toxicity of drugs due to a decreased ability to metabolize them," John Dickerson, Ph.D., professor of nutrition at England's University of Surrey, warned *(Royal Society of Health Journal)*. "Superimposed on this is the fact that illness in the elderly predisposes them to nutritional deficiencies which may be induced by the drugs and also further exacerbate their toxicity."

It's no wonder the number of adverse drug reactions skyrockets with age: The frequency in people age 70 to 79 is seven times that in people age 20 to 29.

Vicious Cycles

Similar vicious cycles are at work in other aspects of the elderly's nutritional problems. Folate deficiency, for example, is common in older people. One study found that 40 percent of elderly subjects had low levels of folate in their blood. A team of scientists led by Herman Baker, Ph.D., of the New Jersey Medical School school of nutrition, showed that older people absorb much less folate from natural sources than younger people *(Journal of the American Geriatrics Society)*. Dr. Baker suggested that the resulting folate deficiency may make the problem even worse by hindering the secretion of an enzyme crucial to the proper breakdown of folate from food.

A vicious cycle is thus begun, according to Dr. Baker. "Aging leads to small-bowel enzyme impairment, which in turn leads to less folate utilization from food, and this intensifies folate depletion." The result: "Because of an inability to utilize food folates, deficiency becomes, if not inevitable, at least common in the elderly."

Life style can also affect nutritional status, particularly in your later years.

In a journal article, Dr. Masud Anwar, consultant physician in geriatric medicine at a hospital in England, described a case history of vitamin D deficiency he had observed *(Journal of the American Geriatrics Society)*. An 80-year-old woman was admitted to the hospital with a history of arthritis that had plagued her for several years. She suffered from swelling of the legs and feet, to the point that she was unable to walk properly, and was chronically depressed. Since she was unable to stand long enough to do any cooking, she lived off canned food, and because of her depression, she often skipped meals altogether.

X rays revealed skeletal structure with low mineral content, and it was apparent from questioning that the woman was getting almost no vitamin D in her diet. She never ate liver, kidney, fish or eggs. She seldom got outside and thus received little vitamin D from natural exposure to sunlight.

The doctors prescribed vitamin D and calcium supplements, and within six months her condition improved markedly. Her bone pains disappeared and she was able to get about on her own, even without the aid of a cane. She became fully independent, able to cook nutritious meals for herself and do her own housework, and she took pride in her independence. Her depression disappeared without any action by the doctors. Physical well-being was obviously the best therapy possible.

"This patient believed that the pain in her thighs was caused by arthritis of the hips," according to Dr. Anwar, "which she considered was due to aging. She did not want to trouble her own doctor. She was afraid to go out, because of inability to walk and lack of confidence, thus depriving herself of exposure to sunlight. Loneliness made her depressed and she lost interest in eating. Thus loneliness, depression and poor eating habits became a vicious cycle which was broken only by admission to the hospital."

The object of the game is to break out of this cycle before you end up in the hospital. It has been estimated that eight million elderly Americans suffer from malnutrition. They are struggling with problems caused by drugs, problems caused by life style, problems caused by changes in the way their bodies work. The sense of taste declines with age, so you want to eat less. The efficiency of digestion declines, so you absorb less of what you eat and need to take in more than a younger person to get the same nutritional benefits.

Modern Diets Are "Diluted"

The peculiarities of the modern diet are no help to older people struggling with all this. Ruth B. Weg, Ph.D., of the Andrus Gerontology Center at the University of Southern California, believes the "dilution" of nutrition in the modern diet poses particular problems for the elderly. In her book, *Nutrition and the Later Years* (USC Press, 1978), she writes, "With the refining and processing of more and more foods, the character of nutrient intake has changed: usually with more sodium than needed, and less potassium, zinc, selenium, chromium, silicon and nickel. Too many extra calories (usually through the addition of sugar and fats) dilute the diet, particularly in relation to minerals and vitamins."

This may have something to do with the fact that, while older people are generally judged to take in fewer calories than the recommended allowance, they are often plagued with obesity. One study found more than 40 percent of its aged subjects to be overweight. The elderly use inefficient digestive systems to consume inefficient fuel.

"Empty calories" are especially dangerous for people who must make the most of everything they eat to stay in decent condition. "Older persons require food intake with higher concentration of micronutrients per calorie than younger individuals," Dr. Weg concludes. "This is especially true as the caloric intake decreases."

So the way out of the malnutrition syndrome is clear. Consume enough calories, but make sure they are nutrient-rich calories. That means the kind of diet that includes fresh fruit, vegetables and low-fat protein like chicken and fish—and an "insurance plan" of supplemental vitamins and minerals to fill in any gaps.

CHAPTER
7

BEATING THE VITAMIN BANDITS

Frank is a middle-aged investment banker, a man whose job is to help people protect their savings against all the things that deplete them in complicated, secret ways. He's very good at what he does, and proud of it. He also is concerned about his health because lately it hasn't been the greatest.

Today he gets up exactly at seven, dresses nattily and goes downstairs for breakfast, ready to conquer inflation. If he only knew the number of ways his health is going to be robbed today. . . . Well, he might even crawl back into bed.

He pours himself a big, cold glass of orange juice to make sure he takes enough vitamin C. A panel on the carton assures him he's getting plenty. But what it doesn't say is that as much as 40 percent of that vitamin C may be in a form that is of no use at all to his body.

Unfortunately, Frank didn't read the study that showed fresh-squeezed orange juice provides up to twice as much *biologically active* vitamin C as pasteurized, carton juice—though total vitamin C levels in the two juices may be the very same (*Journal of the American Medical Association*).

Frank has been robbed even before he has opened his mouth. Next, he pops a slice of whole wheat bread in the toaster, for protein and B vitamins. He doesn't know some of the B vitamins are destroyed by heat and that toasting steals thiamine (vitamin B_1)—the darker the toast, the more you lose—as well as making certain amino acids unavailable to the body. (Actually, 15 to 30 percent of the thiamine originally present in bread dough has been destroyed already by baking.)

Frank's been trying to beat the coffee habit (with middling success), so he pours himself a cup of steaming black tea. It charges his blood—but it also makes off with still more thiamine and iron.

Tannin—the stuff that gives tea its astringent, puckery taste— is believed to be the bandit that steals thiamine. In one study, a thiamine solution was mixed with black tea and allowed to stand for 90 minutes at 86°F. It was discovered that 22 percent of the thiamine was either destroyed or inactivated (*Food Chemistry,* vol. 6, no. 2, 1980–1981).

A report in the *New England Journal of Medicine* (January 4, 1979) suggested that, because of its ability to inhibit the body's absorption of iron, tea might be used to help treat certain anemias in which iron *overload* is the main cause of death.

Poor Frank! He's so proud of himself for drinking orange juice, eating whole wheat toast and avoiding coffee that he treats himself to a sugar-covered doughnut. Bad move, fella.

Refined carbohydrates such as white sugar and flour have most of the B vitamins wrung out of them during the milling process. But because thiamine and others in the B complex are needed to make an enzyme used in the burning of carbohydrates, these vitamins have to be stolen from the liver or other storage places to properly metabolize Frank's doughnut. His little reward is not only deficient in the B complex, it's actually a B-complex thief! (Whole, natural carbohydrates come equipped with their own B vitamin supply, so they don't pilfer the body's store.)

Frank is quite pleased with himself as he strides briskly off into his day. The only trouble is he's got confectioner's sugar on his chin—and a small army of vitamin bandits are already plundering the breakfast in his stomach.

Chemicals That Steal Vitamins

Vitamin antagonists, as they are officially known, are the James Gang of the nutritional world. In one way or another, they either destroy vitamins directly or alter them in a way that makes them useless to your health.

An antagonist may interfere with the conversion of a vitamin to its active, or coenzyme, form—often because the antagonist is so closely related to the vitamin itself. The antagonist may enhance the development of enzymes that destroy certain vitamins. It may cause excessive elimination of nutrients or impair your body's ability to absorb them.

In fact, there are so many different ways your body can be burglarized that it's foolish to think you're actually making use of everything those tidy little nutritional charts promise.

"If we grew all our own vegetables like people did in grandpa's day, we might not have as many problems using all the vitamins we get," says H. Curtis Wood, Jr., M.D., a nutrition-oriented Philadelphia doctor who is the author of *Overfed but Undernourished* (Exposition Press, 1959). "But today, there are more than 3,000 chemicals used in the commercial foods we eat. And in one way or another, many of them can be antagonists."

Insecticide residues and pollutants in the air and water also can raid our vitamin stores, Dr. Wood told us. Even vitamins can sometimes act as antagonists to other vitamins. Large amounts of a single B vitamin actually may increase your need for others in the B complex, Dr. Wood said, so it's best to take the Bs all together.

Life's circumstances also can become antagonists—stress, advanced age, disease, pregnancy, increased physical activity or even lack of sleep all can destroy vitamins at a stepped-up pace.

"Everyone has individualized nutritional needs," Dr. Wood points out. "But a single person may also vary rather widely in his requirements from day to day, depending on stress, exercise, diet and so on. There are so many things that can act as antagonists, it's just unrealistic to think the RDAs [Recommended Dietary Allowances] will give you all the nutrients you need."

Among the most widespread bandits, he says, are drugs.

Drugs Disrupt Your Body's Nutritional Balance

That powerful drugs often cause powerful side effects, altering our metabolism of nutrients in complicated ways, isn't really too surprising. But even "harmless" drugs can take their toll.

"Among the drugs shown to cause tissue depletion of ascorbic acid [vitamin C], aspirin is the most important," writes Daphne A. Roe, M.D., in her book *Drug-Induced Nutritional Deficiencies* (AVI Publishing, 1976). Dr. Roe goes on to point out that diuretics can cause a loss of calcium, magnesium and zinc and that mineral oil, sometimes used as a laxative, may cause deficiencies of vitamins A, D and K.

Some drugs act as antagonists by interfering with the absorption of nutrients through the digestive system. They may actually change the microscopic structure of the villi, or tiny, finger-shaped ridges that line the small intestine. That, in turn, may destroy the enzymes the villi normally produce to break down and absorb nutrients.

The antibiotic neomycin, for example, was shown to cause structural changes in the intestinal villi of people within six hours after it was administered. Neomycin, as a result, interferes with absorption of potassium, calcium, vitamin B_{12}, iron and other substances.

Other drugs, such as certain laxatives and cathartics, greatly speed up the intestinal transit time, causing nutrients to pass through the intestines too rapidly to be absorbed fully.

And some drugs rob your body by binding with nutrients to form a new substance that the body cannot use. For example, a common antacid, aluminum hydroxide, binds with phosphates in the intestines, causing the phosphates to be passed—unused—out of the body. Phosphate depletion, linked with long-term use of these antacids, can be dangerous because it interferes with proper bone formation.

Oral contraceptives, currently used by an estimated 10 to 18 million American women, are among the most nutritionally disruptive drugs. In a review of the medical literature, James L. Webb, Ph.D., reported that contraceptive steroids have been shown to lower the levels of six nutrients in the body: vitamins B_6, B_{12} and C, riboflavin (B_2), folate (folic acid) and zinc (*Journal of Reproductive Medicine,* October, 1980).

Dr. Webb concludes that "females consuming oral contraceptive agents should pay particular attention to vitamin and mineral intake and, if warranted, consume . . . supplements of needed nutrients."

To which Dr. Wood adds a word of general advice: "Doctors are so drug oriented it's unbelievable, but the best thing is to take as few drugs as you possibly can. I'd rather people tried nutritional means [of healing themselves]—calcium or tryptophan instead of sleeping pills, for example. That's the safest way to avoid the nutritional antagonists in drugs."

Smoking and Drinking: A Deadly Duo

You may be careful about avoiding unnecessary drugs, but if you smoke or drink, you are flirting with two of the best-known vitamin antagonists around. In fact, after a two-year study of alcoholic prisoners in California, Jery Meduski, M.D., Ph.D., summed up alcoholism in three scary little words: basic nutritional disaster.

The trouble with alcohol (besides the obvious) is that it provides only "naked" calories, completely bare of nutritional value. And though it's not a nutrient, alcohol is metabolized or processed in the body the same way nutrients are and can interfere with the body's absorption of food.

For example, it has been known for the past 20 years that alcoholism and its offshoot, cirrhosis of the liver, usually are accompanied by zinc deficiencies, though exactly how booze flushes zinc out of the system is not understood. ("Zinc before you drink" is the warning in some circles.)

But zinc isn't the only nutrient drinking destroys. Alcoholics also often show deficiencies of thiamine, folate, vitamins B_6, B_{12}, C, A and D, and calcium, iron and magnesium. "Basic nutritional disaster" is no exaggeration!

But there may be vitamin destroyers awaiting even those who are not long-term heavy drinkers. A researcher at Ohio State University reports that six or seven drinks a day for as little as two weeks can throw the digestive system into reverse, causing the small intestine to begin secreting fluids that flush food from the body before it's used.

Hagop S. Mekhjian, M.D., found that folate supplements could partly correct these alcohol-induced changes—and quitting drinking stopped them completely (*Science News*, March 10, 1979).

To add insult to insult, it appears that heavy drinkers are very often heavy smokers, with one researcher even suggesting that "heavy cigarette smoking constitutes part of the syndrome of alcohol addiction." In addition to the nutritional devastation of alcohol, some researchers warn us, smoking drains your body of vitamin C to the tune of 25 milligrams per cigarette, according to some estimates.

There are hopeful signs, however. Over the past several years, a group of Pennsylvania researchers has been examining natural substances that can block a toxic chemical called acetaldehyde, which occurs in cigarette smoke and is produced in the body when alcohol is consumed.

Herbert Sprince, Ph.D., chief of research biochemistry at the Veterans Administration Medical Center in Coatesville, Pennsylvania, and his associates describe how they gave rats lethal doses of acetaldehyde after first administering large doses of certain nutrients.

The results? A combination of vitamin C, thiamine and an amino acid called cysteine, plentiful in nuts, eggs, soybeans and brewer's yeast, "gave virtually complete protection" *(Agents and Actions)*.

The researchers caution that these were animal, and not human, studies, but they go on to add, "Our findings point the way to a possible buildup of natural protection against the chronic body insult of acetaldehyde arising from heavy drinking of alcohol and heavy smoking of cigarettes."

Life, it seems, is full of "chronic body insults." And the vitamin bandits—hiding just out of sight in a thousand forms—always stand ready to rob your system of the nutrients you need to fight back. Watch your vitamin account!

CHAPTER
8

MEDICINES
THAT CREATE
MALNUTRITION

Headache, runny nose, sore throat—you're under the weather and decide to go "over the counter." But before you visit the shelves packed with fast-relief formulas, stop and pick up some vitamin A.

A recent scientific study shows that ingredients used in common over-the-counter (OTC) pain, cold and allergy remedies lower blood vitamin A levels in animals.

And that could be bad news if the same holds true for humans. Vitamin A protects and strengthens the mucous membranes lining the nose, throat and lungs. These membranes shield you against infection. But without enough vitamin A, they can break down, providing a cozy home for germs and bacteria. The very drugs that are supposed to help you get rid of a cold may actually prolong it!

The researchers who conducted the study—Phyllis Acosta, Ph.D., a dietitian at Emory University in Atlanta, and Philip Garry, Ph.D., a nutritionist at the University of New Mexico in Albuqueruqe—fed rats four common ingredients used in OTC pain, cold and allergy remedies from Allerest to Vanquish.

Dividing the animals into four groups, they fed each group a different ingredient. But not all of the rats were fed the same dose levels. Some were fed one-half, some normal and some two times the normal doses suggested for children. After three weeks, the levels of vitamin A in all four of the groups were tested.

All four ingredients at all dose levels caused a decrease in vitamin A in the blood.

Some of the decreases were over 40 percent, and the average decrease was almost 30 percent.

Dr. Acosta reported her study at the 62nd Annual Meeting of the Federation of American Societies for Experimental Biology. She told us that future research will show if these four OTC drug ingredients decrease vitamin A levels in the blood of people, too.

But there's already plenty of other research that shows drugs can play nasty tricks on a person's nutrients.

All of us take medicine at some time or another, and all of us know that medicine has side effects. Antihistamines can make you drowsy. Aspirin can upset your stomach. But what few people realize (and that includes doctors) is that a side effect of a wide array of drugs is a nutritional deficiency.

That's right, a nutritional deficiency—even if your diet is carefully planned to give you plenty of every vitamin and mineral.

Many drugs either stop the absorption of nutrients or interfere with the cells' ability to use them. That means a drug can cause a nutritional deficiency "even when the diet is adequate," says Daphne A. Roe, M.D., author of *Drug-Induced Nutritional Deficiencies* (AVI Publishing, 1976).

How to protect yourself? Well, the first step is to find out which drugs rob the body of nutrients and what these nutrients are. You already know that aspirin steals vitamin A. But its thievery doesn't stop there.

Aspirin Axes Vitamin C

There's another nutritional reason for keeping aspirin way out of the reach of children—and adults. A study has shown that even a small dose of aspirin can triple the amount of vitamin C the body excretes *(Journal of Human Nutrition)*.

As you probably know, vitamin C is a powerful cold fighter, and researchers have suggested that it be used to treat—and prevent—infections of all kinds. But vitamin C does more than fight colds—a lot more.

If cells are the bricks that hold your body together, collagen is the mortar. But without vitamin C to promote the formation of collagen, your body would be a shambles.

Vitamin C protects you against stress. It's essential to the health of the adrenal gland, the organ which produces the hormones that keep you alert and full of energy.

Vitamin C aids the body in healing. It detoxifies poisons from food and air, such as lead and cadmium. And it's essential for the metabolism of other nutrients: iron, calcium and the vitamin B complex.

So think twice before you take two aspirin.

But sometimes pain can cloud better judgment and taking aspirin may seem like a good idea. Aspirin for a headache. Aspirin for a backache. Or aspirin for aching joints—the searing pain of arthritis or rheumatism. If you're taking aspirin to douse fiery joint pain, take care. Aspirin depletes not only vitamin C, but folate (folic acid) as well. Researchers have found that the routine use of aspirin can lead to a folate deficiency.

Folate is one of the vitamin B complex. Concentrated in the spinal fluid, it's a must for calm nerves and clear thinking. In a study of 51 patients with rheumatoid arthritis, 71 percent had low levels of folate in their blood. All 71 percent were taking aspirin *(Drug Therapy)*.

The Pill: Preventing the Birth of Health

The Pill is a synthetic hormone. It's powerful: It convinces a woman's body that she's pregnant. But the Pill is a reaper of your body's nutrients. It attacks folate and vitamin C, B_6 and B_{12} levels within the body.

The evidence shows that the Pill is very bitter.

An editorial in the *Journal of the American Dietetic Association* reports that half of all Pill users have low levels of vitamin B_{12} in their blood. That could be making these women nervous. B_{12}—like all the vitamin B complex—helps maintain a well-functioning nervous system.

Frequently, women on the Pill are depressed. Many researchers believe this symptom is a result of vitamin B_6 deficiency. In two studies, depression in Pill users cleared up after they took B_6 supplements. But B_6 made these women happy in more ways than one. Without B_6, digestion of protein would go on the blink. A B_6 deficiency can also lower your resistance to infection, and high levels of B_6 help you cope better with stress.

In a study of Pill users and vitamin C, 63 women took the Pill for at least a year and 63 did not. During that time, both groups got the same amount of vitamin C in their diets. But, at the end of the year, the average vitamin C levels in the white blood cells of the women who took the Pill were much lower than the vitamin C levels in the women who did not *(American Journal of Clinical Nutrition)*.

Fighting Side Effects

But all scientific research on drugs and nutrition isn't aimed at finding out which nutrients a drug destroys. A recent study shows that vitamin E can stop the destructive side effects of a drug.

The drug is Adriamycin, an antibiotic. It's also the most commonly used anti-cancer drug, capable of treating at least ten forms of cancer. Trouble is, it can have a devastating side effect: the gradual destruction of the heart muscle.

But a team of scientists at the National Cancer Institute drew up a model of how the drug might damage the heart and theorized that vitamin E could shield the muscle.

To test their theory, they gave two groups of mice huge injections of the drug. One group, however, received vitamin E before the injection *(Science)*. In the group on Adriamycin alone, 85 percent of the mice died within a month. But in the vitamin E group, only 15 percent died.

In a longer study, mice were given Adriamycin once a week for five weeks. Every mouse died. But in a group of mice who got vitamin E along with their weekly Adriamycin, only 60 percent died.

William McGuire, M.D., author of the study, told us that more research is needed before vitamin E can be given to cancer patients on Adriamycin.

But research already shows that vitamin C may protect people—particularly older people—against the toxic effects of drugs.

A group of ten older people who were deficient in vitamin C were metabolizing the painkiller antipyrine very slowly. When eight of these people were given supplements of vitamin C for two weeks, their metabolism of the drug sped up.

"It seems clear that a vitamin C deficiency in man causes a small but demonstrable impairment in drug metabolism that can be reversed by correction of the deficiency," writes the study's author in the *British Medical Journal*.

And another study warns, "Ascorbic acid [vitamin C] deficiency may contribute to the adverse drug reactions found in the elderly" *(Journal of Human Nutrition)*.

Taking extra vitamin C may be one way to guard your body against the side effects of drugs in general. But that leaves the problem of nutritional deficiency. Which, of course, can be remedied.

"A drug-induced nutrient deficiency can be corrected only by giving large enough doses of the deficient nutrient to compensate for the loss caused by the drug," writes Dr. Roe.

But, she continues, "Nutritional side effects are preventable. Most of them occur because physicians are unaware they exist." But you aren't.

9

NUTRITIONAL SUPPLEMENTS DIETERS NEED

At some time in life, just about everybody decides to go on a diet. Young or old, men or women, there comes a point when we aspire to be slimmer or trimmer—if not for life, then at least for a special occasion. The goal may be to lose 5 pounds or 50 pounds, to look better or simply feel better. But always we begin in the same way: by eating less.

Depending on how you go about it, dieting can be either a health-building or a health-destroying process. The important thing to remember is that, while cutting back on your total food intake, you must still be sure to include all the essential protein, vitamins, minerals and other nutrients your body needs to maintain well-being. Wise food selection is imperative, but dietary supplements can also help bridge the gap and provide nutritional insurance.

High-Protein Diets Deficient in Vitamins

Dieting extremes can lead to serious nutrient deficiencies and health problems. In a study conducted by Bonnie S. Worthington, Ph.D., and Lynda E. Taylor while at the University of Washington, 20 overweight women, age 19 to 53, were placed on one of two popular reducing diets. Ten followed the so-called quick-weight-loss diet—a high-protein, low-carbohydrate regimen. The other women were served a more balanced diet. Each group was receiving less than 1,200 calories a day.

As the researchers reported in the *Journal of the American Dietetic Association,* both diets were deficient in certain important nutrients. The first diet, which relied almost exclusively on lean meats, fish, eggs and cottage cheese, failed to supply enough vitamin A, vitamin C, calcium and iron. Vitamin A intake (2,655 international units) was only about half of the Recommended Dietary Allowance (RDA). The vitamin C content of the diet was a paltry 11 milligrams.

The calcium intake of 308 milligrams fell far short of the RDA of 800 milligrams. Iron intake was only 14 milligrams, yet most of the women needed 18 milligrams daily.

The authors concluded, "It is clear that individuals using such a dietary plan should supplement their food intake with appropriate sources of vitamin A, ascorbic acid [vitamin C], iron and calcium."

Even the more balanced reducing diet followed by the other ten women failed to supply enough calcium (only 570 milligrams) or iron (10.9 milligrams). And the supply of important B vitamins—thiamine, riboflavin and niacin—was really only marginally adequate.

There were other problems. "Mild dizziness, headaches and nausea were experienced by four subjects on the high-protein diet and by only one on the balanced low-calorie regimen," the authors noted.

One serious drawback of the high-protein, low-carbohydrate diet that might account for the above symptoms is that it actually forces the body to break down its own protein stores in a frantic effort to keep up levels of glucose, or sugar, circulating in the bloodstream. Especially when combined with moderate alcohol intake, such a diet can lead to hypoglycemia, or low blood sugar, with accompanying dizziness and fatigue.

But any low-calorie diet can cause problems, particularly

when it dips below the 1,200 calorie per day level. At that point, you're just not taking in enough food to guarantee an adequate supply of all the nutrients your body needs.

The sensible and safe way to diet is to cut back moderately on your food intake while making every effort to make every calorie count.

One way to do that is to rely on lean meats like chicken, turkey and veal, fish, lots of salads, cooked vegetables, cottage cheese and fresh fruit.

If you're including eggs, you might want to eat only the whites. That way you'll be getting high-quality protein but with fewer calories or fat. The yolk of one extra-large egg contains 66 calories and 5.8 grams of fat. But the white of the same egg contains only 19 calories and a mere trace of fat.

Following such a sensible slimming diet, you'll be getting adequate protein from the meat and eggs as well as necessary carbohydrates from the fruit and cooked vegetables. The fruit and vegetables will also supply good levels of potassium and vitamin A. For example, 3½ ounces of romaine lettuce contain only 18 calories but provide nearly 2,000 international units of vitamin A and 264 milligrams of potassium. All those greens will also keep you supplied with much of the folate (folic acid) you'll need.

Vitamin C will be provided by the fruits and fresh vegetables, at least at high enough levels to prevent scurvy and meet the RDA. But for larger amounts—200 or 300 milligrams, for instance—you'll have to rely on supplements.

Getting enough of certain other nutrients with such a diet could be even more of a problem, however. For some, you'll definitely need to turn to supplements.

Vitamins for Dieters

If your reducing diet tends to down-play cereals, rice, bread and other baked goods, obtaining adequate amounts of thiamine, niacin, riboflavin and vitamin B_6 could be a problem. Normally, a super food like wheat germ could help out in this department. Wheat germ is a richly concentrated source of B vitamins and other important nutrients. But wheat germ is also relatively high in calories (although those calories are far from empty), more than 360 calories per 3½-ounce serving. So many dieters may not want to eat much wheat germ.

A B-complex supplement seems like the best bet here, especially when you consider that minor nervous aggravation and irritability too often crop up to plague people while they are dieting. The B vitamins, especially thiamine, are important in maintaining sound nerves and good morale.

To sum up, it is possible to successfully take off unwanted pounds with a sensible dieting plan. But the challenge of selecting a balanced and nutritious diet—a challenge we all face every day even when we're not dieting—is even greater when you start cutting calories. You still need the same amounts of nutrients you always did, but you have to obtain them from less food. Careful food selection can help up to a point, but daily supplementation with key nutrients is the best protection.

10

VITAMINS BEFORE AND AFTER SURGERY

Sooner or later, say the statistics, it's almost inevitable that your doctor will suggest for you a surgical solution for some problem. At least 25 million operations are performed on Americans each year, so odds are pretty good that, in the long run, one of those procedures will involve you.

It may be as relatively routine as the removal of wisdom teeth, plantar warts or a gallbladder. Or it could be much more involved and, as surgeons would say, *traumatic*. Open-heart surgery comes immediately to mind.

In any event, after you've sought a second opinion—and it's confirmed the first—take care that your very normal anxiety doesn't ambush your healthy life style!

The best thing you can do for yourself prior to going into the hospital is beef up your body's nutritional front lines so you'll be on the fast track of the road to recovery.

Fortunately, the majority of us are more than halfway there.

"Most patients have to do nothing special," explains James L. Mullen, M.D., of the hospital of the University of Pennsylvania. "Good nutrition—meat, vegetables, fruits—is important," he says. "Stabilize your weight—lose some if you're too heavy. Keep your muscles active and strong. Don't smoke."

George Blackburn, M.D., Ph.D., at the New England Deaconess Hospital of the Harvard medical school, heartily concurs and stresses the importance of both physical fitness and diet.

Give Your Body the Nutrients It Needs

"Our bodies have evolved to hold a supply of calories and micronutrients in reserve," explains Dr. Blackburn. "And long before special diets, the body drew on its stored nutrients to heal itself."

Understanding the healing process helps ensure you'll have your "shelves" stocked with the proper supplies, should the need ever arise.

"When the body is injured, it sets off an alarm system of stress-related chemicals," Dr. Blackburn continues. "In turn, the white corpuscles react to create a fever. If you want to speed up frying an egg, you turn up the heat, right? In much the same manner, fever makes enzymatic processes associated with healing work faster. At the wound site, a clot is created to seal off the open blood vessels, and from it comes *collagen,* the wound-healing tissue."

The protein to make collagen is derived from several sources. Diet is one, but the body can draw on other connective tissues, as well as muscle, if need be. Of course, breaking down one area to rebuild another leaves a net imbalance. Normally, that is corrected during the "get well" stage.

The other point worthy of mention is that healing takes extra energy, which is usually available in the body's "warehouse" of stored sugars.

So far, so good—you are what you eat, and you *are* going to heal well.

But if you're a victim of nutritional deficiencies of various kinds, you could be heading for trouble.

"Recent surveys have demonstrated an alarming incidence of malnutrition in hospital patients. Numerous studies have demonstrated a positive correlation between abnormalities in various objective measures of nutritional status and increased operative morbidity and mortality in surgical patients," writes Dr. Mullen (*Annals of Surgery*, November, 1980).

Vitamins Critical to Healing

Of the vitamins, C plays the best-understood role, for it is critical to the formation of collagen and also helps the body resist infection.

"There is no convincing evidence that wound healing is accelerated by administration of vitamin C when tissue levels of it are normal," says Sheldon Pollack, M.D., chief of dermatologic surgery of the Duke Unversity School of Medicine. "However, seriously ill or injured patients may develop ascorbic acid [vitamin C] deficiency rapidly because ascorbic acid is not stored in appreciable amounts" (*Journal of Dermatologic Surgery and Oncology*, August, 1979).

Dr. Pollack also mentions vitamin A as important for collagen formation and strength. It also exerts a suppressive action on certain infections.

Vitamin E deficiency results in abnormally fast blood platelet aggregation. Such clumping of cells has been implicated in thrombosis (clot formation), a problem that sometimes arises after surgery, according to Peter Thurlow, M.D., and John Grant, M.D., of the department of surgery at the Duke University medical center (*Surgical Forum*, vol. 31, 1980).

And it goes without saying that, while there are certain nutrients that play key roles, all vitamins are doubly important when you're facing the extra stress of surgery—so exercise and eat doubly well.

Not only can such measures help deliver a complication-free convalescence, they can give you the strength necessary to handle some of the toughest hospital procedures.

Nutrition Promotes Turnabout

Dwight Harken, M.D., of the Harvard medical school, reports that some malnourished cardiac patients progressively worsened after surgery. "The analogy to 'running out of gas' may be appropriate—they are patients who behave as if they are running out of energy reserves" (Geriatrics).

Augmenting their nutrition built up protein and muscle, and brought about a "conspicuous improvement" in their appearance, attitude and ability to withstand stress—including major heart surgery.

For cancer patients, having a proper supply of nutritional weapons helps in the fight against that disease and reduces surgical complications.

"Nutritionally replenished patients better tolerate chemotherapy and may have a better chemotherapy response rate," reported Edward Copeland, M.D., and his co-workers at the University of Texas medical school (Cancer, May, 1979).

Clearly then, eating right is your best medicine *before* going into the hospital.

And afterwards, good nutrition is healing insurance and infection protection.

CHAPTER
11

IF YOU MUST SMOKE, AT LEAST TAKE THESE VITAMINS

No one really knows *what* it is in a cigarette that causes disease. But that cigarette smoking *does* cause disease is a well-established scientific fact. In the 70s, the World Health Organization Expert Committee on Smoking and Its Effects on Health met to reconsider the evidence linking cigarette smoking with ill health.

Their verdict?

"Evidence from many countries implicates tobacco smoking as an important causative factor in lung cancer, chronic bronchitis and emphysema, ischemic heart disease, and obstructive peripheral vascular disease. It also shows that smoking plays a part in the causation of cancer of the tongue, larynx, esophagus, pancreas, and bladder; abortion, still-birth, and neonatal death, and gastroduodenal ulcer" *(WHO Chronicle)*.

If you smoke, you probably *know* these facts and *want* to stop. But you're caught between ad campaigns telling you to come "alive with pleasure" and scare-tactic statistics proving that it's more likely that you'll be dead with cancer; caught between a will that wants to say "no" and a nicotine need that is screaming "yes"; caught between tonight's solemn vows and

60

tomorrow morning's humiliating search for butts—well, you're caught in the jaws of an addiction that is chewing up your life piece by piece.

"Three out of four smokers either wish to or have tried to stop smoking, yet only about one in four ever succeeds in becoming a permanent ex-smoker. Thus most people smoke not because they wish to, but because they cannot easily stop." That is the sad pronouncement of M. A. H. Russell of the addiction research unit, institute of psychiatry, Maudsley Hospital, London *(Lancet).*

Is it also your eulogy?

Maybe. But you can do more than start praying for yourself, and you can do it with the right vitamins.

Keeping Your Arteries Clean with Vitamin E

One disease which may be caused or complicated by cigarette smoking is atherosclerosis—a narrowing or blockage within the arteries. And the arteries of the heart, tiny pipes thin as the lead in a pencil, are easily rusted shut by atherosclerosis. So it's no wonder that smokers have a habit of having heart attacks.

And it's the nicotine in cigarette smoke that does the dirty work. For nicotine speeds up a bodily mechanism—platelet aggregation—which may trigger the formation of a nasty blood clot called a thrombus.

An article in the *New York State Journal of Medicine,* exploring previous research in *Circulation* magazine, discusses the link between cigarette smoking, platelet aggregation and arterial disease.

"After smoking a single cigarette, patients demonstrated a marked increase in platelet aggregation, compared to no significant effect after smoking a lettuce leaf filled cigarette. This increase in platelet function could be observed as early as 10 minutes after smoking."

The article concludes, "The data presented a suggestive possible direct causative association between cigarette smoking and arterial thrombotic disease."

But if nicotine is an arterial killer, it just might have met its match in vitamin E.

Two researchers, Manfred Steiner, M.D., Ph.D., and his assistant, John Anastasi, found that vitamin E *decreases* platelet aggregation: the exact opposite of cigarette smoking's effect on platelets.

In his study, Dr. Steiner collected blood samples from several normal, healthy volunteers. He then mixed a test-tube brew: the blood samples, various chemical agents known to trigger rapid platelet aggregation—and vitamin E.

The results?

The more vitamin E that was added to the blood samples, the greater was the reduction in platelet aggregation.

Then Dr. Steiner focused his attention on the "test tube" of the human body. Five healthy men and women were given 1,200 to 2,400 international units of vitamin E with their meals. And again, the more vitamin E given, the less the platelets stuck together. At the level of 1,800 international units, platelet aggregation was cut down by about half. Yet, at 1,800 international units, the platelets also stopped absorbing vitamin E—no more reduction in aggregation took place even when larger doses of the vitamin were given. It was as if a natural mechanism made sure that enough platelet stickiness remained to avert any dangerous hemorrhaging *(Journal of Clinical Investigation)*.

So if you must smoke, it's wise to protect your arteries. And vitamin E seems to be just the protection you need.

Vitamin C Is Highly Protective

But nicotine isn't the only villain in this medical melodrama. Carbon monoxide—or, in its chemical abbreviation, CO—the gas of garage-suicide fame, plays a star role in the harassment of your heart, and its effect on hemoglobin is what puts it under the spotlight.

Hemoglobin is the beast of burden for oxygen in the blood, hauling that life-giving gas to every cell in the body. But hemoglobin actually takes a fancy to the deadly CO. The affinity of hemoglobin for CO is 200 times greater than that for oxygen. So when carbon monoxide is sucked into the circulation during smoking, it chases a lot of oxygen out of the bloodstream.

If you're a smoker, you know the result of this mix-up: shortness of breath, an inability to perform strenuous exercise—perhaps even to climb stairs—without gasping. Day after day, month after month, year after year, you're poisoning yourself with CO.

Is there any antidote?

Yes—vitamin C.

"Very little medical research has been done for finding a simple means of increasing the resistance of the human organism to the irritating, toxic, and carcinogenic constituents of cigarette smoke and detoxicating these constituents in vivo [in the body]. This physiological approach to the smoking problem has been virtually completely neglected."

These are the words of Irwin Stone, D.Sc., a biochemist and author of *The Healing Factor: "Vitamin C" against Disease* (Grosset and Dunlap, 1972), who has devoted much of his life's work to the study and research of vitamin C. It was Dr. Stone who first suggested to Linus Pauling that he begin taking vitamin C, a suggestion that eventually led Pauling to champion vitamin C as a simple and effective means of preventing the common cold. Dr. Stone, writing in *The Journal of Orthomolecular Psychiatry,* suggests that vitamin C can help shield your body against the lethal onslaught of cigarette poisons.

Cleaning Up Tobacco's Act

Dr. Stone explains that, in laboratory tests on guinea pigs, a cancer-causing agent found in cigarettes, called benzpyrene, was detoxified in the liver by hydroxylation, a process in which the oxygen content of a chemical compound is increased, rendering it harmless. And it is vitamin C that activates this hydroxylation. In guinea pigs with a vitamin C deficiency, the detoxification rate was only 10 percent of that in guinea pigs receiving an adequate supply of vitamin C.

But Dr. Stone, a veteran scientist, does not base his opinion on one lone study of guinea pigs. "An important function of ascorbate [vitamin C] in the mammalian organism is the detoxification of poisons, carcinogens, and toxins," he says.

Dr. Stone then cites studies in which vitamin C detoxified carbon monoxide, arsenic compounds and cyanide—all constituents of cigarette smoke. Vitamin C also cleaned up mercury, lead, ozone, nitrates and strychnine. Dr. Stone concludes, "While this is only a small segment of the literature, it is clearly evident that ascorbate is a wide-spectrum detoxicant. . . ."

And Dr. Stone offers sound advice to smokers—take vitamin C: "All this evidence can be used to formulate a simple and inexpensive megascorbic preventive medical regime for the practical use by smokers to inhibit or delay or even possibly prevent the eventual disease consequences of the chronic exposure to high concentrations of the irritating and toxic constituents of tobacco smoke. This regime would comprise . . . the daily intake of sufficient ascorbate. . . ."

But what is "sufficient" vitamin C for a nonsmoker is probably *not* sufficient for the smoker. For in addition to all its other ills, smoking depletes vitamin C.

So when we learn that vitamin C protects us against smoking's poisons, and that smoking depletes vitamin C, it becomes almost suicidal for a smoker not to supplement his diet with vitamin C.

The Special Combination

Acetaldehyde is another killer chemical in cigarette smoke. Herbert Sprince, Ph.D., chief of research biochemistry at the Veterans Administration Hospital, Coatesville, Pennsylvania, and his associates describe how they gave rats *lethal* doses of acetaldehyde and then tested the protective value of various nutrients and combinations of nutrients. The winning combination—vitamin C, thiamine (vitamin B₁) and an amino acid called cysteine—gave "complete protection (zero % lethality) for 72 hours in the 30 rats tested," the authors write *(Agents and Actions)*.

"To the best of our knowledge," they add, "our findings demonstrate for the first time that direct protective action against acetaldehyde toxicity and lethality can be obtained with certain naturally occurring metabolites, namely L-ascorbic acid [vitamin C], L-cysteine, and thiamine, preferably in combination at reduced dose levels."

And although the researchers caution that the findings must be "further evaluated" before they can be extrapolated for human use, they have no qualms in asserting that these laboratory results could "point the way to a possible buildup of natural protection against the chronic body insult of acetaldehyde arising from . . . heavy smoking of cigarettes."

Supplements of vitamin C and thiamine are, of course, readily available. And any good diet including nuts, eggs, soybeans and brewer's yeast will supply the cysteine.

And while you're taking your vitamins, try again to quit smoking. Your supplements will do you a lot more good if they don't have to exhaust themselves fighting smoke.

CHAPTER
12

VITAMIN SUPPLEMENTS: HOW MUCH IS TOO MUCH?

Nutritional therapy is, in many cases, an attractive alternative to conventional medical treatments. One of the main advantages of nutrition is the relative safety with which it can be used. Experimenting with drugs can be hazardous, but it is usually not dangerous to try different nutrients at various doses.

It is a shame that more health professionals are not interested in or well trained in nutrition. Many people have been forced to treat themselves, using what they have learned from books, magazines and friends. It is a testimony to the power of nutrition that millions, even without professional guidance, have been able to improve their health greatly.

On the other hand, it is a mistake to assume that nutritional therapy is totally safe all of the time. Though adverse effects are rare, they can occur. We should be well informed about potential problems with supplements so that we can make better choices about which nutrients to take and in what doses.

The possible hazards of nutritional therapy can be divided into three categories:

1. Self-diagnosis may be overemphasized instead of competent professional advice being sought.

2. Certain nutrients have the ability to change the results of some diagnostic laboratory tests.
3. Some nutrients can have harmful effects themselves.

Let's look at the self-diagnosis hazard first. You may be staying away from the doctor's office because you have no faith in modern medicine. Or else you may fear being ridiculed for taking vitamins and minerals. With all of the popular health books and magazines on the market, it is tempting to try figuring out what is causing your problems and to prescribe your own treatment. Unfortunately, the diagnosis will frequently be wrong, no matter how classic your symptoms appear to be. As a result, a potentially serious but easily treatable disease may be overlooked.

The solution to this problem is easy: Before starting your own nutrition program, get checked out by your doctor to make sure nothing serious is being missed. If some disease is found and you wish to treat it by nutritional means, get the OK from your doctor. Ask him or her to monitor the progress of your disease. In some situations, the benefits of orthodox medicine might outweigh the risks. If your nutrition program is not working, drugs or surgery might be necessary and helpful.

Test Results Altered by Vitamins

Doctors often perform laboratory tests to help them find out what is wrong with their patients. If you are taking large amounts of folate (folic acid) or vitamin C, some of these tests may give incorrect results. You may therefore be treated for a problem that you really do not have. Or else a truly abnormal condition may test normal. It is important that your doctor be aware of these supplements so that no errors are made in diagnosis.

Folate: One type of anemia with serious consequences is called pernicious anemia. Caused by faulty absorption of vitamin B_{12}, it can lead to central-nervous-system damage. Pernicious anemia is easy to discover if the doctor is alerted by a low hematocrit (a measure of red blood cells), which occurs in all anemias. However, if you are taking folate, your hematocrit could be normal even though the B_{12} deficiency might be getting worse. Fortunately, pernicious anemia does not occur often. However, any time your doctor orders a hematocrit, you should inform him if you are taking folate, either by itself or in a B-complex supplement.

Vitamin C: Diabetics who test their urine for sugar may get incorrect results if there is a lot of vitamin C in the urine. Your doctor or pharmacist can recommend a urine testing kit that is not affected by vitamin C.

Doctors frequently do a simple test to look for small amounts of blood in the stool. A positive test suggests bleeding from the bowel, which may occur from cancer or other gastrointestinal diseases. If there is a lot of vitamin C in the stool, the test might not detect the presence of blood.

Toxic Effects of Nutrients

The side effects discussed below are uncommon and usually (but not always) mild. Each person must weigh the risks and benefits in deciding on the proper supplements.

Vitamin A: Since this nutrient is stored in the liver, harmful effects can build up gradually. However, it is extremely unlikely that any problems would occur unless you are taking 50,000 international units or more a day. Even at the 50,000 unit level, you would probably have to continue that dose every day for months to reach a possibly toxic level. Some people can tolerate more. Most people, though, probably take 10,000 to 25,000 international units a day, and at that level there should be no problem at all. Serious side effects of vitamin A can be prevented by heeding early warning signs. These include fatigue, abdominal discomfort, bone and joint pain, throbbing headache, insomnia, restlessness, sweating, hair loss, brittle nails, constipation, menstrual irregularities and swelling of the ankles. If these symptoms are caused by too much vitamin A, then stopping the vitamin will relieve the symptoms.

If you take large amounts of carotene, the vegetal form of vitamin A, which is found in carrots and nonanimal foods, your skin may turn orange. That does not appear to be a toxic effect. The skin change will go away as carotene is stopped.

Vitamin B complex: Because of the many interactions between the B vitamins, large doses of one can lead to deficiencies of the others. When taking a single B vitamin, it is wise to back it up with the entire B complex.

Thiamine (vitamin B₁): Some people become drowsy after taking 500 milligrams or more. But that is an extremely high and unusual dose. No serious side effects have been reported.

Niacin or niacinamide: Niacin may produce an uncomfortable warmth and flushing of the skin when taken in doses higher than 75 to 100 milligrams a day. That is not dangerous. Niacinamide, a form of niacin, will not cause the skin to flush, but it may produce nausea. The dose should be reduced if nausea occurs.

Prolonged use of several grams (a gram is equal to 1,000 milligrams) per day of niacin or niacinamide may cause elevations of blood sugar, uric acid or liver function test results. It is not certain whether these changes are dangerous. However, a few patients have developed yellow jaundice and liver disease after taking 3 or more grams of niacin for a long time.

PABA: This nutrient is safe, but it may interfere with the function of some sulfa drugs.

Folate (folic acid): If you take Dilantin or another anti-epilepsy medication, folate may interfere with it. Check with your doctor.

Vitamin B₆ (pyridoxine): Large doses (200 to 600 milligrams per day) may decrease milk production in nursing mothers. It is unlikely that smaller amounts (10 to 25 milligrams) would cause this problem. However, even small doses of B₆ can interfere with the drug L-dopa (used for Parkinson's disease). There is a substitute for L-dopa which is not affected by vitamin B₆.

Vitamin C: The most common side effects are upset stomach and diarrhea. Usually, that does not occur at levels under several thousand milligrams a day. That can be prevented by decreasing the dose or by taking the vitamin with meals or in the form of sodium ascorbate and calcium ascorbate instead of ascorbic acid.

Past claims that vitamin C destroyed vitamin B_{12} were apparently based on inaccurate measurements of vitamin B_{12}.

Since vitamin C can increase the amount of oxalate in the urine, there is (in theory) a slightly increased risk of developing oxalate kidney stones. Physicians who use large doses of vitamin C in their practice have not yet reported any kidney stones. Vitamin B_6 (25 milligrams or more) seems to prevent vitamin C from increasing the oxalate in the urine. The small risk of kidney stones may, therefore, be reduced even more by taking B_6.

Vitamin C also helps the body get rid of uric acid. In the long run, that may be helpful, since excess uric acid is associated with gout and heart disease. However, in the short run, shifts in the body's uric acid levels can occasionally trigger an attack of gout. That is sometimes seen when drugs are prescribed to lower uric acid. There is no proof yet that vitamin C has caused an attack of gout. If you have a history of gout, though, it is a good idea to build up your vitamin C slowly, rather than taking a large dose from the beginning.

Some scientists believe that large amounts of vitamin C can interfere with pregnancy or fertility. Others disagree.

Vitamin D: In large doses, this nutrient can cause a dangerous elevation of calcium in the blood. At lower doses, vitamin D may increase cholesterol. Some prevention-minded scientists are concerned that too much vitamin D may increase the risk of atherosclerosis (hardening of the arteries). As a general rule, one should not take more than 1,000 international units per day without medical advice.

Vitamin E: This widely used vitamin is usually very safe. However, if you have a vitamin K deficiency, large doses of vitamin E could make it worse. That could impair normal blood clotting. Fortunately, vitamin K deficiency does not occur very often. But if you take an anticoagulant or do not eat vegetables, you might have a deficiency of vitamin K.

Wilfrid Shute, M.D., of the Shute Institute in Ontario, Canada, cautions that those with high blood pressure or rheumatic heart disease should begin vitamin E carefully (about 100 international units per day) and increase gradually (add no more than 100 international units every six weeks). Other doctors, however, have found no problems here.

Diabetes

Some nutrients will improve glucose tolerance; that is helpful for diabetics. However, if you take insulin, you must carefully monitor how much is needed. If good nutrition decreases your insulin requirement and you do not decrease the dose, a low-blood-sugar reaction may result. Supplements to be most aware of are brewer's yeast, chromium, and vitamins E, C and B_6.

All of this is not meant to scare you out of taking supplements.

Nutrients are usually very safe. However, by becoming aware of potential risks, you may develop a better and safer nutritional program.

CHAPTER
13

EVEN "WASTED" VITAMINS HELP PROTECT US

"I can't understand what good it does to take all those high-priced vitamins and minerals," say the nutrition skeptics. "All they do is go right through you. The body hangs onto what it needs and excretes the rest. The only thing you get from taking more than you need is the most expensive urine in town."

You'll hear that type of argument a lot. It's a source of confusion to people who *know* they feel better after taking vitamin supplements. And it raises serious doubts, too: "Am I really popping a bunch of unnecessary pills—and wasting a lot of money, to boot?"

It's true that, when you take a nutritional supplement, some part of it ends up in your urine and is excreted. But that it ends up in the urine isn't bad. There are at least two ways a nutrient can be beneficial to the body even though it eventually gets excreted:

1. Its presence in the urine may promote good health in the bladder and kidneys.

2. The nutrient may perform a useful function somewhere else in the body before it's excreted.

72

How can nutrients in the urine help your bladder and kidneys? Because there are certain ways that urine can harm them. Urine is a body fluid, just like blood or spinal fluid, and bacteria can grow in it and cause infections of the bladder or kidneys. Also, certain compounds in the urine may produce painful kidney stones. And some cancer-causing chemicals you're exposed to pass out of the body through the urine. Since those chemicals come in contact with the bladder, they probably increase risk of bladder cancer.

But there are nutrients that may protect you against each of those problems.

Bladder and Kidney Protection

Vitamin C can kill some bacteria, including *Escherichia coli* *(E. coli),* the most common cause of urinary tract infections. That killing power is especially strong at the uniquely high vitamin C levels that are possible in the concentrated fluid of urine. Doctors have used vitamin C for years to prevent urinary tract infections in people likely to develop them. It's generally assumed that the vitamin works by producing an acid urine which inhibits the growth of bacteria. In fact, vitamin C does a poor job of acidifying the urine. The effectiveness of the vitamin is more likely related to a direct bactericidal (bacteria-killing) action.

The prevention of kidney stones depends in part on the presence of magnesium in the urine. Most kidney stones occur when calcium dissolved in the urine doesn't stay dissolved but forms little pellets made of calcium salts. Any substance that helps keep calcium dissolved will help prevent kidney stones. Magnesium does just that. Edwin Prien, Sr., M.D., emeritus member of the Newton-Wellesley Hospital, Massachusetts, and Stanley Gershoff, Ph.D., director of the nutrition institute, Tufts University, Massachusetts, report that patients with recurrent kidney stones who were given magnesium as part of their therapy had about 90 percent fewer stones.

The kidneys rid the body of various waste products and

environmental poisons, and urine contains a wide range of toxic chemicals, some of which have the potential to cause cancer. However, a few of those chemicals don't become cancer causers until they undergo a chemical reaction called oxidation. A nutrient that could prevent oxidation—an antioxidant—should lessen the number of cancer-causing chemicals the bladder is exposed to. Vitamin C is an antioxidant. It's been shown to prevent the development of bladder cancer in animals exposed to a cancer-causing compound that's often found in human urine. And Jorgen Schlegel, M.D., former chief of staff at the Tulane University medical center, believes that vitamin C may be effective in preventing human cancer, too.

But you have to take enough vitamin C to make sure some of it spills over into the urine. For most people, 300 milligrams a day would do the trick. But people with an increased need for vitamin C—smokers, diabetics, the elderly, the stressed, the allergic and persons taking certain drugs—need more. Other nutrients such as vitamin E, zinc and selenium are also antioxidants and might help prevent bladder cancer.

"Alright," says the skeptic. "Expensive urine may have some value. But most people don't take vitamins and minerals to make healthy urine. They take them in such large amounts to help their nerves, their arthritis, their skin, or any other health problem that's fashionable. And most of what they take ends up down the drain. It seems to me that, if those nutrients just go in one end and out the other, they can't have much effect on the body."

But the skeptic is wrong to believe that any excreted nutrients are excesses the body doesn't need. A simple example will prove the point.

Penicillin Excreted, Too

Doctors often prescribe penicillin for various infections. The goal of therapy is to keep an effective level in the blood and tissues at all times. The larger and more frequent the dose, the more penicillin will be in the body at any one time. On the other hand, the drug is rapidly excreted by the kidneys. In fact, 60 to

90 percent of a given dose will be in the urine within one hour. But doctors don't believe that that penicillin is wasted. They know that high excretion rates can't be helped and that they have to give enough penicillin to stay ahead of losses. The situation is like the water level in a sink with an open drain. If the level is high, the water runs out of the drain faster than if the level is low. To keep the water level high, you need to run the water faster.

As with penicillin therapy, the goal of nutritional therapy is to provide the tissues with effective levels of nutrients at all times. Because of disease, genetic differences, or a chronically poor diet or environment, the body may need nutrient concentrations higher than what is usually considered adequate. And, like penicillin, the only way to achieve those high levels is to take nutrients frequently and in relatively large amounts. That type of supplementation will also stay ahead of the unavoidable urinary losses. For example, when healthy people take 100 to 800 international units of vitamin E over a period of years, blood levels of the vitamin remain higher than normal, even though urinary excretion presumably increases.

There's some confusion in orthodox medical thinking over this point. It's known that the body conserves nutrients in the face of a deficiency—when necessary, the kidneys reduce urinary losses to near zero. So some assume that *any* nutrient excretion means the body has all it needs. What is not well understood is that the kidneys are designed only to prevent severe deficiency from progressing to death. When there is only a mild deficiency, the kidneys are more like a sink with an open drain than one where the drain is sealed off. So when trying for optimal nutrition, you can't expect the kidneys to do much of a conservation job. It becomes a matter of turning on the faucet strong enough to keep the nutrient levels at the amount you want.

The "expensive urine" argument isn't a good reason to reject the thousands of reports about the value of nutritional therapy. Nutrients in the urine may be valuable in their own right, or they may be a reflection of important work being done elsewhere in the body. Yes, vitamins come in and go out. But, as with life itself, it's what happens in between that counts.

CHAPTER

14

VITAMINS: WILL THE SKEPTICS EVER BE CONVINCED?

"Ever since I started taking my vitamins," says the nutrition enthusiast, "I have had much more energy. Whenever I stop taking them, I get tired again. I definitely think my supplements have improved my health."

A physician, skeptical about nutrition, remarks, "A patient begged me for a vitamin B_{12} shot, swearing it gives her more energy. I knew she was not deficient in B_{12}, but it seemed she had a psychological need for an injection of any kind. So I gave her a shot of salt water and told her it was vitamin B_{12}. As expected, the 'vitamin' shot gave her lots of energy."

Another nutrition advocate tells of the pain which followed an injury. His lower back hurt so much that he could barely get out of bed. Because he had read that vitamin C is helpful for disk problems, he increased his vitamin C intake. Within a week, the pain had nearly disappeared, and he was able to lift heavy boxes again.

The skeptic replies that pains from most injuries go away after a week or two, regardless of whether or not any treatment is given. The vitamin C probably had nothing to do with it.

These examples illustrate how difficult it is to prove that any treatment works.

It is well known that, if a person is using a remedy in which he believes strongly, his condition will improve even if the remedy is worthless. That is called the placebo effect, the remarkable influence that mind has over body. Anxiety, depression, chest pain, psoriasis and a host of other disorders are subject to the placebo effect. If the patient has faith in the doctor, he will often get better, even if the doctor's "therapy" is just an inert sugar pill.

In addition, most problems gradually get better by themselves. If this improvement occurs while the patient is following a nutrition program, there is no way to know how much of the benefit was actually due to good nutrition. That uncertainty is why, despite thousands of studies and millions of testimonials, most doctors remain unconvinced about the benefits of nutrition.

Double-Blind Trials: Why Vitamins Get a Hung Jury

For a therapy to be accepted by the pure scientist, research must prove that results are better than one would expect from a placebo effect.

The most convincing way to do that is to perform what is called a controlled, double-blind experiment. In this type of study, half the patients are given the treatment being tested, and the other half (the control group) receive a fake (placebo). To avoid psychological factors, no one knows (until the study is over) who is getting the active ingredient and who is getting the placebo. It is called *double-blind* because neither the patients nor the attending physicians know who is getting what. When the experiment is completed, a statistician compares the results in the two groups and decides whether the treatment has value.

Opponents of nutrition argue that most nutrition studies have not been done in the acceptable double-blind fashion. They assume, therefore, that most reported benefits are nothing more than a placebo effect. Until these studies are done "correctly," they say, nutrition cannot be taken seriously.

The fact is that there have been many well-controlled, double-blind studies in the field of nutrition. These include the use of zinc for rheumatoid arthritis, acne, stomach ulcers and leg ulcers; vitamin B_6 for the carpal tunnel syndrome and for one type of depression; vitamin B_{12} for tiredness; niacinamide (a form of niacin) for acute schizophrenia; vitamin C for the common cold, other viral infections and some psychiatric problems; and vitamin E for intermittent claudication (leg pains associated with hardening of the arteries). And as interest in nutrition increases, the number of well-controlled studies continues to grow.

But what should we do about the thousands of studies that were less well controlled? Should we, as the orthodox suggest, forget them all and wait for double-blind reports to appear? It is true that most nutritional therapy has not been proven conclusively to be effective. But that does not mean claims should automatically be discounted. To reject nutrition is to ignore a half century of experience and accumulated wisdom, to abandon an approach that many nutritionists know is effective. For a number of reasons, it is unrealistic to expect or demand that every piece of nutrition information be studied by the double-blind method.

To begin with, that demand has never been placed upon may of the traditional medical treatments. The use of digitalis, morphine, L-dopa, INH (for tuberculosis) and other drugs is based on the same type of studies that are often rejected in the field of nutrition. Because of years of experience with these drugs, doctors are convinced that they work. The fact that they have not been studied in the "correct" manner has not prevented these drugs from being used widely. If uncontrolled studies are acceptable for potentially toxic drugs, then experiences with relatively safe nutrients should also be taken seriously.

Why has no one demanded that these drugs be submitted for double-blind tests? Doctors argue that it is unethical to do such studies if you already know your treatment works. How can you take a group of heart patients that need digitalis and give half of them a placebo? To perform such a study would deprive half the patients of the best available treatment. And all that would be accomplished would be to prove something that everyone already knows.

The same argument holds for nutrition. If, for example, you are certain that niacinamide helps some types of arthritis, how can you withold it from a patient in pain? Only nutrition skeptics can ethically do a controlled study of niacinamide. They would have no moral objection to withholding the nutrient from half the patients because they do not believe it has any value. But during the 40 years that nutritionists have been using niacinamide for arthritis, none of the skeptics have been interested in doing a controlled study.

The Problems of Designing a Proper Vitamin Experiment

There are more than just ethical factors preventing doctors from doing controlled studies. In many situations, it is literally impossible to design the proper experiment.

Suppose you wanted to prove that bed rest is good for back injuries. You would need a group of patients, half of whom receive bed rest and half of whom do not. But, to avoid psychological factors, no one could be permitted to know whether or not he was in bed. Even to consider such a study is absurd.

Or suppose you wanted to study a new drug for the treatment of cancer. To make sure no one knew if he was getting the real drug, you would have to design a placebo which caused nausea, vomiting, hair loss and possibly death.

With nutrition, as well, there are often major difficulties in designing a placebo. For example, the nutritional approach to diabetes might involve a low-sugar, high-fiber diet, with careful attention to detecting any food allergies. Brewer's yeast, vitamins A, B, C, and E and a number of minerals might also be used. But how, for example, could any scientist fake the high-fiber diet? Or the yeast? And what diabetic would volunteer for such a complicated program, knowing there was a 50-50 chance he would be getting a worthless therapy?

The Cost Is Too Great
to Test Vitamins

Even if the patients can be found and the experiment can be set up, there is another major stumbling block: the enormous cost.

For the results of statistical studies to have meaning, a large number of patients must participate (smaller studies tend to overlook small improvements, which could lead to incorrect conclusions). These large studies cost a lot of money. Researchers recently spent $30 million to find out that aspirin does not prevent heart attacks. Must we design an expensive study to answer each of the many nutritional questions that should be asked? Does thiamine relieve anxiety? How about niacin? Or vitamin B_6? Or folate? Are thiamine and niacin better than thiamine alone? Is the result affected by the amount of protein in the diet? The amount of fat? The number of possible studies is endless, and the cost is unimaginable.

Even if the money were available to do all those studies, there would still be difficulties. Double-blind studies are best suited to testing one nutrient at a time. But nutrients work as a team; individual nutrients do not usually produce dramatic effects. The best results are achieved by a comprehensive nutritional program. Since controlled studies are usually designed to test individual portions of a complete program, they would tend to underestimate the importance of nutrition.

Finally, therapeutic nutrition is based on the understanding that every individual is biochemically different, with different nutritional needs. Double-blind studies, on the other hand, require that everyone (except those in the control group) receive the same treatment. One cannot expect impressive results from a treatment that may be correct for only a small percentage of the patients.

Results We Can't Ignore

Reasonable people should recognize that some studies are important even if there is no placebo control group. For example, James Isaacs, M.D., reported on his use of vitamins, minerals and hormones in the treatment of severe heart disease at the Texas Heart Institute Symposium on Coronary Artery Medicine and Surgery, Houston, Texas. The results were dramatic and far better than anyone else had achieved with a similar group of patients. But the medical community has rejected Dr. Isaacs' work because there was no control group. The experience of other doctors using traditional methods is a built-in control group, however, which can be used at least for rough comparisons. When such a comparison is made, Dr. Isaacs' results are so much better than usual that they cannot be reasonably ignored.

It would certainly be nice if all therapeutic claims were supported by double-blind studies. As research techniques improve and more money becomes available for nutrition research, more such studies will be done.

Knowledge of the value of nutrition will continue to spread until it reaches the mainstream of American medicine. That will occur for a very simple reason: Nutrition works.

BOOK II

A Guide to the Individual Vitamins

INTRODUCTION

Vitamins are designer nutrients.

Sure, they're mass-produced by Mother Nature, Inc. But each "brand" is special, distinctive. Vitamin A helps prevent cancer. Thiamine is a must for good digestion. B_6 specializes in health concerns unique to women. Vitamin C zeros in on your immune system, vitamin D on your bones.

So even though it's best to get *all* the vitamins, it's a good idea to know how each *one* fits into your health plan. (After all, you wouldn't wear pajamas to work or show up at a black-tie affair in a swimsuit.)

That's where book 2—A Guide to the Individual Vitamins— comes in. In it, we'll tell you all you need to know about vitamins—from A to K. And once you've learned *that* alphabet, you'll be able to spell "health."

VITAMIN A

CHAPTER

15

VITAMIN A: A FEAST FOR THE SENSES

It's only fitting that vitamin A should come first alphabetically in the long list of necessary nutrients that science discovered. For no other vitamin or mineral is a more basic building block of good health.

Vitamin A is the foremost example of the awesome versatility nature has packed into vitamins. For, unlike drugs that do just a few specialized things, vitamin A helps to regulate and maintain a whole range of essential functions inside our bodies.

You need vitamin A for smooth, healthy looking skin. And vitamin A helps build resistance to colds. But there's a whole lot more. Vitamin A keeps moist the mucous membranes that line your mouth, respiratory passages and urinary tract—thus ensuring resistance to infection. This nutrient also bolsters your body's natural immunity, which may help the body safeguard itself against cancer. Vitamin A also helps counter the damaging effects of stress and aids in wound healing and detoxifying certain poisonous chemicals.

It's even involved in sexual functioning: A shortage can lead to female problems such as excessive menstruation and also male problems of infertility.

Researchers are continuously expanding our understanding of how vitamin A works and the many ways it helps preserve health. For example, take the housekeeping role vitamin A plays in our ears.

Richard A Chole, M.D., Ph.D., an ear, nose and throat researcher at the University of California at Davis, who in the past has investigated vitamin A's impact on our ability to hear, recently found evidence that vitamin A is necessary for the normal function in the middle ear. Without A, middle ear infection (otitis media) may develop. He also found that cystlike masses of debris, called cholesteatomas, may develop in severely vitamin A-deficient rats.

"Under normal conditions," Dr. Chole told us, "mucus in the ear automatically traps dirt and bacteria and flushes it down the eustachian tube into the throat, where it is swallowed. This is how the ear cleans itself. In a vitamin A deficiency, not enough mucus is produced, and it doesn't get to the right places."

In experiments with rats, Dr. Chole found that depriving them of vitamin A resulted in breakdown of the epithelium—the moist protective layer of cells which lines all body tissues, inside and out—in the middle ear. The epithelium became scaly, stopped producing mucus and lost its ability to flush the ear clean. The result was an ear infection.

"It is reasonable to speculate," reports Dr. Chole, "that the human middle ear undergoes similar changes to those described above [in the rat] during vitamin A deficiency. If this is the case, vitamin A deficiency may be a significant factor in the genesis of otitis media" (*Western Journal of Medicine,* 1980).

In the past, Dr. Chole has shown that vitamin A does much more than perform janitorial services in the ear. In studies with guinea pigs, he has found that the cochlea, the spiral horn in the inner ear, contains vitamin A in concentrations ten times those in most other body tissues. He has gone on to show that sensory receptor cells in the ear, similar to those in the eye that rely on vitamin A, depend on the nutrient for their hearing function.

As Dr. Chole indicates, however, vitamin A's usefulness to the senses is by no means limited to hearing. He cites cases where people regained their sense of smell after taking vitamin A. And researchers at Cornell University have demonstrated that animals deprived of this nutrient lose the ability to differentiate between quinine-flavored, salted and plain water. "These results indicate that vitamin A is required for normal taste function," they note *(Society for Experimental Biology and Medicine)*.

A's Influence on the Eyes

But nowhere is vitamin A's influence on our perceptions more spectacularly evident than in the eyes.

"If the 'lights go out' for a child when dusk approaches, it's quite possible he's suffering from severe vitamin A deficiency . . . ," says Myron Winick, M.D., director of Columbia University's institute of human nutrition. "The primary effect of vitamin A deficiency is damage to the patient's eyes, with problems ranging from night blindness in some cases to irreversible corneal scarring in others" *(Modern Medicine)*.

According to Dr. Winick, prolonged deficiency—which leads to a condition of abnormal dryness of the eye, called xerophthalmia—is the leading cause of blindness in underdeveloped nations. And "although severe manifestations are quite rare in the United States, milder effects are frequently encountered, especially among children."

Another group at special risk for eye damage are heavy drinkers, since alcohol seems to interfere with the liver's ability to store and mobilize vitamin A. And without enough vitamin A being delivered to the retina, the eye can't produce enough of a substance called visual purple, which is necessary for seeing at night.

In one group of 26 patients hospitalized with alcohol-associated cirrhosis of the liver, 14 had problems in adapting their vision to darkness. Daily supplementation with vitamin A helped 8 of those patients overcome night blindness within two to four weeks *(Annals of Internal Medicine)*.

Similar results were reported by a trio of Boston researchers. In one case, a 55-year-old man had a five-year history of progressive night blindness so severe he needed a flashlight to see at dusk. He had been a heavy beer drinker for 25 years. After taking extra vitamin A daily for four weeks, this man regained normal night vision *(American Journal of Ophthalmology)*.

In those rare cases where vitamin A alone fails to help eyesight, extra zinc also may be called for. As Stanley Morrison, M.D., of Baltimore, Maryland, reports, two patients who initially failed to respond to 10,000 international units of vitamin A daily recovered rapidly after taking 90 milligrams of zinc daily *(American Journal of Clinical Nutrition)*.

Poor dark adaptation may be considered more of a nuisance than a serious threat, although it can cause traffic accidents when the affected person attempts to drive at night. A much more serious problem is glaucoma, a condition of increased pressure and fluid buildup inside the eyeball that can lead to total blindness. But here, again, there is evidence that vitamin A may have a protective effect.

Controlling Glaucoma

"In Europe the incidence of primary glaucoma is in the order of 1.5 percent of patients seen in an average ophthalmic practice. . . . In West Africa, the incidence is some 30 times that in Europe," says Dr. Stanley C. Evans of Ibadan, Nigeria *(Nutritional Metabolism)*.

"Whereas in Europe glaucoma does not usually occur below the age of 40 years," he continues, "in West Africa it occurs at all age levels from children of eight years upwards. This evidently is due to the fact that in West Africa the nutritional deficiencies responsible for glaucoma are worse than in Europe, so that not only does it occur in the younger age groups but its progress in development is also very much more rapid."

Although many factors are involved, Dr. Evans says, "Usually the precipitating cause of many eye disorders, including primary glaucoma, is a vitamin A deficiency." When he gave nutritional supplements, including large doses of A, to a group of patients suffering from restricted vision, blind spots and eye pain, their glaucoma was controlled just as effectively as with conventional drug therapies. This was verified by periodic measurements of the pressure inside the eye.

Protector of the Bowel

The epithelial lining of the intestines also needs vitamin A, and physicians in Sweden and Boston think the vitamin might be useful in treating Crohn's disease, a stubborn, unexplained deterioration of the bowel.

At a hospital in Linkoping, Sweden, a 31-year-old woman suffering from Crohn's disease was given large amounts of vitamin A for her psoriasis. The psoriasis began to clear but, surprisingly, so did the chronic diarrhea caused by the Crohn's disease. "The most striking effect was a return to normal bowel function," report the Swedish doctors. "Soon after starting the new treatment the patient found she could eat any food, even plums, without ill effects and with no diarrhea" (*Lancet,* April 5, 1980).

This news from Sweden attracted the attention of Ann Dvorak, M.D., a research pathologist at Beth Israel Hospital in Boston. She had taken electron microscope photographs showing intestinal epithelium damaged by Crohn's disease. The photos offered a possible explanation for vitamin A's success with the woman in Sweden.

Crohn's patients, Dr. Dvorak says, have holes in their intestines. As a result, they might absorb bacteria and food impurities that are normally excreted, and they fail to absorb nutrients, including vitamin A, that they should absorb. When the holes become large enough, the damaged section of the bowel must be removed surgically. She thinks vitamin A might keep tiny holes from becoming big ones by bolstering the epithelium.

"In the past," Dr. Dvork told us, "we thought that the holes were always large enough to see on an X ray. Now we're finding out that the large holes start as microscopic defects in the epithelium. I feel very strongly that, if Crohn's patients took vitamin A after their first operation, they might not need so many operations later on."

The Swedish doctors seem to agree. "It could be that vitamin A restored some previously impaired intestinal-barrier function," they concluded. "If so, and if, as is suspected, the essential abnormality in Crohn's disease is impaired function of the intestinal barrier, other Crohn's patients might benefit from vitamin A."

But vitamin A may do more than reinforce our barriers against disease. Eli Seifter, Ph.D., a professor of biochemistry and surgery at the Albert Einstein College of Medicine in New York, believes vitamin A mobilizes our infection-fighting white blood cells.

In one of his experiments, Dr. Seifter told us, two groups of lab animals, one fed an adequate amount of vitamin A and the other fed ten times that amount, were exposed to gamma radiation. The highly supplemented animals held up better. "The radiation destroys most, but not all, of the animals' white blood cells," he says. "The vitamin A stimulates the rate at which the animals regain a normal number of white blood cells, thereby increasing the rate of survival. The highly supplemented animals are able to recoup in a couple of weeks."

In a second group of experiments, Dr. Seifter's fellow researchers removed the thymus, a glandlike organ that influences production of some kinds of white blood cells, from both groups. Only the highly supplemented animals maintained a near-normal white blood cell count, demonstrating, Dr. Seifter says, that, in the event of injury or infection, vitamin A can reinforce the body's immune response.

Building Healthy Teeth

At the University of Alabama's institute of dental research, two researchers, Juan Navia, Ph.D., and Susan S. Harris, Ph.D., have been investigating the role of vitamin A in the formation of teeth. They've found that infant teeth are prone to decay if they lack vitamin A while they are forming within the gum.

"We're at the very beginning of looking at the possibility that nutrition during tooth formation can affect the development or increase the susceptibility of teeth to decay," Dr. Navia told us.

In the normal construction of teeth, vitamin A is essential for the formation of a scaffolding made up partly of carbohydrates called mucopolysaccharides. If that framework is properly built, calcium and phosphorus lock into place and the result is a healthy tooth.

Without enough vitamin A, however, there will be chinks in the new tooth and bacteria will seep in like rain through a leaky roof.

"Caries [decay] initiated at the enamel surface," Drs. Navia and Harris report, "would meet a less effective barrier at the enamel-dentine [the two outermost layers of the tooth] junction, leading to development of severe, deeply penetrating lesions" (*Archives of Oral Biology,* vol. 25, no. 6, 1980).

CHAPTER

16

VITAMIN A—
INSURANCE AGAINST
CIRCULATORY PROBLEMS

Medical researchers are forever warning about the *bad* effects certain dietary factors can have on our health. We're told that too much fat in our diets can cause heart disease or even cancer, too much salt raises blood pressure and too much refined sugar may promote cavities, not to mention diabetes.

But what about the *good* things we can add to our diets which actually promote health? A major study shows that the amount of vitamin A in our diets may have a profound effect on whether or not we fall prey to heart disease, high blood pressure, stroke or peptic ulcer.

The study, conducted in Israel by Aviva Palgi, Ph.D., analyzed 28 years worth of data in order to determine the cumulative effects of dietary changes on specific disease mortality rates.

Dr. Palgi, who has conducted research in nutrition at the Harvard Medical school and is now at the American Health Foundation in New York City, found that, between 1949 and 1977, the death rate from heart disease in Israel more than doubled while the death rates from high blood pressure, stroke and peptic ulcer also increased significantly. Meanwhile, during that same time, the Israelis had changed their eating habits. By the 1970s, they were consuming 52 percent more fat than in previous years. What's more, they had decreased the amount of calories coming from complex carbohydrates (such as grains) while almost doubling their intake of simple carbohydrates (refined sugars).

But what makes this study special is that Dr. Palgi not only looked at the obvious dietary factors like fats and carbohydrates, she also examined how specific vitamins and minerals can directly affect those same diseases.

And that's where the exciting news about vitamin A comes in.

"Vitamin A," says Dr. Palgi, "consistently had a significant negative association with mortality rates." This means that the more vitamin A individuals in the study consumed, the less likely they were to suffer from heart disease, high blood pressure, stroke and peptic ulcer.

Apparently, while some Israelis were eating more fats, others were enjoying lots of fruits, vegetables and other foods high in vitamin A. And those who ate those foods stayed healthier than those who didn't.

In fact, Dr. Palgi's study concludes by suggesting that reduced total fat intake and increased vitamin A consumption (through fruits and vegetables) may prove beneficial in reducing death rates due to heart disease, high blood pressure, stroke and peptic ulcer (*American Journal of Clinical Nutrition,* August, 1981).

"We are just beginning to see the benefits of vitamin A in the diet," Dr. Palgi says, "and it's very exciting. My study merely emphasizes how much research still needs to be done— especially clinical experiments with human volunteers.

"Right now, we know that 5,000 international units of vitamin A daily is an absolute requirement for health. But for people in a predisease state, more may be needed. I know that in view of the results of my study I am more conscious of my diet, and I try to eat plenty of vitamin A–rich foods while also keeping my total fat intake as low as possible."

Just how vitamin A exerts its protective influence is something scientists are still looking into.

"There have been several studies in the past which have shown vitamin A to be helpful in lowering cholesterol levels, and this may help explain why it aids against heart disease," Dr. Palgi told us. "In one experiment, the vitamin was found to lower blood cholesterol levels in atherosclerotic patients but had no effect on patients whose cholesterol levels were already normal. And another study showed a decreased incidence of cardiovascular disease in patients given vitamins A and D. Still," cautions Dr. Palgi, "vitamin A is not a magic wand."

Maybe it's not a magic wand, but vitamin A is still a valuable diet resource, readily available to anyone willing to invest a little time and thought in planning his diet. The complete form of vitamin A is found only in foods of animal origin, and one of the richest sources is liver. Vitamin A, like vitamins D and E, is a fat-soluble vitamin, which means it is not excreted in the urine, like the water-soluble vitamins, but stored in the body for further use. Vitamin A is stored mainly in the liver, which is why beef liver is rich in the vitamin.

You could easily fulfill your body's need for vitamin A even if you ate nothing but vegetables, though. Substances called carotenes, which are abundant in many vegetables, are readily converted into vitamin A in the human body. Yellow fruits and vegetables like carrots, sweet potatoes, apricots, pumpkins and cantaloupes are rich in carotenes, as are deep-green leafy vegetables like spinach, dandelion greens, beet greens, chard, chicory, turnip greens and kale.

There are a few special tricks you can use to maximize your intake of vitamin A from vegetables.

Researchers have found that the more orange the carrots and sweet potatoes you buy, the more vitamin A they contain. Plant breeding that was originally undertaken to improve the looks of carrots has resulted in strains that are richer in vitamin A. Vitamin A stands up well to cooking, but that's *light* cooking—if you cook too much, you destroy the carotene by oxidation.

Deficiency Is More Common than Overdose

Newspaper articles pointing out the toxicity of vitamin A appear from time to time. One article told of a three-year-old girl given 200,000 international units of vitamin A a day. This is clearly excessive. For adults, a daily intake of 4,000 to 25,000 international units is considered reasonable by the National Academy of Sciences.

But the real problem is a *lack* of vitamin A in our diets, not an oversupply.

"The 1965 household survey of diets showed that one diet in every four failed to supply the recommended allowances [of vitamin A] and that one diet in every 10 supplied less than two-thirds of the recommended allowances," cites one nutritionist (*Normal and Therapeutic Nutrition,* Macmillan, 1977). "Deficiency of vitamin A is not only a major nutritional problem in many developing countries but also in countries such as the United States and Canada," says a National Institutes of Health researcher (*Lung,* vol. 157, no. 4, 1980). Both infants and the elderly are known to have a decreased ability to absorb vitamin A from their diets.

CHAPTER
17

VITAMIN A FOR HEAVY MENSTRUAL BLEEDING

No one likes to get cut up. Yet, more than 670,000 women rushed into hysterectomies in a recent year. What's the hurry?

Well, take the widowed mother of four for an example. As the sole supporter of her family, she can't afford to stay off her feet and miss a couple of days at work every month because of an extremely heavy menstrual flow. Besides, she's been feeling too wiped out lately to give her children the attention they need.

Or what about the young woman who kept her monthly interruptions to a minimum while she was on oral contraceptives. But since she's given up the Pill, she's sacrificed additional days of freedom. Her periods *never* extended beyond six days, she cries to her gynecologist. Now she's strapped for nine or ten.

Undoubtedly, there are thousands more silent sufferers who face such unpleasant confrontations with their femininity each month—tolerating excessive menstrual bleeding and extended bouts with their periods.

In desperation, some will eventually elect surgery as the "ultimate out." Who's to say they made the wrong choice? Certainly not their physicians, who will quickly point to the serious complications of this condition.

96

Menorrhagia—the medical term for either excessive daily bleeding during menstruation, prolonged menstrual flow or both—may lead to anemia, gynecologists warn. Granted. But with complications of its own, surgery is a high price to pay for recovery—particularly when relief can sometimes be had for the cost of a bottle of vitamin A supplements.

According to a study published in the *South African Medical Journal,* menorrhagia may be caused by a vitamin A deficiency. Women who experience heavy menstruation and have lower than normal vitamin A levels in their blood can enjoy alleviation of their symptoms with moderately high doses of the vitamin, the investigators report.

The effect of a vitamin A deficiency on the reproductive system of women has never been clearly documented. But it stands to reason that such a deficiency could alter the menstrual cycle. After all, vitamin A is crucial to the development of the ovaries in animals. In animal tests, a laboratory-induced deficiency of this vitamin can decrease hormone production and suspend the menstrual cycle.

Earlier studies put that theory into human terms when researchers demonstrated that vitamin A levels in women fluctuate in a cyclic pattern during the menstrual cycle. They suggest a strong correlation between vitamin A levels and female hormones.

Keeping these findings in mind, Drs. M. Lithgow and W. M. Politzer, of the Johannesburg General Hospital in South Africa, decided to find out whether vitamin A deficiency causes menorrhagia and whether giving vitamin A would cure the condition. To do this, they tested the vitamin A levels in 71 patients suffering from menorrhagia. These figures were then compared to those obtained from blood tests of 191 healthy women between the ages of 13 and 55.

The results clearly indicated that women with particular menstrual dysfunction have relatively low levels of vitamin A in their bloodstreams. In fact, the women tested had, on the average, only 67 international units of the vitamin per 100 milliliters of blood. In contrast, the women with normal menstrual periods had about 166 international units per 100 milliliters—almost 2½ times the amount measured in the first group!

To define more precisely the role of a vitamin A deficiency in menstrual dysfunction, the records of 103 patients who presented a wider spectrum of the causes of menorrhagia were combined with those of the original group. A vitamin A deficiency was still found to be the primary cause of the menorrhagia in almost 44 percent of the total 174 cases studied. In addition, almost 68 percent of this combined group had lower than average levels of vitamin A in their blood, indicating that a shortage of this vitamin might be a contributing cause of the abnormal bleeding.

A Successful Treatment

Now that the researchers were assured of the cause of the problem, they followed through with treatment using vitamin A supplements. Fifty-two menorrhagia patients were instructed to take 60,000 international units of vitamin A daily for 35 days.

Although a few of these women were lost to follow-up treatment, of the 40 who returned for evaluation one month later, 23 were completely cured. And 14 noted a substantially diminished menstrual flow or a reduction in the duration of their periods. All told, the researchers claimed that close to 93 percent were either cured or helped with vitamin A therapy.

If you've been losing a lot of blood during your menses, you too may gain by increasing your intake of vitamin A. However, the daily dosage of 60,000 international units prescribed by the South African physicians may be more than you'll need. You might want to stick with the amount found in many multivitamins, which is 10,000 international units.

Should you find that the extra boost of A isn't enough to alleviate the heavy or prolonged menstrual bleeding, don't up your intake beyond the suggested amount. Instead, add vitamin E to your nutrition checklist. This vitamin helps improve vitamin A storage and utilization. Or try zinc. An essential mineral, zinc is required to move vitamin A from the large liver reserve to the bloodstream.

The Link with Vasectomy

Interestingly enough, this information may be invaluable to you if you're involved with family planning.

"A syndrome of menorrhagia is now being seen in women whose husbands have had vasectomies," said Dr. Dennis G. Bonham, head of the Auckland University postgraduate school of obstetrics and gynaecology in New Zealand, in *Ob. Gyn. News.* "Like the post-tubal ligation syndrome, the post-vasectomy syndrome appears to be primarily a result of stopping oral contraceptives. . . ." And that, it seems, may be a direct result of a depletion of vitamin A.

For some time now, researchers have suspected that the hormones found in oral contraceptives alter the vitamin A levels in the blood. To test this theory, vitamin A levels in two groups of healthy college women were measured. The first group consisted of 11 women with regular menstrual cycles who had never taken the Pill. The other group consisted of 7 women who had been on the Pill for various lengths of time ranging from two months to slightly over two years (*American Journal of Clinical Nutrition*).

Invariably, the women taking the oral contraceptives had higher levels of vitamin A in their blood than nonusers. This may be due to a stepped-up mobilization of the vitamin stored in the liver. The theory is confirmed by animal experimentation. Rats given oral contraceptives experience a faster liver vitamin A depletion, indicating a higher vitamin A requirement.

Of course, no one knows for sure, but this may explain why women who stop taking the Pill suddenly begin menstruating heavily. While they are taking the Pill, their bloodstreams are pumped full of vitamin A, which assures them a short and uneventful menstrual period. But should they stop taking the Pill, the vitamin A supply in their blood is cut short. The liver reserve which would be called on under normal conditions has become sharply depleted.

So, should you consider giving up the Pill for whatever reason (and there are many), supplement your stores with extra doses of vitamin A. It could protect you from that extreme course of action—hysterectomy.

CHAPTER
18

VITAMIN A CUSHIONS US AGAINST STRESS

We remember when, every August, busloads of city kids would head up north for two weeks of the country life. They came face to face with animals they'd never seen at the city zoo, and they learned that the swimmin' hole was more than a wrench and a fire hydrant. Sending those kids to the country was kind of like hanging sheets out to dry. They could flap around all over the place, and the fresh air did them good.

Today, you wonder how far you'd have to travel to find unpolluted air and water. Chemicals originally designed to improve our lives are doing just the opposite. They're everywhere, but living in wet suits and gas masks is no answer. Eli Seifter, Ph.D., a nutritional biochemist at Albert Einstein College of Medicine, has been doing research on vitamin A and believes the vitamin will help guard against a variety of environmental hazards and stresses.

Chemical hazards in the work place attracted national attention during the last decade. In the mid 1970s, workers in plants manufacturing DBCP, a soil fumigant used to control nematodes, began to complain of sterility and other reproductive deficiencies. Subsequent laboratory studies indicated that exposure to relatively low doses of DBCP could reduce sperm counts enough to cause sterility. When data on the effects on humans were released in 1977, some U.S. manufacturers stopped making it.

Despite efforts by the Occupational Safety and Health Administration and the Environmental Protection Agency to reduce the use of DBCP in the environment, data gathered show unexpectedly high levels of the chemical in drinking water near farming areas. And a lawsuit has been filed by DBCP workers in California who claim that their sons' defective reproductive organs resulted from the workers' exposure to the chemical.

The list of chemicals posing health hazards for both male and female workers has expanded, prompting one labor leader to dub the 1980s the "decade of genetic confrontation."

Even if people aren't working in chemical plants, they are caught in the onslaught. If home is near the freeway or in a highly industrialized area, car exhaust and other pollutants lace the air and water. People also are cleaning their houses, spraying their gardens, refinishing furniture and cooking with chemicals every day.

In a presentation before an American Chemical Society meeting in Houston, Dr. Seifter illustrated how the toxicity of a substance is influenced by the nutritional and the general health status of an animal and how those findings relate to humans in the work place.

Many harmful stimuli, whether physical injury, chemical poisoning or some other factor, will elicit a common response called *stress,* says Dr. Seifter. Stress causes adrenal gland enlargement, a shrinking of the thymus gland and body weight loss. It also can cause stomach ulceration.

In one experiment, Dr. Seifter and his colleagues studied the effects of vitamin A on the toxic compound toluene diamine (TDA). The chemical causes stomach ulceration, which leads to stomach perforation. Death can occur from peritonitis following a leakage from the stomach.

TDA ingestion causes blood to withdraw from the stomach (humans may identify it as a queasy feeling) and from the skin (similar to people turning pale after a type of stress response). The condition is called ischemia, which means a loss of circulating blood that causes blanching or whitening. Ischemia is an early event leading to stress ulceration and delaying healing of the ulcer.

In animals given only TDA, blanching of the stomach occurred. Animals that received both TDA and vitamin A did not show a blanching effect.

Eventually, the animals on TDA alone developed certain stomach ulcerations, while the animals whose TDA intake was supplemented with vitamin A did *not* have the stomach ulcerations.

A toxic compound's ability to produce duodenal and stomach ulcers after diminishing blood supply to those parts of the gastrointestinal tract can be overcome by feeding vitamin A, Dr. Seifter told his audience.

He says that TDA and some other chemicals either directly or indirectly constrict blood vessels to certain organs, like the stomach and skin, while opening up blood vessels elsewhere, especially in muscle. That mimics the fight-or-flight syndrome which prepares the body for intense physical activity or running away. In that instance, blood is diverted from the soft tissues and goes into the muscles. Dr. Seifter and his colleagues speculate that vitamin A prevents that alteration in blood flow pattern from taking place.

Stressed adrenals also become large and swollen and tend to bleed. Vitamin A prevents the swelling and hemorrhage, says Dr. Seifter.

The researchers also have investigated vitamin A in relation to alkylating agents, which, according to Dr. Seifter, are "important agents in industry today, and they affect our health." One of the alkylating agents they looked at, cyclophosphamide, is widely used as an antitumor compound in chemotherapy. The chemical is radiationlike and is known as a radiomimetic chemical.

Cancer Drug Better Tolerated with Vitamin A

"Sick people (and sick animals) cannot take as high doses of some medications as a well person can," Dr. Seifter told us.

"The irony is that it's the sick person who needs the medication. If you give a certain amount of cyclophosphamide to a healthy animal, the animal may not lose weight. Give it to a sick animal, and it may kill him."

The researchers discovered that, if a stressed animal (one that is subjected to experimental surgery, for instance) is given vitamin A along with the cyclophosphamide, it tolerates the drug better. "Vitamin A makes the difference between whether or not the animal survives toxic doses of cyclophosphamide when the animal has some other sickness—and that other sickness can be stress or an implanted tumor," Dr. Seifter told us.

That discovery may be of some importance to employees working with those toxic substances. Alkylating agents are used to combat tumors because they inhibit cell division in the tissues that are turning over most rapidly, like the cancer cells in a tumor, he says.

"In the body, normally among those tissues that are turning over most rapidly are mucosal cells and white blood cells and sperm. And you can be sure . . . if workers are showing low sperm counts, due to working with alkylating agents, they're also showing low counts of certain white blood cells."

Under the stress of a toxicant like cyclophosphamide, mice experience weight loss or a prevention of weight gain, says Dr. Seifter. With vitamin A intake, a good share of that weight loss is avoided.

Protecting the Thymus Gland

One site of immune activity in the body, the thymus gland, reacts to a toxicant like cyclophosphamide by becoming very small or involuted. Part of that involution can be blocked also by giving vitamin A, he says.

Researchers cannot assay the human thymus without causing damage, so they must analyze the blood. "When the thymus is hurt, those circulating blood cells that are influenced by the thymus are also hurt. These are the lymphocytes," Dr. Seifter told us. Lymphocytes that normally constitute more than 20 percent of our circulating white blood cells will drop to 5 or 10 percent and be less active when the thymus is in trouble.

Other Common Stresses

Dr. Seifter maintains that certain jobs are stressful enough to the worker's body to heighten his or her nutritional requirements. He says that, just as society now accepts the idea that people like steelworkers, who perspire heavily on the job, need higher intakes of calories, salt and water, it will in time accept the idea that other jobs increase other nutrient requirements.

"The requirements for other nutrients are dependent on the toxic compounds that we are exposed to. I think the time will come when we'll not only learn that nutrient requirements are increased, but we'll make use of specific nutrients to overcome the toxicity of certain industrial hazards," Dr. Seifter told the American Chemical Society.

There also may come a time when vitamin A will be used to arm someone against another kind of hazard—radiation.

Dr. Seifter and his colleagues discovered that, when X ray treatments were administered to the hind legs of mice, the classic stress responses were recorded. The mice lost weight, their adrenals enlarged, their thymus glands shrank and their white cell counts dropped precipitously.

Mice supplemented with vitamin A fared much better with the radiation treatment. They lost less weight, and their adrenals did not get as large. Perhaps most important, with vitamin A, the thymus gland did not shrink significantly in size. The white cell count remained relatively high, and that's a very good sign, says Dr. Seifter. It's not unusual for a patient who has undergone radiation treatments to develop serious infections, and some of these are fatal. Radiation normally decreases the number of white blood cells, thereby depressing the patient's immune state. Both the tumor and the radiation are immunosuppressive, he says. Vitamin A appears to change some of that.

Animals given vitamin A in advance of the radiation treatment may have had a slight edge over those given the supplement afterward. "What's clear is giving it at all is better than not giving it," Dr. Seifter told us.

"We think that, for people who receive radiotherapy [radiation treatments], vitamin A will contribute to their overall health without decreasing the efficacy of the radiotherapy against the tumor. In fact, vitamin A may increase the efficacy of the radiotherapy. The healthier an animal is—the healthier a person is—the better he can withstand radiotherapy and the better the chance that he will get effective radiation therapy," Dr. Seifter explains.

Some people refuse to believe that something as simple as vitamin A could do so much. But the National Institutes of Health (NIH), for instance, support the use of a kind of vitamin A acid, a synthetic compound for certain clinical uses, Dr. Seifter says. The NIH supports studies involving the use of this analog of vitamin A for tumor prevention, he says, adding that high doses of vitamin A acid are far more toxic than vitamin A. Although they claim they are using vitamin A acid for its vitamin A activity, he explains, they are actually using it in much the same way as they are other toxic agents that cause tumors to decrease in size.

Avoiding "Injury Therapy"

"Practically all of the tumor therapies that we have today are based upon injury . . . injuring both the host and the tumor. People say we've got to blast the hell out of the tumor, but you're also blasting the hell out of the body," says Dr. Seifter. "They tend to favor vitamin A acid because it causes the tumor to get smaller. But the animal gets very sick, and it gets smaller, too. Maybe he'll lose 25 percent or greater of the body weight. Now most people cannot tolerate a 30 percent loss of body weight. That's lethal."

Dr. Seifter believes that it may be unnecessary to totally rid the body of the tumor to obtain survival and a good quality of life. While some tumor cells may live in the body for years, many of them are destroyed by the body's immune system, he says.

"No one is really talking about fully eradicating tumors. That's not a realistic aim at present. The aim is to decrease the tumor cell population size by surgery or other therapy so the body can deal with it. And dealing with it doesn't necessarily mean getting rid of it. If the tumor doesn't get any bigger and doesn't start sending out branches, that would be acceptable."

A Natural Protective Agent

The rift over whether to use vitamin A acid or vitamin A remains unresolved. In 1974, Dr. Seifter proposed to the NIH that studies be initiated to determine if moderate increases in vitamin A given to residents living in an area known as "Cancer Alley" in New Jersey would reduce the incidence of tumors in the high-risk population. The NIH rejected the proposal two years in a row. One of their reasons was that vitamin A was a "toxic substance," says Dr. Seifter. But afterward, research workers at the NIH announced that vitamin A acid would be preferable to use instead of vitamin A for studies of tumor prevention.

Dr. Seifter labels the action "just political," the politics of cancer and cancer research.

He does not promote the use of huge doses of any kind except during extraordinary circumstances. Besides normal supplements, people can get vitamin A by eating organ meats like liver, kidney and spleen, or they can eat foods rich in carotene. Vegetables like squash, carrots, spinach and all greens contain carotene, which the body converts into vitamin as needed.

Whether you choose to get the nutrient through organ meats, vegetables or supplements, vitamin A may cushion you against any number of life's stress-producing elements.

CHAPTER
19

VITAMIN A: A KIND OF INTERNAL GAS MASK

You are surrounded by enemies—ruthless, destructive and invisible as air. Your every breath lays you open to attack by this sinister crew—automobile exhaust, industrial smog, poisonous clouds emitted by smokers who care even less about your health than about their own, tiny particles too small to see, viruses and bacteria.

Individually, they are vicious. Working together, this terrifying pack of marauders can do more to rough up your body than any gang of Central Park muggers. They can lay you low with infection, emphysema, cancer. They can kill you. A black belt in karate won't help you defend yourself against them. And a gas mask is just a bit impractical.

You aren't unarmed against this sea of troubles, though. Deep in your lungs, a complex, highly efficient defense system is always in action to drive out invading chemicals, particles and microorganisms and swiftly undo the damage they cause.

For this, you can thank a special kind of tissue called epithelium, which lines the entire respiratory tract. Some epithelial cells secrete mucus, a thick substance that traps particles and bacteria. Other epithelial cells come equipped with microscopic hairs, called cilia, which constantly sweep invaders up and out of the body.

Most important, this tissue has the ability to repair itself. Every day, epithelial cells are killed by bacteria, poisonous gases and other airborne enemies, and every day they grow back, literally as good as new. Without this power to regenerate, your lungs wouldn't last long in the chemical soup that passes for air in modern cities.

How well your lungs can hold their own in the face of unrelenting assault means the difference between health and very serious disease, so it's natural to wonder if there's anything you can do to strengthen the fortress. In fact, a growing list of studies point to something that can help—vitamin A.

For over 50 years, doctors and scientists have recognized that vitamin A has a special role to play in maintaining the health of epithelial tissue (the skin is largely composed of epithelial cells; this is one reason why vitamin A is so essential for healthy skin). Without enough vitamin A, epithelial tissues become hardened and take abnormal forms. They cannot repair themselves when they are damaged. Abundant vitamin A, on the other hand, promotes the production of healthy new tissue.

With this power, mounting evidence affirms, vitamin A can help lungs protect themselves against the airborne battalions that modern life sends in against them.

Some of the most impressive evidence of this protective ability comes from a study that brought vitamin A into action against a particularly destructive enemy of lung health—a noxious gas called nitrogen dioxide (NO_2) (*Journal of Applied Nutrition*).

The Pollutant That Makes Smog Brown

If you've ever noticed a brownish cast to the smog that seems to be smothering your city, you've seen NO_2. More likely, you've inhaled one lungful after another without even knowing it's there. Automobile exhaust contributes this poisonous chemical to the air you breathe, and so do industrial wastes. It is contained in cigarette smoke and produced when coal or natural gas is burned for heat.

Laboratory tests have shown that NO_2 can damage lung tissue, producing the deteriorated state associated with emphysema. After exposure to NO_2, it has been found, animals are more susceptible to infections of the lung. (In human beings, air pollution in general has been linked to high rates of respiratory infections.) Through a chain of reactions within the body, NO_2 can form nitrosamines, potent cancer-causing chemicals.

What kind of protection can vitamin A offer against this poison gas? At the Delta Regional Primate Research Center of Tulane University, James C. S. Kim, D.V.M., Sc.D., exposed three groups of hamsters to NO_2 for five-hour periods once a week for eight weeks. The conditions, he told us, were "comparable not only to industrial pollution found in an urban-suburban environment, but also to the exposure of the respiratory tract of a habitual smoker."

The first group of hamsters received a diet lacking in vitamin A. The second ate what Dr. Kim called a "vitamin A–adequate" diet. The third was fed a "vitamin A–high" diet—twice what the second group received. After eight weeks of exposure and observation, the hamsters were killed and their lung tissues examined.

The vitamin A–deficient animals, Dr. Kim noted, responded poorly to NO_2 exposure: "Rapid and often labored breathing appeared immediately and continued throughout the five hours. Recovery was slow." By the fifth week of the experiment, they had started to decline visibly. When they were killed, "all exposed animals without exception were in poor condition."

Microscopic examination of their lung tissues revealed severe damage. The epithelial lining, it was found, had degenerated badly. The cilia, so necessary for defense against bacteria, had been impaired, in some cases destroyed. Cells in the alveoli (the little sacs where oxygen passes from the air into the bloodstream) had hardened and were unable to function properly. In many animals, there were signs of pneumonia. And instances of abnormal cell growth—the kind that is associated with the development of cancer—were widespread.

The hamsters that received a vitamin A–adequate diet fared a good deal better. NO_2 made them breathe rapidly, but they showed no signs of distress, and afterward their breathing quickly returned to normal. They remained in good condition throughout the eight weeks of the experiment and were "healthy and alert" at its end.

When the lungs of these animals were examined, there were no signs of pneumonia or the severe inflammation that had afflicted the deficient group. The gas had caused damage, certainly, but normal lung tissue had apparently grown back to repair it. "There appeared to be an increase in cell regeneration in animals supplemented with vitamin A, in contrast with those not supplemented," Dr. Kim noted. The epithelial lining, for the most part, was intact, and there were few abnormal cells.

The animals that received double doses of vitamin A survived their polluted environment equally well. Observation and microscopic examination showed them to be much like the vitamin A–adequate group *(Environmental Research)*.

How A Protects the Lungs

In a telephone interview, Dr. Kim summed up the significant implications of his experiment: "High concentrations of NO_2 destroy the epithelial lining. With enough (or a little more than enough) vitamin A, regeneration of the lung is rapid and successful. But with a low dose, this protective response is retarded—and the animal suffers."

Too little vitamin A in the face of NO_2 exposure can raise the risk of disease, he explained. "Without vitamin A, ciliated epithelium doesn't form. Instead, you get squamous cells—precarcinoma-type cells. You get abnormal mucous cells, which mean clogging in the respiratory tract and danger of infection. If the epithelium doesn't form properly, it can lead to emphysema and chronic bronchitis.

His findings should be of special interest to commuters, Dr. Kim says, because they subject themselves to conditions much like those of his experiment. "If you commute, you have intermittent exposure to NO_2. You may be exposed to urban pollution for five hours, eight hours, then you come back to your house in the suburbs, where the air is cleaner. The next day you go back to the city. The epithelium in the lung has to repair itself accordingly, after each exposure."

Vitamin A can help the lungs adapt to this less-than-perfect world, Dr. Kim says. "But a commuter who doesn't get enough vitamin A is going to suffer."

In general, the effects he observed in his lab led Dr. Kim to regard vitamin A highly as a preventive measure for safeguarding lung health. Even the lung problems that we associate with old age, like emphysema, may be forestalled with the early, regular use of vitamin A supplements, he speculates.

CHAPTER
20

THE NUMBER ONE
ANTI-CANCER VITAMIN

The evidence has been piling up higher than a bumper crop of corn in August. Eating green and yellow vegetables just may be your buffer against cancer.

Actually, it's not so much the vegetables as what's in them that seems to be doing the trick. The good guy's name is beta-carotene, a natural pigment found in these vegetables and even some fruits. Once inside our bodies, beta-carotene is converted to usable vitamin A. Carrots, sweet potatoes, dark leafy greens, apricots, cantaloupe and winter squash are excellent sources of this important nutrient.

While all this may seem like a mouthful in itself, there are reams of research to indicate that those who eat carotene-rich foods on a routine basis are a lot more successful at avoiding cancer or beating it down than those who don't.

The evidence is so impressive, in fact, that the conservative National Research Council, convinced that there's a link between diet and cancer, has gone public with a list of dietary recommendations designed to reduce the risks of developing cancers, especially those that attack the lungs, stomach, throat, skin, bowel and bladder. The council recommends that all Americans significantly reduce consumption of fats, fat-laden meats and dairy products; eat less cured, pickled and smoked foods; convert to whole grains on a daily basis; and eat plenty of vitamin C and foods rich in beta-carotene.

And that's not all. The news about beta-carotene is so promising that the National Institutes of Health are now funding what is believed to be the biggest population study ever undertaken to test the hypothesis that beta-carotene, known also by the name provitamin A, does prevent cancer. The two-pronged study (the other half deals with aspirin and heart disease) is being conducted by the Harvard medical school and involves approximately 25,000 physicians throughout the country. The doctors are taking either a beta-carotene supplement or a placebo (dummy pill) every other day. Questionnaires concerning their dietary intake and current health status are being tallied at six-month intervals. At the end of the five-year study, the incidence of cancer in both the placebo and supplement groups will be measured.

"We hope the Harvard study will show exactly how important beta-carotene is in preventing cancer," Micheline Mathews-Roth, M.D., the beta-carotene consultant for the study, told us. "The studies to date show that there is something in beta-carotene-rich foods that has an effect on cancer. But whether it's the beta-carotene or some other component of the vegetables isn't known for sure yet."

That doesn't mean you have to get rabid about rabbit food, either. "The studies to date show that those who benefited from the beta-carotene in fighting cancer weren't eating huge amounts of vegetables," says Dr. Mathews-Roth, whose own studies have found a link between beta-carotene and skin cancer. "What it does show is that people aren't even eating the 3 ounces a day or so that they should be getting."

Eat Your Vegetables

So the bottom line is that it's a good idea, in fact a wise idea, to get your full allowance of those wholesome greens and yellows each and every day. "We think it is prudent for all apparently healthy adults to include in the daily diet one or two servings of the vegetables or fruits that are rich in beta-carotene," says Richard B. Shekelle, Ph.D., an eminent researcher in diet and health at Rush–Presbyterian–St. Luke's Medical Center in Chicago. "The weight of evidence at this time suggests that people who eat these kinds of foods on a regular basis run a lower risk of getting cancer than those who don't."

Dr. Shekelle sent the cancer research community into a spin with the results of his long-term study on beta-carotene and its effects on the deadliest of malignancies to man—lung cancer.

Dr. Shekelle's study actually began as a long-term investigation into coronary heart disease on 2,107 workers of a Chicago-based plant of the Western Electric Company. One aspect of the study was to take dietary records of the participants. When it came to plotting vitamin A intake, Dr. Shekelle and his colleagues decided to divide the vitamin intake into that which came from animal sources (whole milk, liver, cream, butter and cheese) and that which came from beta-carotene-rich fruits and vegetables.

Over the next 19 years, 33 of the men developed lung cancer—all positively related to cigarette smoking. However, Dr. Shekelle and his colleagues noticed something else very significant in those who developed lung cancer. The rate was highest in those who ate the least amount of beta-carotene foods and lowest in those who ate the greatest amount. The result: an eight-to-one difference in risk between the lowest and highest carotene-intake groups (*Lancet,* November 28, 1981).

Also of major significance is the work of Eli Seifter, Ph.D., Guiseppi Rettura, Ph.D., Jacques Padawer, Ph.D., and Stanley Levenson, M.D., of Albert Einstein College of Medicine in New York City, who have published studies pinpointing the benefits of beta-carotene and vitamin A in fighting cancer in animals.

"Our studies show that, if you inoculate mice with low doses of tumor cells, about 50 percent of them will develop tumors. However, in those pretreated with beta-carotene supplements, only 10 percent develop tumors," Dr. Seifter told us. "We also did a study in which we let the tumors grow to a certain size before we started beta-carotene supplementation. With beta-carotene, the tumors grew more slowly than normal and the animals survived longer.''

Vitamin A Strengthens Cancer Therapy

Perhaps the team's most dramatic experiment is a two-year study concerning the effects of radiation therapy, beta-carotene and vitamin A supplementation on induced cancer in mice. The mice were inoculated in the leg with cancer cells, which were permitted to grow. The mice were then divided into six treatment groups. Dr. Seifter explains:

"The radiation dose we used was comparable to the dose used in many cancer patients. That is, it was enough to reduce the tumor but not make it disappear. The dosage needed for that is too powerful. In the case of our mice, it would have burned off the leg.

"The first group got no diet therapy and no radiation therapy. The tumors grew and the animals died in 41 days. The second group got vitamin A but no radiation therapy and died in 60 days. The third group got beta-carotene and no radiation therapy and died in 61 days. And the fourth group got radiation therapy and no dietary supplementation and survived 83 days.

"So far, radiation therapy proved to be the best of the single treatments, but when it was combined with dietary supplementation, life expectancy was much geater.

"In the group that received radiation and vitamin A therapy, the tumors got smaller to the point where you couldn't feel them any more. Only one animal regrew the tumor and died. The others lived out the first year. The same results were found in mice given radiation therapy and beta-carotene.''

The benefits of beta-carotene became even more obvious in the second year when these survivors were again divided into groups. "Of the animals kept on vitamin A, none redeveloped their tumors and they lived a normal mouse life of two years. However, five of the six taken off of vitamin A regrew their tumors and died.

"In the beta-carotene group, those kept on the supplements also remained tumor free. And of those in which the beta-carotene was held back, only two redeveloped their cancers. And this is where the significance lies. The vitamin A–deprived mice got their tumors back in 66 days. But it took the beta-carotene-deprived mice 204 days to regrow their tumors." Even after developing cancer twice, they managed to survive 654 days—the natural life span of a mouse.

"It appears that the beta-carotene-fed mice retained a sufficient supply in their bodies to protect them from cancer even after they stopped taking the supplements," says Dr. Seifter.

There is also a human element in the chemotherapy–vitamin A cancer connection. This was found at the Wisconsin Cancer Center in Madison during a study of 37 women with breast cancer who were scheduled to undergo chemotherapy.

The study showed that 36 percent of the patients with low vitamin A levels improved with treatment, compared with 83 percent of those with normal or high vitamin A levels. Twenty-four percent of the patients in the low–vitamin A group remained stable and 40 percent worsened, while only 17 percent of the patients with normal or high vitamin A levels were listed as stable. What's more, none of these women grew worse (*Proceedings of American Association for Cancer Research*, 1981).

These studies come on the heels of other research, from such diverse sites as Norway, Japan, Singapore and Great Britain, that shows a correlation between foods rich in vitamin A or beta-carotene and a low cancer rate.

In many cultures, a particular plant or group of plants accounts for a large share of the people's dietary intake. In Japan, yellow and green vegetables are a mainstay of the diet. In West Africa, people eat a lot of red palm oil, the richest source of beta-carotene. In Singapore, it's dark green leafy vegetables. And North Americans are known to like their carrots.

One of the largest population studies to date was a five-year look into the smoking and eating habits of 8,278 Norwegians. Researchers found that, of the smokers, those who ate the least amount of beta-carotene had more than twice as great a chance of getting cancer as those who ate more *(International Journal of Cancer)*.

While the evidence strongly suggests that beta-carotene may be a safeguard against cancer, the final decision is still pending—at least until the Harvard study results are in. In the meantime, it's good to keep up your stock of beta-carotene.

"I think that beta-carotene, like vitamin E, is a good measure of what you're eating," says Dr. Seifter. "If you're not eating much, you're not getting enough. In terms of measurements, daily intake should be from 5 to 10 milligrams." That's equivalent to 8,375 to 16,750 international units of vitamin A a day.

But you needn't stop there if you don't want to. And that's the great thing about beta-carotene. Although it converts into beneficial vitamin A in the body, it doesn't lead to the side effects that taking too much vitamin A can produce. Most people know that taking too much vitamin A, more than 50,000 international units a day, can be toxic. Not so with beta-carotene.

Sure, you can get too much. A warning indication would likely be a coloring of the skin, like that of the 50 orange-faced people who were diagnosed in 1942 as having severe carotenemia after consuming 5 to 8 pounds of carrots a day! Getting over that required their getting off beta-carotene.

The other nice thing about beta-carotene is that finding the vegetables and fruits rich in it is simple. Spinach; dandelion, beet and collard greens; cantaloupe; broccoli and squash are just a slim picking of the edibles that are rich in beta-carotene. And they're the very things you can easily grow in your own back yard.

So remember the name beta-carotene. It's a friend you just might want to keep close to home.

THE B VITAMINS

CHAPTER

21

REAP THE REWARDS OF NUTRITIONAL TEAMWORK

Teamwork is something special.

It's a cooperative magic that happens when talented individuals get together and bring out the best in each other. No doubt you can come up with countless examples, from a major league baseball club to your favorite singing group. Regardless of your choice, you know that the team wouldn't work as well—it might not work at all—if someone decided to take the day off.

Just like the B vitamins.

Thiamine, riboflavin, niacin, vitamins B_6 and B_{12} and folate (folic acid), along with the lesser-known, but still vital, nutrients biotin, pantothenate (pantothenic acid), para-aminobenzoic acid (PABA), inositol and choline—there's the roster of a winning nutritional team.

Roger Williams, Ph.D., D.Sc., a University of Texas chemist and pioneer vitamin researcher, places special emphasis on the teamwork principle.

"Each B vitamin fits into different parts of the metabolic machinery of every living cell. And like cogs on a wheel, each has a specialized function," he told us.

But to prevent or cure disease, Dr. Williams explains, nutrients must also work cooperatively.

"When human beings are fortunate enough to maintain health by consuming wholesome food, this is accomplished by reason of the fact that they consume regularly every one of about 40 nutritional essentials. . . . We utilize in our bodies all nutritional elements simultaneously every day," a paper coauthored by Dr. Williams points out *(Proceedings of the National Academy of Sciences)*.

Unfortunately, try as we might, many of us can't meet all our B vitamin needs from food alone. So when we look for a helping hand, Dr. Williams notes, the way to "follow in nature's footsteps" is to choose a supplement containing each member of the B team.

"That way, they can work together," he says.

An Ideal Supplement

But how much of each is enough?

"In the body, B vitamins function as coenzymes," says Rebecca Riales, Ph.D., nutrition consultant from Parkersburg, West Virginia. Coenzymes are keys that unlock an enzyme's effectiveness and allow it to take part in a biological reaction.

Dr. Riales explains that very small amounts of the B vitamins are stored in the body, and what isn't used is soon excreted.

"The ideal B-complex supplement is one that provides the Recommended Dietary Allowance of all the vitamins. That way, you're covered in the event that you occasionally don't eat right," Dr. Riales told us.

As a good, natural B vitamin source, many people swear by brewer's yeast (although they may have less than lofty things to say about its taste), and Dr. Riales concurs.

"As a supplement, brewer's yeast provides a nice mix of B vitamins," she says, "but remember, all yeasts are not the same. Natural products can vary, so you have to read labels. For example, unless the yeast is enriched, folate may not be present. Even with the most gentle processing, this vitamin is very easily lost."

Dr. Riales points out that the RDAs for B vitamins can change at different times in an individual's life.

Pregnancy, of course, has its own special demands, and people under constant stress may have increased requirements.

"Anyone on long-term drug therapy should talk to the doctor or a good dietitian to find out if what they're taking may bring on a deficiency," she adds.

Because biochemical individuality is a fact of life, a number of doctors recommend taking many times the amounts suggested by Dr. Riales.

"The basic B complex is a foundation," says Harold Rosenberg, M.D., a New York physician who often prescribes megadoses of nutrients to help his patients cope with the stress of high-pressure living. "We can build on it to meet individual needs."

But might there be a problem with nutritional imbalances brought on by too much of a good thing?

Dr. Rosenberg doubts it and talks instead about the body's "wisdom."

"We find our own physiological balance," he says. "The body takes what it needs, stores what it can and throws the rest away."

So what's the ideal B vitamin supplement?

We know the cast of characters, but beyond the sometimes shifting RDAs, the jury's still out on the optimal amount of each nutrient required to ensure high-level health.

However, there's no doubt about the wide-ranging consequences of B vitamin insufficiency.

"The biological reactions dependent on the vitamin B complex are numerous," William Shive, Ph.D., researcher at the Clayton Foundation Biochemical Institute of the University of Texas, told us.

As an example, he described just one part of the amazingly intricate process by which our bodies utilize carbohydrates.

"This particular series of reactions requires five of the B vitamins. And it's a case of the chain being only as strong as its weakest link."

If one of the nutrients isn't in the proper place at the proper time, the work stops—like a construction project that suddenly finds itself short of mortgage money.

"We can now explain and treat a number of conditions that baffled us because we were used to thinking in terms of single nutrient deficiencies," says Howerde E. Sauberlich, Ph.D., chief of the division of nutrition technology at California's Letterman Army Institute of Research.

"Pellagra, for instance, is usually thought of as a niacin-deficiency disorder," says Dr. Sauberlich, "but the disease may not be due directly to a lack of this one nutrient. You see, the manufacture of niacin by the body requires the concerted action of riboflavin and vitamin B_6."

If any of these players don't make it to the field, the biological ball game could be over. Pellagra, though now quite rare, is often fatal. B vitamins team up in other ways, too.

A riboflavin deficiency may rear its ugly head in the form of mouth lesions, but Dr. Sauberlich writes that treatment with that one vitamin alone may not do the trick.

"Patients . . . [may] require supplementation with vitamin B_6 or other B-complex vitamins," he states (*Micronutrient Interactions: Vitamins, Minerals, and Hazardous Elements,* New York Academy of Sciences, 1980).

In the same paper, Dr. Sauberlich lists a number of other interacting partnerships vital to your well-being, including vitamin B_6 and B_{12}, B_{12} and folate, and biotin and pantothenate.

Is the Modern Diet Inadequate?

A deficiency of all members of the team is undoubtedly very rare, but because of their interaction, it's vital that every one fills its proper position.

Before modern food processing, it was reasonably possible to eat hearty and satisfy your B vitamin needs. But when white bread became the staff of life, the nutrient team came up short on a number of key players.

"Milling removes a significant portion of wheat's B vitamins," Paul LaChance, Ph.D., professor of nutrition at Rutgers University, told us. "What gets added back and what gets left behind depend both on federal regulation and company policy."

He explains that niacin and thiamine are restored to roughly the same amount as would be found in whole wheat. And enriched white flour actually has more riboflavin in it than does the original grain.

"Enrichment helped eradicate beriberi and pellagra," notes Dr. LaChance. "The public health benefits have been very real."

But he admits that white-as-the-driven-snow refined flour is but a pale echo of the whole wheat original. Depending on the degree of refinement, significant amounts of B_6, folate, pantothenate and other nutrients may be lost—and not restored.

"I'm not against enriched products in one sense—they're gap fillers and certainly better than a lot of meals people throw together on the run."

But since enrichment is partial at best, it offers a false sense of security. Better by far would be a diet rich in complete B vitamin sources.

Liver, milk products, whole grains, lean meats and many vegetables are tasty ways to eat your way to vitamin self-sufficiency.

And add a B-complex supplement as a kind of nutritional insurance.

You might be interested to know our astronauts bank on a supplement despite a well-thought-out menu. "They're free to eat what they want along certain lines—they can exchange items on the menu for other things they like. But remember, there's no fresh fruit, meat or vegetables in space—it's all thermostabilized or freeze-dried," explains Rita Rapp, dietitian and food-system coordinator at the Johnson Space Center in Houston. "Some of our pilots feel they can't survive without that multiple vitamin to supplement their meals!"

CHAPTER

22

THE THIAMINE THIEF MAY BE STEALING YOUR HEALTH

It's been said that good nutrition is like money in the bank. And to those of us who are in the know, it may seem a relatively easy matter to balance our nutritional "deposits" and so have a healthy personal economy.

But suppose for a moment that your bank has unknowingly hired a rather sneaky teller who has found a way to embezzle thiamine (vitamin B_1) from your account. In fact, this guy is so clever that he can skim your thiamine deposits without your being the wiser. Even the bank examiner—in this case, your doctor—might not detect the shenanigans of this underhanded teller.

Then one day comes the crunch. Suddenly you're having a little trouble sleeping, or you've lost your appetite. Maybe you're itching to pick a fight with your spouse. Maybe your chest hurts and you're scared that your heart's acting up.

What's going on? This: You've overdrawn your thiamine account, and your checks are bouncing all over the place.

If you think this sounds a bit farfetched—if you think it couldn't happen to you—maybe it's time to think again. Scientific evidence is mounting that an alarming number of people,

124

both young and old, are to one degree or another deficient in thiamine. Consider:

- A 1979 New Jersey study showed that 25 percent of 146 elderly people living at home were deficient in thiamine (*Journal of the American Geriatrics Society,* October, 1979).
- In a 1980 Irish study, up to 35 percent of the elderly surveyed had a thiamine deficiency (*Irish Journal of Medicine,* vol. 149, no. 3, 1980).
- In Australia, "thiamine status determined by biochemical assay was abnormal in one in five apparently healthy . . . blood donors" (*Medical Journal of Australia,* May, 1980).
- In a California study, Joseph D. Walters, M.D., and Richard P. Huemer, M.D., found that "the most common vitamin deficiences in our series were low serum B_1 and D," each of which occurred in 32 percent of their patients. Drs. Walters and Huemer conclude, "subclinical, but biochemically significant, vitamin deficiencies occur quite commonly [and] may be significant elements . . . that contribute to a disease state" (*Journal of the International Academy of Preventive Medicine*).

We Need Only a Little Thiamine

In light of the fact that thiamine was the first member of the vitamin B complex to be identified chemically and is thus so well known, it is somewhat ironic that so many people are deficient in it. Perhaps doubly ironic is the fact that the human need for the vitamin is relatively low. The National Research Council recommends only 0.5 milligram of thiamine per every 1,000 calories that we take in. The daily Recommended Dietary Allowance is set at 1.0 milligram for most women and between 1.2 and 1.4 milligrams for most men.

If the vitamin is so well known and our daily requirement for it apparently so low, why are so many deficient in it?

Part of the problem lies in the very nature of thiamine. Like vitamin C, thiamine is one of the water-soluble vitamins, which means that we can't store it in our bodies. We have to make new thiamine "deposits" every day because we are continually writing checks against our account.

Another part of the problem, according to Sue Rodwell Williams, M.P.H., author of *Nutrition and Diet Therapy* (C. V. Mosby, 1973), is the fact that "thiamine is less widely distributed in food than some other vitamins." To be sure, thiamine is available in fairly high quantities in such foods as pork, beef, liver, whole grains and legumes, but many people do not eat these foods regularly, and thiamine is hard to come by in other foods. "Therefore," says Mrs. Williams, "a deficiency in thiamine is a distinct possibility in the average diet."

But the big rub with thiamine gets back to that weasel of a bank teller. He takes every opportunity to snitch some thiamine, and all sorts of factors give him just the opportunity he needs.

Age: A number of dietary studies have suggested that our requirements for certain nutrients increase with age. In the case of thiamine, one study indicates that this may be due not to any malabsorption of the vitamin but to our inability, as we get older, to utilize what we do absorb, in effect raising our daily requirements (*Journal of the American Geriatrics Society,* October, 1979).

Eating foods with empty calories: Thiamine is essential for metabolizing sugar, and eating too much sugar-laden food and beverages not only depletes the thiamine we do have, but adds no new thiamine to our diet.

Unknowingly eating foods low in thiamine: In one study, 25 volunteers were allowed to continue their normal diets with a few seemingly minor exceptions: They were to eat no pork (high in thiamine but, unfortunately, high in fat as well) or vitamin-enriched cereal, bread or breakfast drinks. Even such mild restrictions produced a "significant fall" in thiamine in only 14 days (*Importance of Vitamins to Human Health,* University Park Press, 1979).

Overcooking foods: Thiamine is fragile, and too much heat or prolonged cooking can reduce or even destroy the vitamin.

Drinking alcoholic beverages: This can destroy thiamine or reduce the amount the body can absorb.

Dieting to reduce weight: With dieting or any reduced intake of food, your thiamine supply may fall 40 percent.

No Symptoms—At First

Now, none of the above would probably result in a big-time, clinical thiamine-deficiency disease such as beriberi. No, what we are talking about here is not Bonnie and Clyde knocking over your bank, but just a teller with a mean streak who is stealing a little too much of your thiamine each day.

Such a condition is called a subclinical deficiency. That means it's serious enough to be concerned about, not serious enough to kill you, and perhaps most important, so well hidden that neither you nor your doctor may suspect that anything is abnormal.

The hidden nature of subclinical deficiencies was vividly demonstrated in a recent study in which 19 medical students volunteered to go on a partially thiamine-restricted diet. Using chemical analysis of urine samples, the investigators could easily identify students who were low in thiamine. But every other commonly used method of diagnosing the deficiency was considered a failure. Those methods included asking the students how they felt, psychological testing, nerve conduction studies and work performance studies (*American Journal of Clinical Nutrition,* April, 1980).

As the researchers themselves put it, their study "casts some doubt on the long-held belief that certain subjective signs and symptoms herald early thiamine deficiency." In other words, lots of people are walking around with subclinical thiamine deficiencies and don't know it. And it might not take too much more of a deficiency to push them into a category where they'd know it more than they'd like to.

One step below subclinical is chronic, mild deficiency of thiamine. The problem here is that, although the condition is no longer hidden, it's nonetheless very hard to diagnose. Why? Because the symptoms are so general and vague. Lack of appetite, indigestion, nausea, severe constipation—do those sound like symptoms of chronic, mild thiamine deficiency? Well, they are but a few, and they might even cause you to eat less, which would only aggravate the deficiency!

How a Deficiency Affects the Nervous System

Other, more serious thiamine-deficiency problems can be heart muscle weakness and edema (an abnormal accumulation of body fluids). Also, thiamine deficiency can cause neuropathy, a degeneration of the nerves that can lead to paralysis.

But perhaps the most noteworthy instances of mild, chronic thiamine deficiency have to do with a symptom not normally associated with it: neurotic behavior.

In a study of 65 patients found to have neurosis, the subjects were tested for thiamine deficiency. The researchers concluded that the "neurosis was associated with thiamine deficiency and with consumption of foods poor or practically lacking in this vitamin." Unfortunately, the researchers did not give the patients thiamine to see if it would cure or lessen their neurosis (*Nutrition Reports International*).

However, in another study, thiamine was administered—with surprising results.

In a remarkable case, 20 patients with such symptoms as sleep disturbances, personality changes (sometimes hostile), fevers of unknown cause, intermittent diarrhea and lack of appetite were studied. As the researchers point out, many of these symptoms "would represent a trap for the unwary physician since he would be unable to find any objective physical sign other than variations of normal, which would be easily classed as the effects of a chronic state of anxiety. Thus some of the physical signs that [were] observed were the classical signs which have generally become associated with 'neurotic tension.' " Of course, these symptoms were not life threatening, but they were "nevertheless debilitating and extremely frustrating since many of [the patients] had already received conventional therapy unsuccessfully" (*American Journal of Clinical Nutrition*, February, 1980).

Could low thiamine be the culprit here? Apparently so, for the researchers report that "all of the 20 patients noticed marked symptomatic improvement or lost their symptoms completely after thiamine supplement." It's also interesting that many of the patients had been consuming large quantities of junk foods, notably soft drinks.

Fortunately, after thiamine therapy, "some patients lost their craving for sweet-tasting foods and beverages."

As you can see, even a mild thiamine deficiency can have important consequences, and that scoundrel of a bank teller is going to keep on embezzling his share. But you can keep ahead of the little rascal by keeping up your thiamine balance. That way, you'll never have to worry about getting a check returned for insufficient funds.

CHAPTER

23

MAKE UP YOUR MIND— EAT MORE THIAMINE

Thiamine might have saved her.

An elderly woman was admitted to the hospital from a nursing home. Her body was dehydrated. Her mind, too, was seared and desertlike, empty of life. Given fluids, she became more alert. But still too lethargic and confused to drink anything herself, she was fed intravenously. Four weeks later, she was well enough to go back to the nursing home—but she never went back to solid foods.

At the home, they hooked her up to an intravenous solution of sugar, salt and water and spoon-fed her clear liquids. Two months passed. Then, she lapsed into a stupor. Taken to the hospital, she died in four days.

An autopsy showed the causes of death. A major cause was Wernicke's disease—a brain disease caused by a severe lack of thiamine.

Without thiamine—vitamin B_1—the brain and nervous system collapse. Arms and legs lose their coordination. Eye muscles freeze in paralysis. The mind blackens into amnesia, coma, death. But even a slight deficiency of thiamine wounds the brain. Irritability, depression, lack of initiative, insomnia, inability to concentrate: Those are the symptoms of a mild thiamine deficiency, symptoms too often diagnosed as senility or neurosis.

Improving a Too-Short Memory

Working with rats, Japanese researchers have found, for example, that thiamine deficiency erases memory. They took two groups of animals—one maintained on a thiamine-supplemented diet and the other on a diet deficient in thiamine—and timed them individually in an enclosed alley maze. After 20 days, those deprived of thiamine appeared to forget the pattern that would lead them out the other side. They groped around the maze and made repeated wrong turns so that it took them an average of 55 seconds to get through the maze, compared to 20 seconds for those on a thiamine-rich diet. It wasn't until they were put back on a high-thiamine diet that their memory and timing improved (*Journal of Nutritional Science and Vitaminology*).

And this seems to be one finding that's not limited to animals. Mounting evidence suggests that the loss of memory—as well as other symptoms normally associated with senility—may in fact be a result of a thiamine deficiency.

One such study, published in the *International Journal of Vitamin and Nutrition Research,* tested 18 geriatric patients, suffering from dementia, irritability and loss of appetite, for possible vitamin deficiencies. Fifteen of the 18 oldsters were rated deficient in thiamine.

Who knows how many more miserable grandmothers and grandfathers are hopelessly condemned to mind-boggling drugs and disrespect when all they may need is a daily dose of thiamine? The problem is, vague symptoms of an early deficiency—including poor memory, unsteadiness, alterations in blood pressure and pulse rate, and heart complaints—are easily overlooked and may be misdiagnosed.

Lack of Thiamine
Causes Mental Problems

In a study of the thiamine levels of 154 psychiatric patients, researchers found more thiamine deficiencies among those patients with severe disorders (such as schizophrenia) than among those with milder illnesses (*British Journal of Psychiatry*, September, 1979).

How can a physical lack, a lack of a vitamin, cause mental problems?

Thiamine is central to carbohydrate digestion. Carbohydrates break down into simple sugars, such as the glucose which fuels the brain. Missing thiamine, the body fails to churn out enough blood sugar, and intelligence fades. Also, when blood sugar metabolism goes awry, acids build up in the blood and irritate the nervous system.

But that explanation, while based on the facts of thiamine metabolism, is still only a theory.

Some researchers believe that a thiamine deficiency causes mental problems by cutting down the availability of serotonin, a chemical in the brain that helps regulate emotions.

In a study investigating that theory, researchers from the Mount Sinai School of Medicine in New York City divided rats into separate groups. They fed one group a diet containing pyrithiamine, a chemical that drains the body of thiamine. Another group got a normal diet. During the study, the researchers took samples from the brains of both groups and measured them for serotonin.

Turning Seizures On and Off

For the first eight days of the study, the pyrithiamine rats had no change in either their behavior or their average serotonin level. Then the rats began to have "dramatic behavioral changes"—they went into spasms and convulsions and had little or no coordination—and their serotonin levels dropped 60 percent below the level of the normally fed rats. But when the pyrithiamine rats were given massive doses of thiamine, their seizures stopped within 24 hours and their serotonin levels returned to normal *(Neurology)*.

Millions of human beings weren't as lucky as those rats. When they lost their coordination, when their arms and legs were paralyzed, no scientist replaced the thiamine in their diets. They were the victims of beriberi, a disease once epidemic in Asia, where polished rice—stripped of its thiamine-rich bran—was the dietary staple. But those millions didn't die of paralysis. They died of heart failure. In the final stages of beriberi, the heart swells, stretches—and stops.

Few Americans die of beriberi heart disease. But many Americans have a heart problem—a problem they might solve if they upped their intake of thiamine.

When researchers measured the thiamine blood levels of over 125 elderly people, they found that 32 percent were deficient in thiamine—and that heart pain was more common among those with a deficiency *(Nutrition and Metabolism)*.

In another study, researchers from the University of Alabama medical center in Birmingham measured the daily thiamine intake of 74 people and then had them fill out a questionnaire in which they listed their cardiovascular (heart and circulatory system) complaints.

Dividing the people into a high-intake and a low-intake group, they found that those with a low intake of thiamine had almost twice as many cardiovascular complaints *(Journal of the American Geriatrics Society)*.

In a third study, researchers compared the levels of thiamine in the heart muscles of 12 patients who died of heart disease to the levels of 10 patients who died of other causes. They found that the heart patients had an average thiamine level 57 percent lower than the other patients *(Nutrition Reviews)*.

Fewer Heart Spasms with Thiamine

A study from Japan provides more proof that thiamine strengthens the heart. There, in the 10 days before their open heart surgery, a group of 25 patients received thiamine while another group of patients did not. When their hearts were artificially stopped to perform the operation, only 10 percent of the thiamine group had abnormal heart spasms, compared to 30 percent of the other group. And when their hearts were revived at the end of the operation, 30 percent of the thiamine group had heart spasms, compared to 95 percent of the other group (*Medical Tribune*).

The body's two most important organs—the heart and the brain—need thiamine. But the rest of the body demands a fair share, too. If the system lacks thiamine, any part can rebel: Studies link many diseases to a thiamine deficiency. One of them is cancer.

Thiamine against Cancer

Scientists from the University of Surrey in England studied a group of 17 people with breast cancer and 25 people with bronchial cancer. Sixty-five percent of those with breast cancer and 52 percent of those with bronchial cancer had a thiamine deficiency—compared with only 13 percent of a group without cancer (*Oncology*).

That a lack of thiamine causes cancer has yet to be proved. But that an abundance of thiamine treats the disease—at least in laboratory animals—is a fact.

Tumors, transplanted into laboratory animals, were treated with an anti-cancer substance. When the animals received thiamine, the "antitumor activity" of the substance increased (*Cancer Research*). In other animals with cancer, the growth of tumors slowed in those receiving yeast, and a researcher theorized that "the effectiveness of the yeast could well be due to its content of thiamine" *(European Journal of Cancer).*

Eye problems have also been linked to thiamine deficiency.

Measuring the thiamine blood levels in 38 patients with glaucoma, an eye disease that can lead to blindness, researchers found the glaucoma patients had a "significantly lower" average level than 12 healthy people *(Annals of Ophthalmology,* July, 1979).

Two children who developed severe eye problems while being treated for seizures were given 50 milligrams of thiamine a day for six weeks. Their vision returned to normal *(British Journal of Ophthalmology,* March, 1979).

Beneficial in Liver Disease

Studies show that thiamine deficiency may complicate liver disease.

Measuring the thiamine levels of patients with chronic liver disease, doctors found that 58 percent of the patients had a deficiency of thiamine. When they supplemented the patients' diets with 200 milligrams of thiamine a day for one week, the disease improved.

"High doses of thiamine," the doctors wrote, "should be included in the routine nutritional management of patients with severe chronic liver disease" *(Scandinavian Journal of Gastroenterology).*

A Common Deficiency

But it's not only sick people who need more thiamine. Measuring the thiamine levels of diabetic patients and healthy people, researchers found that many people in both groups had low levels of thiamine. "Fifty percent both of our control subjects and

patients would benefit from increasing their intake of thiamine,"
said the researchers *(American Journal of Clinical Nutrition)*.

Fifty percent. Either you or your spouse? A thiamine deficiency is one of the most widespread of nutritional problems,
particularly among the elderly.

When researchers from Colorado State University measured
the blood levels of various nutrients in 70 older women, they
found that a lack of thiamine was the most common deficiency
(American Journal of Clinical Nutrition).

In a study measuring the thiamine levels of 35 older men,
more than 25 percent were found to have a deficiency *(New
Zealand Medical Journal)*.

Not only older people lack thiamine, however. When the
daily thiamine intake of a group of college women was calculated,
it was found that 75 percent had an intake below the government's Recommended Dietary Allowance *(Journal of the American Dietetic Association)*. Pregnant women, too, run the risk
of a deficiency. A study showed that 25 to 30 percent of pregnant
women were "thiamine depleted" *(American Journal of Clinical
Nutrition)*.

But a thiamine deficiency is easy to correct. Measuring the
thiamine levels of 153 men and women, researchers found that
23 percent had a deficiency. Giving them 20 milligrams of thiamine a day for 12 days brought their levels up to normal *(Clinica
Chimica Acta)*.

But why is a thiamine deficiency so common? Why are
supplements necessary? Can't you get enough of the nutrient
from your diet?

Thiamine Is Destroyed by Chlorine

You can. But it's not easy, especially if you use tap water.

Most people do, of course—tap water that contains chlorine.
And recent evidence indicates that chlorine destroys thiamine.
Researchers cooked rice in either chlorinated tap water or dis-
tilled water and then measured the amount of thiamine in the

rice. The rice cooked in tap water had 36 percent less thiamine. When the researchers added more chlorine to the tap water, rice cooked in it contained even less thiamine (*Journal of Nutritional Science and Vitaminology*, August, 1979).

It's hard to avoid chlorine. It's even harder to avoid polychlorinated biphenyl (PCB), a chemical pollutant that has contaminated the globe. Researchers from Kyoto University in Japan have unfortunately found that, when rats are given PCB, the chemical destroys much of the thiamine in their bodies. "Administration of PCB," they write, "resulted in a thiamine deficiency, even when dietary thiamine levels were normal" (*Journal of Environmental Pathology and Toxicology*, March, 1979).

Chlorine and PCB—two strikes against thiamine. Do you drink coffee? Strike three.

In a study on coffee and thiamine, volunteers drank seven cups of coffee in three hours. Eight days later, they drank the same amount of water. On both days, researchers measured the amount of thiamine excreted in the volunteers' urine. The amount was 45 percent less on the coffee day than on the water day— good evidence, say the researchers, that coffee destroys thiamine in the body (*International Journal of Vitamin and Nutrition Research*). And decaffeinated coffee is no way out. It's not caffeine that destroys thiamine, but another coffee ingredient, chlorogenic acid. Should coffee lovers switch to tea? Just as bad.

Volunteers drank four to six cups of tea a day for a few weeks. And even though they ate a diet designed to provide enough thiamine, all of them developed a deficiency within a week (*Federation Proceedings*).

You may be able to have your tea and drink it too, however. Researchers have discovered that the ingredient in tea that causes a thiamine deficiency is tannic acid but that vitamin C protects the body against tannic acid, allowing absorption of thiamine (*American Journal of Clinical Nutrition*). If you must drink tea, drink it with a squeeze of vitamin C–rich lemon, or take a small amount of vitamin C with each cup.

CHAPTER
24

KEEP IN THE PINK
WITH RIBOFLAVIN

It may be bad form to stick out your tongue—but a good idea. This organ of speech, even when silent, can tell many a tale about your nutritional status.

It might clue you in on whether you need more riboflavin (vitamin B_2), a deficiency of which can open the door to a host of problems (like cataracts, conjunctivitis, fatigue, dermatitis, birth defects and even, according to some researchers, the most dreaded of all diseases—cancer).

If your tongue is pink and velvety, chances are you are well supplied with B vitamins, including riboflavin.

But if your tongue has a purplish cast, more like fuchsia or magenta than pink roses, then, indeed, you may need more riboflavin.

Maybe you also have lines radiating from your lips, oily hair, blurred vision in poor light, a tendency to whip out your sunglasses at the first ray of golden sun, frequent tearing of the eyes, red inflamed eyelids or flaky areas around your nose, eyebrows or hairline. Many of these conditions respond to riboflavin and are due to a dietary deficiency of this nutrient, according to a survey of the scientific literature *(Progress in Food and Nutrition Science)*.

In the United States, where there is plenty of meat and milk (two primary sources of riboflavin) and where bread is enriched with this vitamin, there are, nevertheless, shortages. As many as one family out of every seven has a diet deficient in riboflavin, according to a *World Health Organization Report.*

You may consume what you think is a well-balanced diet and still suffer a deficiency of riboflavin. In your food, this water-soluble nutrient is quickly destroyed by light. In your body, drugs like oral contraceptives and tranquilizers inhibit absorption. As an enzyme activator, riboflavin is so busy that it is sometimes completely used up before it has completed its metabolic chores. And that's too bad because, as a part of coenzymes and enzymes necessary for the transport of oxygen, riboflavin participates in the respiration of every single cell.

Defense against Cancer

That makes riboflavin a very important member of the nutritional team that can help you build a better defense against cancer. As Nobel prize winner Otto Warburg, a biochemist who was director of the Max Planck Institute for Cell Physiology in Berlin, explained to the Nobel laureates at Lindau in 1966, though there are hundreds, perhaps thousands of secondary causes that stimulate cancer growth, there is only *one primary cause,* and that is replacement of the respiration of oxygen (energy for normal cells) by a fermentation of sugar (energy for cancer cells).

Therefore, Dr. Warburg continued, what we need in order to have the best possible chance of avoiding cancer are those factors that are involved in the health of cell respiration. Those factors are iron and three of the B vitamins—riboflavin, niacin and pantothenate (pantothenic acid)—found in brewer's yeast and liver.

Earlier studies reported by the late Boris Sokoloff, M.D., Ph.D., director of the Southern Bio-Research Institute, Florida Southern College, Lakeland, revealed that, when riboflavin is added to a diet that includes cancer-causing chemicals, it reduces the incidence of cancer in laboratory animals. Other vitamins of the B family used singly had no noticeable effects (*Cancer—New Approaches, New Hope,* Devin-Adair, 1952). This does not mean that the other members of the B family are not helpful when used with riboflavin. They help each other.

But it is riboflavin which takes part in cell respiration, providing oxygen for the cell to breathe and go about the business of duplicating itself in a normal, orderly fashion. Without riboflavin, the oxygen supply is reduced.

As little as a 35 percent reduction in the available supply, according to Dr. Warburg, causes the cell, in its efforts to stay alive, to make a metabolic switch. Since it can no longer derive energy from the oxidation, or burning, of food, it turns for energy to an alternate process that requires no oxygen, thus initiating the uncontrolled growth process we know as cancer.

Dr. Warburg believed so strongly that the B vitamins and iron would enhance the body's defenses that he went so far as to suggest that, following surgery for cancer, a sufficient supply of these nutrients would help prevent the spread or recurrence of malignant growths.

Laboratory research seems to justify Dr. Warburg's faith in the efficacy of the B vitamins—especially riboflavin.

For instance, Lionel A. Poirier, formerly of the National Cancer Institute, reported at the American Chemical Society national meeting that riboflavin inhibits the production of liver cancer in laboratory animals injected with cancer-causing chemicals.

Henry Foy and Athena Kondi of the National Public Health Laboratory Service, Nairobi, Kenya, point out in a letter to the editor of the *British Medical Journal* the important role of riboflavin in maintaining the integrity of the epithelial, or body-lining, tissue—particularly in the esophagus. They suggest that riboflavin should be considered—along with vitamin A—as a nutrient whose deficiency may lead to precancerous conditions. They base their conclusions on a study involving eight baboons fed a diet deficient in riboflavin. Even though the baboons received an otherwise adequate diet completely balanced with protein, as well as vitamins A and D and all the members of the B family except riboflavin, they developed, after 160 to 300 days, profound changes in the skin of the face, hands, legs and feet as well as more sinister changes in the esophagus.

Very Important in Pregnancy

Along with her prayers for a normal healthy child, every expectant mother should include a good riboflavin source such as brewer's yeast or desiccated liver in her daily routine.

Laboratory experiments have indeed shown that a deficiency of riboflavin in pregnant mammals causes malformations in their offspring. When Bruce Mackler, M.D., and colleagues at the school of medicine of the University of Washington, Seattle, created riboflavin deficiencies in pregnant rats, a very large proportion of the fetuses—greater than 95 percent—developed malformations *(Pediatrics)*.

Most of the defects, Dr. Mackler reports, were skeletal—abnormal development of the bones. The most common problems were incomplete development of the bones of the extremities. Dr. Mackler also mentions cleft palate as an example of "a wide number of other anomalies" that have been produced in the fetuses of rats with riboflavin deficiency.

Since the effects of riboflavin deficiency are similar to, but less severe than, those produced by the drug thalidomide, it has been postulated by investigators that the drug may be a riboflavin antagonist, either causing a deficiency of riboflavin or preventing its metabolism.

Adequate amounts of riboflavin are essential for the mind as well as the body. They may not ensure that your child will be an Einstein but, "a number of important enzymes in the brain require riboflavin to function," says Richard S. Rivlin, M.D., chief of nutrition service at Memorial Sloan-Kettering Cancer Center in New York. "It is likely, therefore, that a deficiency of riboflavin during a critical period of time probably would impair the normal development of the brain to some extent."

The Sensitive Nutrient

Riboflavin is found in a variety of foods including yeast, liver, wheat germ, eggs, milk and green leafy vegetables, but it's often tough to get your family to eat these foods. Then, too, we've seen that riboflavin is as sensitive as a prima donna. It is easily destroyed by exposure to light, as when milk is stored in glass jars, for example. It can also be destroyed in cooking because it is water soluble.

How can you be sure of a good supply of this vitally important nutrient? If the milkman leaves milk in bottles on your doorstep, make sure he sets them in an opaque, covered container. Bottled milk loses up to 70 percent of its riboflavin in four hours when exposed to sunlight.

Cover your pots when cooking. Exposure of food to light during cooking causes even greater riboflavin losses than heat. And be sure to use all your pot liquor left after cooking—it's rich in B vitamins. If you soak seeds and grains for sprouting, use the soak water in soups or to cook vegetables. It's another good source of B vitamins.

Remember that you lose some riboflavin when you soak vegetables or fruits in large quantities of water. You also lose some during cold storage, whether in supermarkets and warehouses or in your own refrigerator or freezer. In addition, frozen meat develops a "drip" when thawed which contains approximately 9 percent of the protein, 12 percent of the thiamine, 10 percent of the riboflavin and 15 percent of the niacin. So repeated freezing and thawing may result in considerable losses of the original nutrient content—not to mention flavor.

How much riboflavin do you need?

The Recommended Dietary Allowance (RDA) is 1.6 milligrams for an average adult male and 1.2 for a female. The need is higher in pregnant and nursing women. Because riboflavin participates in the metabolism of protein, the need is also higher when the diet is high in protein.

Since riboflavin is so vital, and because it is rarely toxic, it would be nutritional wisdom to get even more than the RDA. How? A convenient source is brewer's yeast, which contains a minimum of 0.3 milligrams of riboflavin per tablespoon. And don't say you can't stand the taste. Shop around till you find some that is to your liking. Then use it in soups, stews, casseroles, or mix it with flour to thicken gravy. In baked goods, add two tablespoons to every cup of flour and no one will know it's there—except your body's cells, which will probably stand up and cheer.

Some people start the day with a yeasty tomato shake—a glass of tomato juice, 1 or 2 tablespoons of brewer's yeast and a dash of basil, nicely blended. Take a yeast break instead of a coffee break for a lift without a letdown.

Liver, kidney and heart are all excellent sources of riboflavin, but you can't expect your family to eat them every day. So are milk, cheese, eggs, green leafy vegetables and whole grains.

Make an effort to step up your intake of riboflavin. You'll be ensuring yourself a steady supply of the nutrient that can help keep not only your tongue, but your whole body, in the pink.

CHAPTER
25

RIBOFLAVIN IS READY TO HELP

Just before her second birthday, a very ill little girl named Christina was brought to the Medical College of Georgia in Augusta. For no apparent reason, the child seemed to be losing her abilities to see, hear and walk, and she had life-threatening anemia. She was put in the care of three doctors: Patricia Hartlage, M.D., Dorothy Hahn, M.D., and Robert Leshner, M.D.

The doctors were puzzled. In spite of an adequate diet and even a daily multivitamin with iron, Christina's anemia wouldn't quit. "We were keeping her alive with transfusions," Dr. Hartlage told us. "She was a pretty sick little girl."

Searching for an effective treatment for the anemia, the doctors turned to B vitamins. Under the microscope, Christina's red blood cells were disfigured by funny little bubbles called vacuoles; B vitamins are known to promote the production of healthy red blood cells.

The doctors narrowed the choices down to vitamin B_6 (pyridoxine), thiamine (B_1) and riboflavin (B_2) and decided to give Christina high doses of each of them, alone, for one month. They tried vitamin B_6 and thiamine, but neither had any effect. Then, almost as a last resort, they gave her riboflavin. Five days later,

"Whammo!" recalls Dr. Hartlage. "Christina started to produce healthy red blood cells."

"We just happened to try riboflavin last," Dr. Hahn told us. "We gave her the vitamins in sequence. Riboflavin was the last we tried, and lo and behold, she responded to it. If we had tried riboflavin first, we would never have known whether thiamine or pyridoxine [vitamin B$_6$] would have worked or not."

Even more amazingly, riboflavin began to reverse the neurological damage done to Christina's eyesight and hearing. Riboflavin deficiency is known to affect the blood and skin, but not the nervous system in humans. "We haven't been able to find any similar reports in the medical literature," Dr. Hahn said. "We've talked to hematologists, neurologists and pediatricians."

Christina's illness is an extreme and unique case. Her diet contained all the riboflavin most of us would need, but she has a rare need for large amounts of it. Her response to riboflavin, and riboflavin alone, however, shows that the vitamin has what Dr. Leshner calls a "niche of its own" among the B vitamins. For various reasons, riboflavin has not received much attention in the past. "We know a lot about the other vitamins," Dr. Hartlage told us, "but there's not a lot on riboflavin."

A Clue to Cataracts?

Not that there isn't a lot of interesting work on riboflavin going on. Two researchers at the University of Alabama, Harold W. Skalka, M.D., and Josef Prchal, M.D., are pursuing a scientific lead that might make some of the 400,000 cataract operations performed in the United States every year unnecessary.

"Riboflavin might not prevent cataracts," Dr. Skalka told us, "but it may be able to help retard their formation. That is, instead of a person developing cataracts at 50, you could hold it back to age 60 or 70 or 80 in some cases."

In a study of 173 patients at the Eye Foundation hospital in Birmingham, Alabama, the two doctors found that 20 percent of a group of cataract patients under age 50 were deficient in riboflavin, and 34 percent of a group of cataract patients over 50 were deficient in the vitamin. On the other hand, all 16 of a group of people over 50 with normal vision and clear lenses had high levels of riboflavin—higher, even, than the levels in young, healthy people who served as controls in the experiment.

The doctors did not conclude from this evidence that riboflavin can prevent cataracts. But they were intrigued—and totally surprised—by the fact that the older people with good eyes all had a lot of riboflavin in their systems.

"What is perhaps surprising is the lack of any riboflavin deficiency in our older clinic patients with clear lenses. The possibility that dietary riboflavin supplementation (beyond current recommended levels) may be useful in retarding the formation of senile cataracts is currently under investigation," the researchers reported (*Metabolic and Pediatric Ophthalmology,* vol 5, no. 1, 1981).

The vitamin is believed to help protect the eye through an intricate chain of chemical reactions, culminating in the release of a substance called glutathione, which apparently shields the proteins in the lens of the eye from the kind of damage that causes cataracts.

"There are so few good, solid leads in the treatment of cataracts, which are a major public health problem in the United States," Dr. Skalka told us, "that anything is worth investigating. In this case, riboflavin therapy makes sense theoretically and there are also some laboratory suggestions that it will work."

Dr. Skalka and Dr. Prchal are starting experiments with animals to test their idea. They are optimistic. "In 5 to 15 years," they say, "we may have several ways to slow down the development of cataracts."

Riboflavin Builds Healthy Blood

There has also been some significant research into riboflavin's beneficial effects on the blood, including some that might explain why riboflavin helped little Christina in Georgia. Riboflavin lengthens the lives of red blood cells and boosts the action of folate (folic acid, another B vitamin) in the production of new red blood cells in bone marrow. The vitamin also seems to help maintain a high level of iron in red blood cells.

In London, two researchers found that riboflavin protects red blood cells the same way it protects proteins in the lens of the eye—by promoting the release of glutathione. Their findings are important because an estimated 30 percent of Britons over age 65 who live in their own homes are mildly riboflavin deficient (*British Journal of Nutrition,* September, 1981).

The researchers found that red blood cells in riboflavin-deficient people have a shorter life span. The deficiency in each cell seems to weaken its ability to resist damage from highly reactive oxidants. The cells die before their time and are filtered out of the blood.

A researcher from the University of Ghana in West Africa—where diets are commonly low in riboflavin—found a special relationship between riboflavin and folate. Knowing that folate is responsible for the production of red blood cells, the professor found that folate works much better if it's reinforced by a dose of riboflavin. "Riboflavin may be exerting its effect through its involvement in folate metabolism," he notes (*International Journal for Vitamin and Nutrition Research,* vol. 50, no. 3, 1980).

The researcher also found that, by a separate process, "riboflavin is involved in the absorption and utilization of dietary iron" in the blood. He suggests that riboflavin supplements should accompany iron therapy, adding that "in pregnancy, iron and folate deficiencies are common and the addition of riboflavin to iron and folate used in treatment may be advisable."

Deficiency—How Common?

Clearly, we all need riboflavin. But how much do we need, and under what conditions may our requirements be higher?

Jack M. Cooperman, Ph.D., director of nutritional education at New York Medical College in Valhalla, has studied riboflavin levels in several groups of Americans. He says, "In this country, 60 percent of our riboflavin intake comes from milk or skim milk and other dairy products such as yogurt and cheese." He has found that people who don't consume much milk—such as urban teenagers—tend to be deficient in riboflavin.

In a study of 210 white, Hispanic American and black youths between the ages of 13 and 19 in New York City, Dr. Cooperman found that 26 percent were deficient in riboflavin. The teenagers with the highest levels were those who drank the most milk— up to three cups a day—and those with the lowest vitamin levels drank the least—one cup a week. He found that black youths were especially susceptible to riboflavin deficiency. As a group, they often get cramps or diarrhea from milk and tend to avoid it (*American Journal of Clinical Nutrition*, June, 1980).

Few people are seriously short of riboflavin, Dr. Cooperman told us, but many may be marginally deficient and may suffer subtly. "With a marginal deficiency, no one knows exactly what the symptoms might be," he says. "Children may fail to grow properly. Adults may feel slightly ill. They might not be able to do a full day's work. They'll be mildly anemic and lackadaisical. That's all we know right now."

Diabetics, women using oral contraceptives and infants are other high-risk riboflavin-deficiency groups Dr. Cooperman has studied. He told us that it has been only ten years since a reliable test has been available for measuring riboflavin levels in people. It was developed in Switzerland and is usually called EGR for short.

And that test had found that a program of vigorous physical exercise may increase a person's riboflavin needs. Daphne Roe, M.D., of Cornell University, says that the recommended daily intake of 0.6 milligrams for every 1,000 calories in the diet, which was set in 1943, may be obsolete for today's active women.

Using the EGR test, Dr. Roe studied a group of women age 21 to 32 and found that they needed 0.7 milligrams of riboflavin per 1,000 calories to replenish themselves. (A normal diet contains 2,000 to 3,000 calories per day.)

Affected by Drugs

There are other factors that can affect riboflavin levels. Richard Rivlin, M.D., editor of the book *Riboflavin* (Plenum Press, 1975), says hormone levels and drugs also make an impact.

"A riboflavin-deficient state physiologically may result not only from inadequate dietary intake of this vitamin, but also from disturbances in endocrine control and as sequelae of treatment with certain pharmacological agents," he writes (*Nutrition Reviews,* August, 1979).

In particular, Dr. Rivlin says, people with either hypothyroidism or hyperthyroidism may need extra riboflavin, based on findings in experimental animals. In hyperthyroidism, the body processes so much riboflavin that it becomes hungry for more, and in hypothyroidism, it processes too little.

John Pinto, Ph.D., Yee Ping Huang and Dr. Rivlin, all of the Memorial Sloan-Kettering Cancer Center, have shown that chlorpromazine, imipramine and amitriptyline, all psychiatric drugs, can block the action of riboflavin in animals. Dr. Rivlin also suspects that pregnant women and women using oral contraceptives need more of the vitamin. "Inasmuch as riboflavin deficiency may occur with considerable frequency in pregnant patients," he says, "and shortage of this vitamin causes congenital malformations, at least in experimental animals, a reasonable case can be made for administration of riboflavin supplements in pregnancy."

Boric acid may also drain riboflavin from the system. "Boric acid, which is present in some 400 home products, such as mouth washes, suppositories and a number of imported foods, claws onto the sugar portion of riboflavin, binds it, and takes it out into the urine," he writes.

Insidiously, a riboflavin deficiency feeds on itself. "When there is an inadequate amount of riboflavin in the diet, you may lose that ability to utilize what you have. It's a vicious circle," Dr. Rivlin wrote in a paper presented to the Vitamin Nutrition

Issues Symposium in Boca Raton, Florida, in October, 1979. "The less you have, the less you are able to utilize; once the body gets sick, it gets sicker, because it lacks this enzyme and therefore cannot utilize what little vitamin there is in the diet."

Large as some people's riboflavin deficiencies might be, the needs of little Christina in Georgia are much higher. (By comparison, the adult Recommended Dietary Allowance ranges from 1.0 to 1.7 milligrams, depending on age and sex.) Her riboflavin therapy started at a massive 75 milligrams per day. At four years old, she used only 25 milligrams per day, but her doctors didn't know whether she still needed so much of the vitamin or not.

"Someday I'll be gutsy enough to take her off the supplements," Dr. Hartlage says.

Christina's doctors are excited by the idea that their breakthrough might help other children who may be suffering from the same riboflavin-dependency disease without knowing it and that the problem could be averted entirely in future cases. "This is the first documented case, as far as I know, of a non-experimentally-induced riboflavin-dependency disease in a human," Dr. Leshner told us. "I'd like to believe it could be diagnosed earlier and prevented."

"I'm very anxious that people know about this," added Dr. Hartlage, who is particularly optimistic about Christina's recovery, though it is still far from complete. "She has not failed to show progress," Dr. Hartlage said. "We thought her deafness was irreversible, but her hearing is slowly coming back. And her eyesight is coming back. She was just in today for physical therapy, and she gets better every time."

CHAPTER
26

NIACIN FOR BRIGHTER MOODS AND BETTER MEMORY

Are you a lame brain?

Sorry for the insult. But before you turn the page in a huff, turn the other cheek instead and let us ask you a few more questions about your brain—and the B vitamin niacin.

Is your first hour or so in bed at night ever a "witching hour," with your thoughts cackling out a spell to keep you tossing and turning? Insomnia can be a symptom of niacin deficiency.

Are you ever so far down in the dumps that the whole world looks like a junkyard? Depression can be a symptom of niacin deficiency.

When you want to take a stroll down memory lane, do you sometimes find yourself falling flat on your face? Forgetfulness can be a symptom of niacin deficiency.

Or are you irritable? Anxious? Easily distracted? Yes, all of them can be symptoms of niacin deficiency.

The brain—as psychiatrists and psychologists too often forget—is part of the body, the crown of the central nervous system. And just as a calcium deficiency can make a bone so fragile that it breaks with the slightest bump, so a deficiency of niacin can make your brain so "lame" that thoughts are weak and emotions shaky.

Way back in 1947, Tom Spies, M.D., in his pioneering book *Rehabilitation through Better Nutrition* (W. B. Saunders), detailed the many mental problems that can accompany, not an out-and-out deficiency of niacin, but merely an inadequate intake. The list of symptoms he compiled reads like a passage out of a neurotic's diary: irritability, depression, memory loss, insomnia, nervousness, distractibility, apprehension, morbid fears, mental confusion and forgetfulness.

And if a lack of niacin in the diet can make you fall apart, it follows that extra niacin can help you keep it all together.

That thought occurred to Abram Hoffer, Ph.D., M.D., president of the Huxley Institute for Biosocial Research in New York City. In his book *Niacin Therapy in Psychiatry* (Charles C. Thomas, 1962), Dr. Hoffer describes how he and his colleagues gave large doses of nicotinic acid (a form of niacin) to 15 middle-aged and elderly people. "Perhaps," wrote Dr. Hoffer, "if it was given early enough, it would stop senile changes from occurring or slow them down greatly."

Of ten people suffering from senility who got niacin, five "recovered," and two had "marked improvement." Three others did not benefit from the niacin. Four people who were normal when the therapy began remained well.

One middle-aged woman spoke enthusiastically of niacin's many benefits:

"Since we began taking 12 nicotinic acid tablets daily, we have noticed a decided improvement in sleeping. We have more energy and find we can do a good day's work without undue fatigue. Prior to taking the tablets, Martin was subject to headaches and took aspirin nearly every day. Now, he very seldom complains of a headache. I never have one. Our outlook on life seems to be much more optimistic and we have cheerful, happy dispositions."

So it seems that niacin can spark the brain back into working order. And when we say spark, we mean it.

The Spark of Life

Oxygen-laden red blood cells have a "spark"—a negative electrical charge. Like the negative poles of two magnets, two red blood cells will repel each other. They have to—to carry their oxygen to the brain's tissues, they must crawl single file through tiny blood vessels called capillaries. But if—because of disease or old age—the red blood cells lose their charge and bunch up, a microscopic traffic jam is created. The brain gets less oxygen. Senility—or any of a dozen other varieties of dullness and irritability—can set in. But niacin restores the red blood cells' electrical charge. Your brain can take a breath of fresh air.

But not only your brain. Your heart, too.

The late Edwin Boyle, M.D., a clinical professor at the Medical University of South Carolina, Charleston, was called "North America's foremost expert on niacin and heart disease." For good reason. Dr. Boyle treated heart disease with niacin for over 20 years. In a telephone interview several years ago, Dr. Boyle told us that a five-year study of over 8,000 men revealed that those who took niacin regularly—1,000 men—had 25 percent fewer nonfatal heart attacks.

Doctors have long known that niacin can help lower the level of blood fats like cholesterol and triglycerides that can muck up arteries and cause heart attacks. In his practice, Dr. Boyle used niacin to help those who had very high levels of blood fats.

Not only did niacin lower their cholesterol levels, but it eliminated *sludging*—the bunching up of red blood cells that we mentioned earlier. Once sludging was gone, Dr. Boyle prescribed proper diet and moderate exercise to restore a heart patient's health. "There is a proper sequence of treatment, and niacin fits into that sequence," he told us.

"People with elevated cholesterol and clinical vascular disease do as well with niacin, diet and exercise as with any other regimen," he said.

A Prescription for Good Moods

Though using vitamins marks a doctor as unconventional, Dr. Boyle was hardly alone in prescribing niacin. William Kaufman, M.D., Ph.D., a retired doctor living in Bridgeport, Connecticut, treated many of his patients with niacinamide, the chemical that niacin changes into before it goes to work in the body.

"When I began practicing in 1941, I found it striking that patient after patient came in with a group of symptoms which were quite similar. They might have other symptoms besides, but in these certain symptoms, such as the lack of ability to concentrate, depression, irritability, joint complaints, excessive fatigue, bloating and intestinal complaints, there was fingerprint similarity. Many patients were so easily startled they jumped when the phone rang. A number had black and blue marks on their bodies where they had bumped into things, since their sense of balance was far off.

"I began tabulating symptoms and physical abnormalities and very soon recognized that this strange syndrome was probably a form of pellagra, or niacin deficiency, that had not yet reached the degree of severity to cause the classic combination of skin rash, diarrhea and dementia. I reasoned that if this was a form of pellagra, then niacinamide—which had just been discovered as a preventative—might provide useful treatment.

I administered 100 milligrams of niacinamide as a test dose. If the patient had no adverse reactions to the test dose, I prescribed 100 milligrams three to four times a day. Male and female patients would return a few days later and . . . I didn't believe it! They looked different. They acted different. They told me that their symptoms had vanished, they felt a new zest for life. I decided to test it. I gave a few of these improved patients calcium tablets instead of niacinamide. They were unaware of the change. At the end of ten days they were right back to where they had been when they first saw me. When they resumed niacinamide treatment, they once again improved.

"But even though I had good therapeutic results with this group of patients, I wasn't satisfied with this. I wanted to have a way of measuring improvements objectively. I needed some new standards of measurement. So I designed some simple instruments I could use to measure joint mobility and adapted other instruments for measuring muscle strength and working capacity. With these devices I could show, for example, how niacinamide properly used was enabling people to turn their heads further, as well as move their other joints through wider ranges of motion."

"The 100 milligram per day dose of niacinamide would be ineffective in producing sustained results, though. The daily dose I prescribed since 1944 ranged from 900 to 4,000 milligrams a day in divided doses. These amounts were calculated by taking special measurements of patients' joints to test their mobility and are not recomended for individual treatment without a doctor's supervision."

Fatigue and Stiffness Helped

One of the many people Dr. Kaufman helped with niacinamide was a 78-year-old woman. "When I first saw her, she was feeble, exhausted all the time. When she wasn't in bed, she sat in her rocker. To make matters worse, her joints were stiff and painful. She was too tired to go anywhere or do anything. She was downhearted all the time, weepy and looking forward to dying as her only release. After more than a year of continuous treatment with high doses of niacinamide, her joints greatly improved and she was virtually free from pain and stiffness.

"The measurement of her joint mobility showed that she now had the ranges of joint movement that one would expect in an 11- to 15-year-old girl. Her strength had increased markedly, too, more than double what it was a year earlier. She no longer felt feeble. Her state of mind also greatly improved. She felt much happier and once more enjoyed living. She looked forward to going out and to the doings of the next day. And, of course, she continued taking niacinamide in the doses I prescribed for her.''

Dr. Kaufman doesn't put much stock in statements that most people get all the vitamins they need from their food. ''You know, people aren't getting as much of the vitamins in their diets as they think they are. Processing, cooking and storage can destroy a high percentage of many of the vitamins originally present. For this reason alone, for many people just having meals that seem to supply the 'minimum daily requirement' is not enough. Generally, my patients could be termed middle or upper class economically and educationally. They had no problems with money as far as food was concerned. They were getting enough food, without a doubt. Still, the vitamins I prescribed helped them.''

But you don't want to wait until you find yourself in the waiting room of a general practitioner (or a psychiatrist) before you begin making sure you're getting enough niacin. How much is enough? The Recommended Dietary Allowance—a level set by the government's National Academy of Sciences, aimed at suggesting a healthful intake for the ''average'' person—is 13 to 19 milligrams of niacin a day.

OK. Let's say for a moment that 19 milligrams a day *is* enough. Could you get this much from an ''average'' diet? Probably not.

''I think the fact that the American public has gone from eating 7 or 8 pounds of refined sugar a year to 175 pounds is causing a tremendous rash of ill health,'' Dr. Boyle asserted, ''part of which could be attributed to the lessened intake of niacin and chromium. People have replaced the calories that would have come from whole grain cereals, a rich source of niacin, with sugar's empty calories.

''I think there is ample reason to believe that the amount of niacin a person should be getting for good health is not the amount most Americans are getting on a so-called normal diet. The diet is greatly shortchanged on all the water-soluble vitamins, and niacin is one of the most important.''

As Dr. Boyle pointed out, replacing high-niacin foods with low-niacin foods like sugar is a raw deal for your health. But sugar gets you in double trouble. Niacin fuels digestion. Carbohydrates such as whole wheat bread and brown rice contain niacin; even as they are digested they put more fuel on the digestive fire. But sugar is almost nothing but sucrose. It uses up niacin but puts none back. The result: a niacin deficiency.

That's a health problem you don't need. But how much niacin do you need to stay healthy, really healthy?

That depends—on what you eat, on what you do and on your personal history. In a telephone interview, Dr. Hoffer, whose study of senility we talked about earlier, told us a dramatic story of prisoners of war rescued, not by lightening-strike missions, but by niacin.

"Most of those who were POWs in Japan or in Vietnam are still sick—except for those who are taking large quantities of niacin. Niacin has healed the ravages of months of severe malnutrition and mistreatment.

"Every year in captivity can hasten senility by five years. Fifty-year-old men are blind, senile and arthritic with severe psychotic problems. Niacin can stop this from happening."

Well, that's one end of the spectrum. At the other, says Dr. Hoffer, are people who are eating a sugar-free, high-fiber diet. Chances are they won't need any niacin supplements to feel at their best.

Probably you're somewhere in between. Maybe you need to take two or three times the RDA to keep your chin up and a smile on your face.

But if you do need niacin and you take as much as 100 milligrams of it, you may have an unusual side effect—frightening, perhaps, but harmless: flushing. Your skin will tingle and turn red, as if you had an instant sunburn. Dr. Boyle described this reaction as the "initiation ceremony." But unlike sunburn, flushing fades rather quickly. Both Drs. Hoffer and Boyle pointed out that flushing, caused by the release of histamine and heparin into the bloodstream, is no cause for concern.

And Dr. Boyle added that if you take niacin regularly—four times a day—flushing will eventually disappear. Niacin, said Dr. Boyle, is preferable to niacinamide (which does not cause flushing) because niacinamide is not effective in lowering the level of fats in the blood.

Dr. Hoffer agrees that niacin is one up on niacinamide and suggests, "Taking 50 milligrams twice a day will seldom cause flushing." He suggests that the best time to take niacin is after meals. But the niacin you "take" *during* meals is important, too.

Inviting Niacin to Dinner

Niacin is part of the vitamin B complex. And the B complex likes to hang out together. So most of the foods rich in other B vitamins will also be rich in niacin. One such food is liver. A typical serving supplies 14 milligrams of niacin.

Other meats are good sources, too. And so are shelled, roasted peanuts. One-quarter cup has a whopping 6.2 milligrams of niacin. Other nuts and seeds are also good sources.

But if you're a dieter and those peanuts have you worrying about putting on the pounds, skip them. Eat plenty of tuna, a dieter's delight, instead. Tuna has 21 milligrams of niacin in every cup.

Whole grains are also good sources. Peas and beans are fair. And the king of the B-complex foods, brewer's yeast, supplies a hearty 3 milligrams of niacin in every tablespoon.

Scientists often tell us the brain is like a computer. Niacin may keep your computer programmed for happiness.

CHAPTER
27

WHY THIS EPIDEMIC OF VITAMIN B$_6$ DEFICIENCY?

Until recently, vitamin B$_6$ (pyridoxine) was considered something of a second-line vitamin. Unlike niacin, thiamine and vitamin C, which can dramatically cure certain life-threatening deficiency diseases, B$_6$ has never attained the status of "magic bullet."

Of course, even nutrition skeptics know that vitamin B$_6$ can help a few rare genetic disorders of metabolism and an uncommon type of anemia. They are also aware that this vitamin can prevent some of the side effects of a few prescription drugs, including oral contraceptives. But aside from these uses, traditionalists do not believe B$_6$ supplementation has much value.

Research over the past decade has been forcing a change in this opinion. Numerous reports indicate that vitamin B$_6$ can be beneficial in a wide range of apparently unrelated medical conditions. Furthermore, a substantial percentage even of healthy people are now believed to be low in this nutrient.

Nutrition-oriented doctors have begun using B$_6$ in the treatment of hyperactive children, asthma, diabetes mellitus, so-called autoimmune diseases, infertility, recurrent calcium oxalate kidney stones and for prevention and treatment of toxemia during pregnancy. In addition, according to an editorial in the prestigious journal *Lancet,* B_6 may benefit heart patients by reducing the tendency of their blood to form dangerous clots.

Carpal tunnel syndrome, a nerve disorder that produces numbness, tingling, pain and weakness in the hands and some fingers, is a problem of particular interest. For while vitamin B_6 is only one part of a comprehensive treatment program for the above maladies, carpal tunnel syndrome is usually controlled by B_6 alone.

Why should B_6, nearly a half century after its discovery, suddenly become such a versatile therapeutic weapon? The obvious explanation is that modern scientists have made discoveries that were overlooked in earlier research. In other words, B_6 has always been valuable; it's just that no one realized it.

B_6 Deficiency: A New Problem?

That explanation, however, is not entirely satisfactory. Our predecessors in nutritional science were too good to have missed the boat so badly on vitamin B_6. They were shrewd observers with fertile minds. For example, 25 years before Linus Pauling, Ph.D., wrote his book on the subject, they recognized that vitamin C might help the common cold. They advocated allergy elimination diets for the treatment of migraine headaches 50 years before this method was "discovered" by modern scientists. They knew that essential fatty acids could improve eczema before most modern nutrition doctors were even born. And they discovered countless other nutritional pearls that are only now coming back into vogue. But about vitamin B_6 there was hardly a word.

If we accept that scientists of yesteryear were good at what they did, we are forced to conclude that B_6 deficiency was not much of a problem back in their time. The reason that B_6 has only recently become so useful must be that widespread deficiency of this vitamin is a new problem.

Is this logic farfetched? Not really. Consider carpal tunnel syndrome: It is caused by pressure on a nerve that passes down the arm, through a structure at the wrist called the carpal tunnel and into the hand. Vitamin B$_6$ somehow relieves this pressure and the symptoms that go with it. Even George Phalen, M.D., the man who discovered this syndrome, now believes that B$_6$ therapy may soon replace the more widely used hand surgery.

But what does this have to do with a new epidemic of vitamin B$_6$ deficiency? The fact is that carpal tunnel syndrome appears to be a new disease. When Dr. Phalen presented his first 11 cases in 1950 at the 99th Annual Meeting of the American Medical Association, he noted that very few of the doctors attending that meeting were familiar with this syndrome. Today, however, most doctors see it frequently.

So carpal tunnel syndrome is a new disease, becoming prominent in the past 30 years. It is a disease that usually can be traced to lack of sufficient vitamin B$_6$. It stands to reason, then, that B$_6$ deficiency has also emerged in our population during the last three decades.

Inadequate B$_6$ can manifest itself not only as carpal tunnel syndrome, but as a contributing factor in many cases of asthma, diabetes, hyperactivity, heart disease and other problems. And, as mentioned, B$_6$ deficiency is a time bomb that may be ticking in many healthy individuals.

What has happened since World War II that could have caused so many of us to become low in this important nutrient? Is our overrefined, overcooked diet doing us in? If you analyze our modern food supply, you indeed find that many of us are getting the Recommended Dietary Allowance (RDA) for vitamin B$_6$. On the other hand, a sugar-laden, nutrient-depleted diet has been with us for quite some time, and marginal B$_6$ intake is nothing new. If we are eating less B$_6$ than we did 50 years ago, the difference could not be much more than few tenths of a milligram.

Could such a small change in dietary B$_6$ be the straw that broke the camel's back, plunging millions of us into a state of deficiency? That is an unlikely explanation, because the epidemic of B$_6$ deficiency looks like something more than just a simple dietary shortage. The RDA for vitamin B$_6$ is only 2 milligrams per day. If all we are doing with B$_6$ therapy is correcting a deficient diet, then a few milligrams daily should do the job. But some doctors are prescribing extremely large doses: anywhere from 20 to 500 times the RDA.

These amounts cannot possibly be obtained from food alone, even if you consume the most well-balanced, nutrient-rich diet imaginable. Smaller doses, however, don't seem to work—so it's not that we are getting less B_6 than before. What has apparently happened is that many of us have come to need a lot more of this vitamin than our grandparents did.

An increased need for a vitamin could occur because of either a genetic mutation or exposure to some chemical that interferes with the function of that vitamin. The genetic theory is unlikely, since mutations take thousands or millions of years to have a major impact on the human race. There may, therefore, exist some antivitamin to which we are being exposed, a substance which might either prevent us from absorbing our vitamin B_6, destroy it in our bodies or in some way prevent it from carrying out its usual tasks. If there is such a chemical, then we would need to increase our B_6 intake in order to counteract its effects.

Such antipyridoxine compounds do indeed exist, and we have been exposed to them in increasing amounts during the past 30 to 40 years. These vitamin B_6 antagonist belong to a class of chemicals called hydrazines.

Bela Toth, Ph.D., of the University of Nebraska, who has studied hydrazines extensively, points out that the high chemical reactivity of these substances makes them ideal for a very wide range of uses.

"In agriculture," Dr. Toth writes, "many of these compounds are used as plant growth regulators and herbicides. Numerous hydrazines are extensively used in medicine as pharmaceutical agents for a broad variety of diseases. They are used industrially in high energy fuels . . . as antioxidants in the petroleum industry and as plating materials and antitarnish agents, etc., in metal manufacturing."

The first indication that hydrazines interfered with vitamin B_6 was the discovery that an antituberculosis drug, isonicotinic acid hydrazine (INH), could produce a disorder which is similar to carpal tunnel syndrome. But large amounts of B$_6$, given along with INH, can prevent this disorder.

Later on, two other hydrazine medications, hydralazine and phenelzine, also were found to be vitamin B$_6$ inhibitors. Dr. Toth studied numerous other hydrazine compounds and found that most of them greatly increased the need for B$_6$. F. Buffoni, an Italian researcher, extended the list of B$_6$ antagonists even further and suggested that most, if not all, hydrazine compounds are capable of interfering with vitamin B$_6$.

Unfortunately, the story doesn't end there. Not only must we deal with the hydrazines, we must also face other chemicals that our bodies can convert to hydrazines. The chemical of greatest concern in this regard is tartrazine, also known as FD&C Yellow No. 5. This widely used coloring agent is added to hundreds of different foods and medications. In 1970, 21 years after its patent was approved, nearly a million pounds of tartrazine were being used annually.

Although tartrazine is not itself a hydrazine, at least 30 percent of it is converted by the body into a hydrazine compound. So it's likely that this food dye is another vitamin B$_6$ inhibitor— and we cannot rule out the possibility that other food additives of similar structure may also be converted by the body into hydrazine.

Is it possible, then, that more and more people need more and more B$_6$ because B$_6$ antagonists are sprayed on our food, spewed into the air and used widely in manufacturing?

Ways to Avoid Exposure to Hydrazine

It can be depressing to think about the many environmental chemicals that may be interfering with the normal functioning of our bodies. Nevertheless, rather than throw our hands up in despair, there are a few things we can do to try to deal with the hydrazine problem. One is to minimize avoidable exposures to these chemicals. If you can find produce that has not been chemically treated, by all means use it. If no such food is available to you, then at least wash your fruits and vegetables thoroughly. Try to avoid unnecessary exposure to food dyes. There are lists available that tell you which foods and medications contain FD&C Yellow No. 5.

Another positive step you can take is to stay away from foods that have been fried at high temperatures. When vegetable oils are exposed to high temperatures in the presence of air, toxic by-products are created, and these by-products are known to increase the need for vitamin B_6.

Of course, it's not possible to avoid all hydrazine compounds completely. For this reason, it's a good idea to make sure you're getting enough vitamin B_6 in the first place. At present, unfortunately, there is no way to determine exactly how much B_6 the average healthy person should use. But since B_6 is a vitamin with very little risk of toxicity, it would probably be better to err on the side of too much rather than too little. A conservative, rough estimate is that the average, healthy person might be wise to ingest 10 to 20 milligrams daily. (Amounts over 50 milligrams should only be taken under a doctor's supervision.)

If you have some disorder that might be helped by vitamin B_6, then larger amounts should be used. Of course, before undertaking a program of vitamin therapy, you should obtain the approval of your doctor. In a few special situations, notably insulin-dependent diabetes and Parkinson's disease, B_6 therapy should be monitored by someone familiar with its effects. In addition, nursing mothers should be careful with B_6, since massive doses may cut off the milk supply.

28

VITAMIN B$_6$ FOR CARPAL TUNNEL SYNDROME

Ask a traditional doctor about vitamin C deficiency, and the topic of scurvy will surely come up. Niacin will summon a response about pellagra, and thiamine will be linked with beriberi. In fact, if a vitamin doesn't have its very own specific deficiency disease, the vitamin's importance and its Recommended Dietary Allowance may be hotly disputed.

Of course, there are those who know that vitamins do more than just cure one particular ailment. They know that vitamins are intimately involved in any number of the enzymatic and metabolic workings of our bodies.

But if a specific disease is needed to wake up the traditionalists to the wonders of a vitamin, then we've got some news about one of our favorites, vitamin B$_6$, or pyridoxine.

Even though some researchers have suspected for years that there is indeed a specific disease associated with B$_6$ deficiency, only recently has hard scientific data been able to back up that suspicion. That's what Karl Folkers, Ph.D., says and, since he conducted the experiments, he should know. Dr. Folkers, director of the institute for biomedical research at the University of Texas at Austin, announced his findings at a symposium honoring his contributions to medical science.

Dr. Folkers told the conference held at Lehigh University in Bethlehem, Pennsylvania, that biochemical research conducted over the last five to six years has led to the conclusion that a human vitamin B_6-deficiency disease does in fact exist. The disease is a neurological disorder commonly known as carpal tunnel syndrome. (We talked about this disease in the last chapter, but here we'll discuss it in a little more depth.) *Carpus* is the medical term for your wrist. The bones and ligaments in your wrist form a tunnel through which pass the tendons and the nerve that make it possible for you to move your fingers and that control your sense of touch.

"When the disease strikes, an accumulation of fluid inside the carpal tunnel puts pressure on the nerve," explains Dr. Folkers. "This, in turn, leads to numbness and tingling in the tips of the fingers. Sometimes patients will tell me that at night their arms or hands 'fall asleep.' It's true that they may have, indeed, been sleeping on their arm, but I suspect that a more likely explanation is that they have carpal tunnel syndrome."

Because the nerve is being compressed, other, more serious symptoms may also develop—painful elbows or shoulders and very weak handgrips, to name a few. Somtimes symptoms are so severe that patients have to quit their jobs.

For years, patients with this disorder were routinely subjected to hand surgery to relieve compression on the nerve. But it's no secret that the surgery may be only partially successful and that any relief gained is likely to be lost in a few short months.

Now, permanent relief of carpal tunnel syndrome is perhaps only a B_6 supplement away, thanks to the research efforts of Dr. Folkers and his associates. They were able to reach that conclusion by using a new and better blood test which can detect and accurately measure deficiences of vitamin B_6 on a patient-by-patient basis. Working in conjunction with John Ellis, M.D., of Mt. Pleasant, Texas, the doctors discovered, for the first time, that patients with carpal tunnel syndrome actually had a previously unrecognized severe deficiency of vitamin B_6. What's more, B_6 supplements always corrected the deficiency and led to disappearance of the signs and symptoms.

Their next step was to repeat this research, using the highly respected double-blind crossover technique. That means neither the patients nor the doctors conducting the experiments know which patients receive the actual vitamin and which receive a nontherapeutic, look-alike placebo pill—until the testing is completed.

Results? Patients responded well to the B_6 and not at all to the placebo. But when the patients on the placebo were given B_6, they, too, showed the same marked improvement.

"We've gotten as far as relating the disease to a B_6 deficiency and showing that the disease, if it hasn't progressed to the point of atrophy [wasting away], responds well to B_6," Dr. Folkers told us. "And what I think is almost unbelievable (but seems to be true) is that individuals who have had symptoms for years—a decade, even 15 years—show such remarkable reversal and improvement of their condition. I don't mean to say that the symptoms are 100 percent reversed, but they are improved *so much* that the patients do not need orthopedic surgery for their hands."

RDA Is "Far Too Low"

"It doesn't even take huge doses of B_6, either," Dr. Folkers assured us. "However, I *am* convinced that the Recommended Dietary Allowance [RDA] of 2 milligrams is far too low. Our research shows that a very high percentage of the population in this country appears to have a deficiency of B_6. I believe that an effective RDA would be around 25 milligrams or possibly even 35 milligrams. That means a supplement of B_6 will be needed to ensure health. In fact, the risk to health in *not* taking a B_6 supplement is far greater than the risk of taking it. Besides, it's virtually impossible to get that much B_6 in your daily diet"— even if you eat foods rich in this nutrient, such as bananas, salmon, chicken, liver and sunflower seeds.

But that's not all the interesting news about B_6.

B$_6$ and "Chinese Restaurant Syndrome"

Maybe you've heard of the notorious "Chinese restaurant syndrome." It comes on about 20 minutes after eating a meal spiced heavily with monosodium glutamate (MSG). Headache, feverish flush and a detached or distant feeling overcome those who are susceptible.

According to Dr. Folkers, it is people deficient in B$_6$ that develop Chinese restaurant syndrome. He proved his theory by showing that supplemental B$_6$ could effectively prevent a recurrence of the MSG reaction, whereas a placebo had no effect.

Because of that study, Dr. Folkers began to wonder if those with carpal tunnel syndrome might also be sensitive to MSG since they, too, have a B$_6$ deficiency. An opportunity to test such a correlation became available in the case of a student who was known to be severely affected by carpal tunnel syndrome and extremely deficient in B$_6$.

Dr. Folkers was afraid the student might overreact to the 8.5 grams of MSG usually given in the test, so he cut the dosage to 4 grams, even though 4 grams rarely produced a response with other volunteers. Neveretheless, after 20 minutes, the predictable signs of Chinese restaurant syndrome appeared.

"The carpal tunnel syndrome reveals a vitamin B$_6$ deficiency over months and years," says Dr. Folkers, "but the Chinese restaurant syndrome reveals a deficiency over a period of 20 to 60 *minutes*. In principle, the underlying cause of both syndromes appears identical."

B$_6$ and Kidney Stones

Even though vitamin B$_6$ can now claim exclusive rights to its own deficiency disease, we don't want its other newly found benefits to go by without at least a little fanfare. That's why we want to tell you it can also help people who suffer from recurrent kidney stone formation, especially of stones that are composed mainly of oxalates. So say doctors at St. Peter's Hospitals and Institute of Urology in London. They tried 200 milligrams of B$_6$ twice a day on one man who had been plagued with kidney stones for years. He took the vitamin for five months during 1977 and hasn't had a stone since.

The same success story can also be told for another patient. She was passing an average of one stone every *month* until B$_6$ was started. Now she has been free of stones for almost three years. "These two patients did not relapse, even after long periods of time," write the researchers, who say the patients have "an apparently permanent remission on pyridoxine [B$_6$]" (*British Medical Journal,* June 27, 1981).

You may be wondering how B$_6$ can have an effect on kidney stone formation. Well, you're not alone. In fact, doctors at the University of California at Los Angeles school of medicine think they may have a possible explanation.

Since both magnesium and B$_6$ had been reported as successful in preventing kidney stones in susceptible patients, the scientists felt that B$_6$ might in some way mimic the effects of magnesium. They weren't sure how, but they suspected that B$_6$ increased the utilization of magnesium by aiding the transport of this mineral across cell membranes.

To prove this theory, they gave nine volunteers 100 milligrams of B$_6$ twice a day for one month and then compared their magnesium levels after treatment to their levels before the experiment.

The results thoroughly supported their ideas. Following vitamin B$_6$ administration, the magnesium levels were significantly elevated in all the volunteers, with more than a doubling of the levels after four weeks of therapy (*Annals of Clinical and Laboratory Science,* July–August, 1981).

Vitamin B$_6$ seems to be one of those vitamins that's especially versatile. It can cure carpal tunnel syndrome, help keep blood clots at bay and may even stop kidney stones from making encore appearances. Now doctors are saying that B_6, which is also known for keeping the immune system healthy, may even help keep cancer from recurring.

In research done at the Imperial Cancer Research Fund Laboratories in London, patients undergoing treatment for breast cancer were studied to determine the likelihood that their cancer would return. What the doctors did was analyze the patients' urine for a by-product of vitamin B_6 metabolism known as 4-PA. Low urinary amounts of 4-PA reflect a vitamin B_6 deficiency, and the results of the study showed that patients who excreted lower levels of 4-PA had a significantly greater probability of recurrence of breast cancer than patients who excreted higher levels (*European Journal of Cancer,* February, 1980).

So, to help keep your health from becoming "bad news," just remember all the good news about B_6—and that it makes more sense than ever to make sure you're getting enough.

CHAPTER
29

B₆—MAYBE THE ANSWER TO HEART DISEASE

What causes arteriosclerosis?

Is it cholesterol, a high-fat diet, hypertension, stress, smoking?

All of those factors do play a role.

But according to a theory put forth by Kilmer McCully, M.D., former professor of pathology at the Harvard medical school, not one of them is the cause. They are all risk factors, true. But not one of those risk factors is responsible for the initial injury in the artery which ultimately escalates to a blocked artery.

Every disease must have a prime cause, one that is found in every case of the disease. Until now, scientists have assembled quite a few risk factors associated with arteriosclerosis but have never been able to pinpoint one basic chemical cause.

Dr. McCully, on the basis of extensive laboratory studies and many years of studying the scientific literature, is convinced that the original injury (or *lesion,* as scientists call it) in the arteries is caused by a series of events initiated by a deficiency of our old friend vitamin B_6 (pyridoxine).

We know that B_6 is a very special member of the family of B vitamins, that a deficiency can cause anemia, kidney stones, convulsions, neuritis, skin problems and even mental illness.

Could it be that vitamin B_6 is the missing element in the causation of the disease that kills twice as many people as cancer? We considered this theory so important, we invited Dr. McCully to discuss it with us.

Question: If it isn't cholesterol or any of the other risk factors which initiates the disease, what is the cause?

Dr. McCully: The original lesion in the arteries is caused by a toxic substance, homocysteine, which is a breakdown product of the amino acid methionine. But when pyridoxine [vitamin B_6] is present, homocysteine is unable to do its destructive work. B_6, acting as a coenzyme, facilitates the enzyme reaction, which quickly converts homocysteine to cystathionine, which is not toxic and is safely used by the body in other pathways.

Since pyridoxine is necessary to prevent the buildup of homocysteine in the blood, this vitamin can do much to prevent the original lesion leading to arteriosclerosis and to atherosclerosis, the advanced form of the disease.

Q: In what way does homocysteine initiate the process?

Dr. McCully: Homocysteine, which is formed in metabolism from methionine, is a toxic amino acid which causes the cells lining the artery to degenerate and slough off. The artery responds to this damage by synthesizing new cells and new connective tissue substance which accumulate lipids, especially cholesterol and triglycerides. Now we have what is known as an atheroma. An atheroma is something like a cyst. It is composed of connective tissue cells, fibers and lipoproteins which are deposited from the blood. We now have an impediment, a sort of roadblock in the artery which slows down the flow of blood. When the blood flow is severely restricted, the tissues beyond the blocked area die from lack of oxygen. The result here could be a heart attack or stroke.

When the same process affects the renal arteries supplying the kidneys, then the kidneys react by releasing renin, a hormone which reacts on the blood plasma to form angiotensin, a vasoconstrictor which raises the blood pressure.

Q: Then high blood pressure may be a consequence of the initial lesion, rather than the cause. What role does cholesterol play?

Dr. McCully: Another consequence sometimes associated with the increased blood pressure is a rise in blood cholesterol. The original theory was that cholesterol somehow caused the damage to the artery. Because of the association of high blood cholesterol with arteriosclerosis, it has been hypothesized for many years that somehow cholesterol, or the lipoproteins which carry the cholesterol, damage the artery walls. But this has never been proven. As a matter of fact, there are many experiments in which investigators have injected lipoprotein directly into the arterial wall and it is immediately cleared without any sign of damage. There's never been any proof that cholesterol, as it is carried in the blood, actually initiates the lesion.

However, once the lesion is initiated by homocysteine damage, then the blood cholesterol tends to increase.

Q: Then cholesterol and hypertension are associated with the disease as a result of the initial lesion, but are not the cause of the lesion?

Dr. McCully: Right. Arteriosclerosis is not an overnight phenomenon. It is a long-term process that could begin in childhood. Arteriosclerosis may be the first clinical sign of a marginal B₆ deficiency. Very careful studies have been done in Israel of the different populations. The bedouin tribes have very little arteriosclerosis, and their children have practically no arteriosclerotic lesions. However, the populations that come from Eastern Europe have a high incidence of arteriosclerosis, and their children show early arteriosclerotic lesions.

Q: What is the difference in their diets that contributes to this difference?

Dr. McCully: The difference is in both animal protein and animal fats. The bedouin diet is practically pure vegetarian, relatively few animal products. Being pure vegetarian, it would be high in B₆ and comparatively low in the amino acid methionine. Animal protein eaten by the Ashkenazi Jews has two to three times as much methionine as plant protein, on a weight basis, and it is relatively lower in pyridoxine. One of the reasons that it has less pyridoxine is that it is rich in fats. Pyridoxine is a water-soluble vitamin; the more fat in the diet, the less pyridoxine one consumes.

Food processing destroys vitamin B_6. In a diet that is rich in fats and contains processed foods, there is a very poor intake of pyridoxine to protect against the large quantities of methionine that are eaten with the animal products.

Q: What about sugar? Does it contribute to arteriosclerosis?

Dr. McCully: It might. Dr. John Yudkin about 15 years ago came out with a very important series of epidemiological studies in which he showed that arteriosclerosis and coronary heart disease are highly correlated with the consumption of sugar and refined carbohydrates. Yudkin felt that somehow sugar was causing the disease. But one could also interpret it in another way, that populations which consume much of their caloric intake in the form of sugar are depriving themselves of pyridoxine.

Q; Is there any laboratory evidence linking homocysteine to the original lesion?

Dr. McCully: There are several studies revealing that arteriosclerosis develops in animals when they are treated with homocysteine or methionine. We did some studies in 1970 showing that injecting homocysteine into rabbits produces arteriosclerotic lesions.

Then later, Harker and Ross at the University of Washington in Seattle showed that intravenous infusion of homocysteine into baboons also produces arteriosclerosis.

The relationship between pyridoxine deficiency and arteriosclerosis was discovered by Rinehart and Greenberg in the late 40s, when they showed that monkeys made deficient in vitamin B_6 rapidly develop atherosclerosis.

Monkeys made deficient in other B vitamins did not develop it.

At that time, it was not appreciated how significant their work was because they could not say what the biochemical steps and the intermediate pathways were which lead to arteriosclerosis. What I am doing is building on their observations. I'm showing, and published studies have indicated, that the monkeys deficient in pyridoxine maintained by Rinehart and Greenberg probably developed arteriosclerosis because they accumulated homocysteine. And it has been found more recently, both in human volunteers and in animals, that a vitamin B_6 deficiency leads to homocysteine accumulation when large doses of methionine are given.

Q: Could B_6 help reverse the damage to the artery?

Dr. McCully: It is possible. Moses M. Suzman of Johannesburg, South Africa, carried out a study on 17 patients with coronary artery disease. Animal protein was reduced to approximately one-quarter to one-half of their customary intake and each patient received 100 milligrams pyridoxine daily with a potent preparation of vitamin B complex. The patients were observed for an average of 13 months. All patients claimed a notable increase in exercise tolerance with complete or partial relief of angina, a gain in energy and a heightened sense of well-being. Glucose tolerance increased to almost normal in two of the patients who were diabetic. This study suggests that the lesions may be partially reversible with B_6.

Q: Does B_6 have any effect on cholesterol levels?

Dr. McCully: Yes, it does. Rinehart and Greenberg observed that monkeys supplemented with B_6 had lower levels of cholesterol. It has also been shown by other investigators, using rabbits and other models, that vitamin B_6 deficiency tends to elevate the blood cholesterol. The other point is that fat metabolism is impaired by B_6 deficiency so that an animal or a person who is deficient in B_6 is less able to metabolize fats, which then accumulate in the plasma. So this gives you a direct correlation. It begins to explain why persons with arteriosclerosis have elevated blood cholesterol and other lipids, including triglycerides. Pyridoxine appears to be necessary for the normal metabolism of these lipids.

Q: Does stress play an important role in the disease?

Dr. McCully: Stress is not a major factor in arteriosclerosis. Diet is by far the most important factor. An argument against stress as a major factor is that Japan, a crowded and highly industrialized nation, has a very low incidence of the disease, while Finland, a quiet, peaceful, rural community, has the highest incidence in the world. During both World Wars, when the population of Europe was coping with stressful wartime conditions, meat was scarce, vitamins were not refined out of the flour and there was a dramatic decrease in arteriosclerosis.

Q: What about physical exercise?

Dr. McCully: There is conflicting evidence about the importance of a sedentary life style and physical conditioning. These are minor factors which may contribute to decreased or increased survival but do not by themselves explain the cause of the disease.

Q: What about smoking?

Dr. McCully: Cigarette smoking is associated with a twofold to threefold increase in the risk of arteriosclerosis. Nicotine and carbon monoxide, which are among the 600 to 1,000 toxic components of cigarette smoke, are probably the atherogenic substances. It is highly possible, though it has never been proven, that some of the toxic elements in tobacco may be B_6 antagonists. Many drugs are known to interfere with the utilization of B_6. The birth control pill is one, and it has been shown that women who smoke and take the Pill place themselves in double jeopardy.

Q: B_6 is found in a great many foods. Why don't we get enough in our diets to prevent homocysteine damage?

Dr. McCully: B_6 is sensitive to heat and is water soluble. It is destroyed by the cook, the canner and the food processor. It is removed from most grains in the refining process. Even though this vitamin is widely distributed in a variety of foods, the amount consumed by a weight-conscious population may be marginal. Foods such as beans, peas, nuts, grains, bananas and avocados contain reasonable amounts of this vitamin. Meats, eggs and milk are also good sources, but they contain high levels of methionine. Hence, someone eating a high-protein diet, while he needs more of the vitamin to prevent homocysteine formation, is actually getting less.

Q: Have you made any changes in your own diet as a result of these findings?

Dr. McCully: Oh, yes. We have cut down considerably on meat and increased consumption of vegetables, grains and beans. Grains have half as much methionine as meat. Beans have one-third as much methionine as meat.

Bear in mind that methionine is a necessary amino acid, especially important to growth. We can't live without it. What we must do is strike a good balance between methionine-containing foods and foods rich in B$_6$.

Q: Why do so many older people suffer from arteriosclerosis?

Dr. McCully: For some reason, there is a clear decline of B$_6$ with age. Also a dramatic decline of B$_6$ in diabetes, a disease frequently complicated by arteriosclerosis. This may be due to inadequate intake, though this has not been proven.

Q: With this theory, many pieces of the cholesterol puzzle begin to fall into place. For want of a nail, the battle was lost. Do we have a parallel here?

Dr. McCully: The theory illustrates how interdependent all these processes are—nutrition, physiology, biochemistry—and that, if the first event in a cascading series of changes is prevented, then the whole disease can be prevented. The theory predicts that if one prevents the initial lesion due to homocysteine effect in the cells of the arteries, one can prevent all the consequences and complications of the disease.

Rating Foods for Heart Health: The McCully Thesis

Both vitamin B_6 and the amino acid methionine are essential elements in the diet, and a good balance between the two may be the answer to preventing arteriosclerosis, according to Dr. McCully. That balance can be expressed as the ratio of B_6 to methionine. A ratio of 15, for instance, means the food has 15 times more B_6 than methionine. Foods with a high ratio contain a desirably high level of B_6 with a low level of methionine. Here are the levels of some common foods.

Food	Ratio	Food	Ratio
Bananas	46	Toasted wheat germ	3
Carrots	15	Beef liver	2
Onions	10	Chick-peas	2
Kale	9	Corn	2
Spinach	7	Peanuts	2
Sweet potatoes	7	Soybeans	2
Asparagus	5	Walnuts	2
Cauliflower	5	Chicken	1
Turnip greens	5	Salmon	1
Broccoli	4	Beef	0.9
Brewer's yeast	3	Mushrooms	0.7
Lentils	3	Cod	0.5
Peas	3	Eggs	0.3
Sunflower seeds	3		

CHAPTER
30

B$_6$ FOR COMMON AND UNCOMMON AILMENTS

Every vitamin has its limitations. Vitamin B$_6$ will not walk the dog, chauffeur the kids or do windows. But scientists are finding that B$_6$—pyridoxine—may do a lot of other things that might previously have been considered impossible. Research indicates that vitamin B$_6$ is not only tackling some common medical ailments, but some extraordinarily uncommon maladies as well.

Gyrate atrophy is about as rare as a disease can get. It is a hereditary eye disease that may start as tunnel vision when the cells in the eye begin to degenerate and die. Night blindness can follow, and cataracts may occur in mid life between the ages of 40 and 60. The disease has been considered incurable, and eventually blindness ensues.

"Probably no more than 20 cases of gyrate atrophy have existed in the United States, and maybe only 50 cases have appeared in the world's literature," says Richard Weleber, M.D., at the University of Oregon health sciences center in Portland. "But by studying rare diseases, we better understand how the body works, and we get information on how to help people with more common problems, too."

Together with biochemist Nancy Kennaway, Ph.D., and pediatrician Neil Buist, M.D., Dr. Weleber has observed a startling discovery about gyrate atrophy. The scientists have seen that patients with the curious malady may respond favorably to high doses of vitamin B_6. Three of their four patients with the disease have done so.

"Our patients with gyrate atrophy do *not* have a vitamin B_6 deficiency," says Dr. Kennaway. "They have a vitamin B_6 *dependency*, which means they have inherited defects of the biochemical process which may be modified by large doses of vitamin B_6."

Patients with gyrate atrophy all have elevated levels of the amino acid ornithine in their blood. That elevation occurs because an enzyme which normally converts ornithine to glutamate is not working, Dr. Kennaway explains. So the patients' ornithine levels are high. Vitamin B_6 is a *cofactor* which works with the enzyme. Before it can change ornithine into glutamate, the enzyme needs small amounts of B_6 in healthy individuals. But small amounts of B_6 just won't do in some patients with gyrate atrophy. They need much larger doses of the vitamin before the enzyme is jolted into action.

Why a Little B_6 Isn't Enough

"It's like saying you can't open the door unless you push very hard," Dr. Buist told us. "A goodly number of enzymes within the body require a vitamin cofactor to work. That vitamin cofactor plugs itself into a very special hole of the protein enzyme in order for the enzyme to do its job. If, because of a hereditary defect, the hole is distorted or misshapen, teensy amounts of the vitamin, which normally would be sufficient, are not enough. Therefore, if we flood the system with the vitamin, we may be able to get the enzyme to work better."

While some gyrate atrophy patients apparently respond to vitamin B_6 therapy, not all of them do. So patients are broken down into two categories: B_6 responsive and B_6 nonresponsive.

object to giving multiple vitamin supplements because it's "shotgun therapy." But shotgun therapy is preferable to "machinegun therapy"—which is what one drug after another is. And a number of drugs also interfere with B_{12} absorption, including certain medications for high blood pressure, tuberculosis, Parkinson's disease, gout and excess cholesterol. Alcohol also adversely affects B_{12} absorption, just as it does the absorption of other B vitamins.

If you have a history of stomach surgery or are taking drugs and have any reason to suspect a B_{12} deficiency, you should certainly discuss that situation with your physician. In general, though, older people are the ones most likely to be deficient.

Because the most widely used B_{12}-deficiency test is so unreliable, it's difficult to say how many older people are actually deficient or on the verge of being deficient. But we can get some indication from a study published by three doctors from Denmark (*Acta Medica Scandinavica*). These doctors used a very reliable microbiological B_{12} test to measure levels of the vitamin in 349 patients admitted to a geriatric center. Low values of vitamin B_{12} were found in one out of every three of these patients. Dr. L. Elsborg and colleagues urged other physicians to study B_{12} levels in older patients much more frequently than it is now done and to treat deficiencies before they have turned into major medical problems.

If you rarely eat meat, don't like liver and eat a lot of noodles, rice, potatoes and vegetables, you should do *something* to protect your B_{12} status.

One common-sense step is to make sure your vitamin B supplement contains B_{12}. Since it is inexpensive and safe, there is almost no need to worry about taking too much. The important thing about B_{12} is to be sure.

CHAPTER
34

FOLATE, THE GOLD IN THE COOKING WATER

Vegetables are the most important dietary source of folate (folic acid), a member of the B-complex family of vitamins. Folate is essential for a host of functions inside our bodies, including maintaining the integrity of the blood and the nervous system. Yet, you'll find precious little of it in meat or in fish or eggs or milk and other dairy products. So there's a lot of wisdom in that old entreaty "eat your vegetables"! Ironically, though, there's evidence that mother's best efforts to nourish us may have been compromised, depending on how long and how hard she cooked those vegetables.

Fresh cauliflower cooked for as little as 10 minutes in vigorously boiling water loses 84 percent of its folate, Joseph Leichter, Ph.D., and two co-workers at the University of British Columbia's division of human nutrition in Vancouver report. Other vegetables fared little better, with substantial portions of their folate content leaching into the cooking water. Broccoli lost 69 percent of its folate, spinach 65 percent and cabbage 57 percent. Only asparagus and Brussels sprouts came through the cooking experience relatively unscathed, parting with just 22 and 28 percent of the folate, respectively (*Nutrition Reports International*).

"The boiling of vegetables for 10 minutes in a salt solution was chosen because it is close to the usual circumstances of food preparation and consumption at home," the Canadian researchers note. "With the exception of asparagus and Brussels sprouts, the cooking water contained more folate than the cooked vegetables. This and other studies indicate that the loss of folate from vegetables during cooking is caused by extraction of the vitamin into the cooking water rather than by destruction."

What about microwave cooking? A recent study indicates that folate losses are even greater—an ominous finding given the ever-increasing trend toward microwave heating, both in restaurants and at home.

According to Rayna G. Cooper, R.D., various forms of folate are destroyed at markedly different rates during microwave heating. But one of the forms found in high concentration in foods (and, interestingly, in human blood also) is the most rapidly destroyed.

Dietitian Cooper, who was formerly associated with Mira Loma Hospital, Lancaster, California, found that this form of folate was 90 percent obliterated after 28 minutes inside a microwave oven set at 212°F, whereas the same destruction required 65 minutes of conventional heating at the same temperature *(Journal of the American Dietetic Association).*

Even microwave heating at a lower temperature (187°F) resulted in quicker destruction of folate than conventional cooking at 212°F.

So much for folate's ability to squeak past the perils of the kitchen. Now add the fact that as much as *half* of the folate in a normal diet may not be fully absorbed by our bodies because of digestive enzyme insufficiency, and you begin to sense the magnitude of the problem.

Sunlight Destroys Folate

There's even some evidence that oridinary sunshine can deplete our folate stores. Researchers at the University of Minnesota have discovered that, when samples of human blood are exposed to strong sunlight, they lose 30 to 50 percent of their folate in about an hour *(Science)*.

Of course, in real life we have several layers of skin shielding our insides from the sun. But that protection appears less than total. The same scientists found that some patients who had been undergoing lengthy ultraviolet light treatments for skin problems had unusually depressed levels of folate circulating in their bloodstreams.

The Minnesota researchers point out that many tropical populations suffer a high incidence of severe anemia, infertility, dangerous birth complications and other folate-deficiency problems. And excessive sunlight exposure may aggravate that situation.

Those of us in better-fed, more temperate nations don't face those kinds of risks. But there is evidence that marginal amounts of folate in the diet are catching some people unawares.

For example, M. I. Botez, M.D., and co-workers at Montreal's Clinical Research Institute report a number of cases of central-nervous-system abnormalities linked to folate deficiency *(Archives of Neurology)*.

Folate and the Nervous System

In one instance, a 62-year-old woman was hospitalized because of weakness in both legs. For the previous 13 years, she had complained of burning feet, cramps and tingling feelings in her limbs. Examination revealed some loss of sensation and sensitivity to pain in both legs, which were now partially paralyzed. There was also evidence of spinal-cord degeneration.

This woman had low blood folate levels, and she admitted that she had not eaten fresh vegetables for many years. Because of the extremity of her situation, doctors began giving her 15 milligrams of supplementary folate a day by mouth along with periodic injections—far in excess of the estimated daily requirement of about 400 *micro*grams or 0.4 milligrams. Within two months, symptoms started to abate. After 12 months, she was almost walking normally.

Another woman, age 76, suffered with lightning stabs of pain along with episodes of numbness during the night—symptoms which awakened her nightly without fail. She was unable to walk alone. Supported by two people, she could manage a few steps. Standing with her eyes closed, she would lose her balance.

Because of allergic migraine headaches, this woman had not eaten fresh vegetables or fruits since she was 14 years old. Eight weeks after beginning to take daily folate supplements, she was able to walk alone with the aid of a cane. After nine months, she didn't need the cane.

No wonder the authors speak of folate's "spectacularly beneficial effect."

Dr. Botez believes there may also be a correlation between lack of folate and a condition known as the restless legs syndrome in pregnant women. Those afflicted with the syndrome complain of creeping, irritating sensations in the lower legs, which can often be relieved by walking or moving.

For one thing, estimates of folate deficiency among expectant mothers run as high as 60 percent. And restless legs often occur in the late stages of pregnancy just when folate deficiency is most pronounced. When Dr. Botez and an associate examined two groups of pregnant women, they found that 8 out of 10 not receiving supplemental folate had restless legs syndrome. But only 1 of 11 taking folate had the problems *(Nutrition Reports International)*.

When three women with severe restless legs syndrome were given 10 milligrams of folate daily, their symptoms disappeared after eight days.

Folate Foils Senility

As you may have guessed from its central-nervous-system role, folate is especially concentrated in the fluid of the spinal column—the switchboard of the central nervous system that relays messages between your brain and body.

Dr. Botez has found that many of the signs of approaching senility may actually be caused by a folate deficiency "short-circuiting" the nervous system.

Speaking to an annual meeting of the Royal College of Physicians and Surgeons of Canada, the neurologist reported that four of his patients complained of fatigue, weight loss, insomina and severe constipation. They also had cold, numb legs and poor reflexes. Testing them, Dr. Botez found that they had low blood levels of folate. He started them on supplements and injections of this vitamin. After three months of treatment, their subjective symptoms disappeared, they gradually put on weight and their reflexes normalized. These improvements coincided with rises in the concentration of folate in their blood *(Clinical Psychiatry News)*.

These patients, who had been under psychiatric care for an extended period and had been unresponsive to various medications taken before the study, did not know they were receiving folate, Dr. Botez told the meeting.

In Scotland, ten elderly patients—five of them diagnosed as senile—had nervous-system disorders so severe that their spinal cords were thought to have degenerated. Upon closer investigation, they were found to be folate deficient. Folate treatment led to an improvement in mood of all of the patients. The condition of two patients with severe mental illness was "dramatically resolved" *(British Medical Journal)*.

Vital to Newborn

Now let's trace folate back from the nursing home to the nursery. For folate is vital not only in ensuring the health of an adult's nervous system, but also in protecting the health of a newborn. To find out why, let's take a look at genes.

Genes are found in every cell and are responsible for passing down physical and biochemical traits from generation to generation. Every living thing, from the mighty whale to the tiniest amoeba, is built up from a blueprint of genes. Tall or short; small-boned or heavyset; blond, brunet or redhead—genes make us what we are.

And it is folate that makes genes what *they* are.

When scientists make a diagram of the complex metabolic pathways that create a chemical substance, such as a gene, out of folate and other nutrients, the drawing often looks to a layman like a map of the New York City subway system as finger painted by a two-year-old. So without going into the somewhat mystifying details of *how* folate helps to produce a gene, let's just say that it's a critically important contributor to gene formation. Without folate, the "blueprint" of a gene could not be designed with any accuracy; the "building" built up from such a blueprint would be a shambles. Tragically, this sometimes happens.

Scientists examined 805 women in early pregnancy. Low folate levels were found in 135. Among these women, the frequency of malformations among their offspring was four times greater than among the 670 women whose blood levels of folate were normal *(South African Medical Journal)*.

In a study of 35 mothers whose children had birth defects, 23 of the mothers had abnormal folate metabolism *(Lancet)*.

In a South African study, 57 percent of the children born to mothers who were severely deficient in folate during pregnancy showed abnormal or delayed development *(Nutrition Reports International)*.

Lower Resistance

A Massachusetts Institute of Technology (MIT) scientist, Paul M. Newberne, D.V.M., Ph.D., has suggested that even a marginal deficiency of folate in a mother-to-be could severely hinder her child's ability to fight off disease later in life. In laboratory tests, offspring of mother animals fed diets with marginal amounts of folate were less able to overcome a common food-poisoning bacterium than rats whose mothers received adequate amounts of folate *(Technology Review)*.

Besides causing a greater chance of birth deformities or slower development in the child, folate deficiency also creates a greater likelihood that the mother will develop:

- toxemia of pregnancy,
- abruptio placentae (premature separation of the placenta from the wall of the uterus),
- anemia.

The most marked symptom of a severe folate deficiency is megaloblastic anemia. In this anemia, red blood cells become *megaloblastoid*. They are too large, oddly shaped, and have a very short life span. Robert L. Gross, M.D., formerly of the department of nutrition and food science at MIT and currently practicing in San Francisco, found that, in folate deficiency, the cells responsible for fighting infection *also* become megaloblastoid and lose their ability to defend the body against viruses and bacteria. This inability is reversed by folate treatment *(American Journal of Clinical Nutrition)*.

But you don't have to be newborn, long ago born or pregnant for a folate problem to hit you like a ton of bricks, suggest William E. Thornton, M.D., and Bonnie Pray Thornton, R.N. The Thorntons, formerly associated with the Medical University of South Carolina in Charleston, report evidence of a relationship between lack of folate and forgetfulness, apathy, irritability, disturbed sleep, depression and even psychosis *(Journal of Clinical Psychiatry)*.

The two investigators concluded, after examining the records of 269 patients hospitalized for psychiatric problems, that the mentally disturbed were more likely to have low levels of folate than were normal individuals, regardless of sex or age.

Since dietary surveys revealed that the disturbed patients were consuming reasonable amounts of folate, it may have been that some inner problem of metabolism was responsible. Such individuals might need folate in extra-large amounts.

Can folate deficiency affect the brain in more subtle ways? To find out, Dr. Botez and another researcher kept a group of young rats on a folate-deficient diet for three weeks. Then, one at a time, the animals were placed in a special box. To avoid being subjected to a mild electric shock, the rats had to learn to recognize a warning signal (in this case a light) and escape to the safe corner of the box.

Those animals deprived of folate required significantly more trials than folate-fed rats before they learned to associate the light with impending shock and take appropriate action *(Tohoku Journal of Experimental Medicine)*.

Such results suggest that "folate deficiency could be responsible for a deleterious effect upon the growing nervous system," the Montreal researchers warn.

Eat Your Vegetables and Save Your Cooking Water

Given folate's well-documented susceptibility to destruction between farm and fork, how can you still be sure you're getting enough of this essential nutrient?

Vegetables, despite their potential vulnerability to having folate hijacked in the kitchen, remain the best source—provided you take certain precautions.

Brussels sprouts, you'll recall, come through the cooking process with flying colors as far as their precious folate cargo is concerned. According to Scottish researcher J. D. Malin of the University of Strathclyde in Glasgow, that's because Brussels sprouts, being dense and compact, have a relatively small surface area. There's less opportunity for folate to leach out into the cooking water.

At the same time, Brussels sprouts are exceptionally rich in vitamin C (as much as 140 milligrams in 3½ ounces of sprouts), which protects the folate from oxidative destruction.

According to Malin, "An average helping of sprouts could provide almost half of the average daily intake of total folate" for many people *(Journal of Food Technology)*.

If Brussels sprouts are not to your taste, other vegetables can be excellent sources, provided you don't overcook them. "Cooking vegetables for a shorter time would reduce folate loss," Dr. Leichter of the University of British Columbia told us. "And using less water would definitely decrease the amount that leaches out."

A cup of cooked spinach supplies 164 micrograms; a cup of cooked beets 133 micrograms. But be sure to keep cooking water and cooking time to a minimum.

Better still, try eating more vegetables in their raw state. Tables compiled by the U.S. Department of Agriculture (USDA) indicate that romaine lettuce, parsley, broccoli and collard greens all provide more than 100 micrograms of folate per 3½-ounce portion when served raw (*Journal of the American Dietetic Association*).

Another suggestion: Use your leftover cooking water for steaming rice or, as Dr. Leichter suggests, add it to soups and stews. That way, whatever folate is leached into the water will be regained.

Grains in the diet can supply some additional folate, but here wholeness is the key: 3½ ounces of whole wheat flour contain 54 micrograms of folate; the same amount of white flour contains less than half that amount. Toasted wheat germ is an outstanding source. A 1-ounce serving provides 120 micrograms.

We mentioned that meat is a poor provider of folate. Liver is an exception to that rule, however. A 3-ounce serving of cooked liver contains about 123 micrograms.

A real sleeper in the folate sweepstakes is black-eyed peas. USDA scientists consider them a better source of folate than even liver or wheat germ, since a normal 6-ounce serving supplies about 230 micrograms (*Journal of Food Science*).

Probably the surest way to meet your folate requirements on a day-to-day basis would be to take this vitamin in supplement form. If you're already taking a B-complex formula, check the label for folate (or folic acid). Be sure it doesn't skimp. Remember that the normal adult RDA for folate is 400 micrograms.

One final thing to keep in mind: Researchers at the University of California at Berkeley have found that *zinc* deficiency interferes with the intestinal absorption of some forms of folate. Among a group of six healthy male volunteers, such reductions averaged 53 percent *(Federation Proceedings)*. So don't let a zinc oversight undermine your folate quest.

And if "eat your vegetables" is a plea you've always ignored, try substituting "take your folate." Either way, you'll be helping yourself immeasurably.

35

FOLATE: A WOMAN'S BEST FRIEND

"Diamonds," goes the song, "are a girl's best friend." Now, while we're not songwriters, we respectfully suggest that, if *folate* were substituted for *diamonds*, the song might be even more true.

For folate is a nutrient of extraordinary powers. From your head to your toes—literally—you need folate to keep you functioning at peak performance, especially if you're a woman.

As far as your whole body is concerned, a serious folate deficiency could result in severe anemia. You'd feel weak and weary, and your skin might take on an ashen pallor.

The use of oral contraceptives has been implicated in such folate deficiencies. The case of a 29-year-old executive illustrates the point. She was admitted to a hospital because of pounding pulse in her ears, easy bruising, fatigue and a sensation of weakness. Diagnosed initially as having an inflamed gallbladder and gallstones, she had her gallbladder removed.

After her operation, she was found to have not only anemia, but also hemorrhages in the retina of her right eye. Apparently, no one had ever asked if she was taking the Pill, but finally a physician discovered she had been taking it for three years.

As the physician in charge noted, "The contraceptive was stopped and the patient was started on oral folic acid [folate] . . . . She was subsequently followed as an outpatient, and on continued folate therapy her blood counts and morphology have normalized and the retinal hemorrhages have disappeared" *(Minnesota Medicine)*.

Your gums may need folate therapy, too. During pregnancy, many women suffer from inflamed gums—estimates range from as low as 30 to as high as 100 percent of them.

A recent study of 30 women done during their fourth and eighth months of pregnancy showed that those who rinsed their mouths twice daily for one minute with a folate mouth wash experienced a "highly significant improvement" in the health of their gums during the eighth month *(Journal of Clinical Periodontology*, October, 1980).

Link with Depression

Nowadays, too, more and more physicians are looking into folate deficiency as a cause of depression. A study at McGill University, Montreal, examined the folate levels of three different groups of patients: those who were depressed, those who were psychiatrically ill but not depressed and those who were medically ill. Six of the patients were men, 42 were women, and their ages ranged from 20 to 91 years.

The researchers discovered that "serum folic acid [folate] levels were significantly lower in the depressed patients than in the psychiatric and medical patients . . . . On the basis of our results, we believe that folic acid deficiency depression may exist" *(Psychosomatics*, November, 1980).

Would folate therapy help clear up depression?

To find out, we spoke to A. Missagh Ghadirian, M.D., of the department of psychiatry, McGill University, the head researcher in the study. "Based on my clinical observations, it seems that people whose depressions are purely due to folate deficiency do get better with folate therapy," Dr. Ghadirian told us. "To make absolutely sure, we will have to wait for the results of the second phase of our study, in which folate therapy is used."

Such positive findings for folate therapy may explain the remarkable case of a young woman with "baby blues," or post-partam depression. Her pregnancy and the delivery of her baby were uncomplicated. However, several weeks after delivery, she became progressively withdrawn and emotionally unstable.

Soon she became disoriented, panicky, and had hallucinations about large, ugly figures that intended harm to her and her new baby.

Hospitalized in two different psychiatric facilities for a period of 19 months, she received shock treatments and various tranquilizers. She also tried to commit suicide three times.

According to the physician who saw her as a result of her third suicide attempt, "She was an attractive but very distressed-appearing young woman who was extremely frightened, whining and literally withdrawn into the corner of her hospital room" (*American Journal of Obstetrics and Gynecology*). Three blood tests for folate levels were performed on her, one of which was reported as very low and two of which were reported as "none detectable."

The doctor's report continues: "She was treated for anemia with five mg. of folic acid twice a day . . . for 10 days [a large therapeutic dose]. On the seventh day of folic acid treatment, an improvement in the mental status was noted; by the tenth day a complete remission had occurred. The patient was discharged on one mg. of oral folic acid daily.

"She has been followed for the past 2½ years without evidence of any psychiatric disturbance. She is presently an active student in nursing school and doing very well academically."

Some scientists now think that it's possible not only to be generally deficient in folate, but also to have a localized deficiency—a deficiency in a certain spot in the body. One such scientist is C. E. Butterworth, M.D., professor and chairman of the department of nutrition sciences at the University of Alabama.

According to Dr. Butterworth, one kind of problem that may be due to a localized folate deficiency is cervical dysplasia—a condition in which abnormal cells, thought to be precancerous and identified by Pap smear, are found in the cervix. In an investigation performed by Dr. Butterworth, 47 young women who were on the Pill and who had mild to moderate cervical dysplasia were studied. Some of the women received oral supplements of 100 milligrams of folate daily while the others received placebos.

The results of the study are impressive. The women taking therapeutic doses of folate improved significantly while the unsupplemented women showed no change.

Furthermore, says Dr. Butterworth, "There were four cases of apparent regression to normal among subjects receiving folic acid supplementation, but none in the unsupplemented group." There were four cases of apparent progression to cancer among the unsupplemented subjects, but none in the group receiving folate supplementation. "The data is interpreted as indicating that oral folic acid supplementation may prevent the progression of early cancer to a more severe form and in some cases promote reversion to normalcy" (*Contemporary Nutrition*, December, 1980).

A Very Common Deficiency

How common are folate deficiencies?

One physician has said that "primary folic acid deficiency is probably the most common vitamin deficiency in man," and, indeed, more and more evidence is piling up that it's true.

At the Florida Symposium on Micronutrients in Human Nutrition, held at the University of Florida in February, 1981, several papers were presented that detailed the evidence of low levels of folate in various groups of people.

Lynn B. Bailey, Ph.D., assistant professor of nutrition, University of Florida, pointed out that both "folacin [folate] and iron status were less than adequate" in a large group of adolescents she had studied. And according to Patricia A. Wagner, Ph.D., associate professor of nutrition, University of Florida, 60 percent of the elderly living in a low-income area of Miami had low folate concentrations in their bloodstreams. Also at risk for folate problems are alcoholics, those taking certain anticonvulsive, antibacterial or diuretic drugs and, as we've mentioned, women on the Pill and women who are pregnant or nursing.

Studies carried out by the World Health Organization in various countries outside the United States have suggested that up to *a third of all the pregnant women in the world* have a folate deficiency. And it seems that here in America we're no exception.

Victor Herbert, M.D., of the Veterans Administration Hospital, Bronx, New York, and several colleagues testing 110 pregnant women from low-income families in New York City found that 16 percent had definite folate deficiency. Another 14 percent had only marginal levels *(American Journal of Obstetrics and Gynecology)*.

And in a study of 27 women of "better economic circumstances"—patients in a private obstetrical practice—over half had a mild folate deficiency *(American Journal of Clinical Nutrition)*.

That's not the best of news, because even a mild deficiency can limit the formation of genes.

But it's not only pregnant women and their children who suffer from a folate deficiency. "Quite apart from pregnancy, folate deficiency is a real problem in the U.S.," writes Ronald Girdwood, M.D., Ph.D., of the university department of therapeutics, Royal Infirmary, in Scotland in the *American Journal of Clinical Nutrition*. A spate of studies bear out his opinion.

Charles A. Hall, M.D., of the Veterans Administration Hospital in Albany, New York, and his co-workers tested the folate levels of 106 "essentially healthy persons" and found 31 percent of them had folate blood levels on the borderline of deficiency *(American Journal of Clinical Nutrition)*.

Who Is at High Risk?

Older people run a great risk of folate deficiency. British researchers found abnormally low folate levels in the blood of

80 percent of 51 people entering an old persons' home *(British Medical Journal)*.

A large volume of research suggests that oral contraceptives interfere with folate metabolism and lead to a lowering of levels in the blood. The World Health Organization has recommended that those on the Pill—as well as pregnant women and the aged—should receive more folate.

Taking antibiotics can cause a deficiency. Folate is thought to be manufactured to some extent by bacteria in the intestinal tract; prolonged use of antibiotics kills these bacteria.

Excessive alcohol consumption also robs the body of folate. Ninety percent of alcoholics suffer from folate deficiency.

But most of us are not on antibiotics, the Pill, or a bottle a day of Old Crow. If we're deficient, how come?

"This deficiency may result from inadequate intake or secondary disease," says Carl Pfeiffer,Ph.D., M.D., in *Mental and Elemental Nutrients* (Keats, 1975).

Secondary diseases (that is, diseases not *directly* caused by folate deficiency) can impair our ability to use the folate we take in. An African study found that patients with bacterial infections could not absorb folate as efficiently as healthy persons *(Lancet)*. Psoriasis, a skin disease, may cause folate levels to fall *(Skin and Allergy News)*. An article in the *British Medical Journal* reports that severely injured or ill hospital patients often need extra doses of folate. That's because it's so crucial to bodily repair.

How about inadequate intake?

A study of adolescents found that 85 percent of boys, 90 percent of girls from families of low-income status and 100 percent of girls from families of upper-income status took in *less than half* the Recommended Dietary Allowance for folate *(American Journal of Clinical Nutrition)*. The RDA for adults is 400 micrograms; for children under 10, 300 micrograms.

In a study of black school children in Mississippi, the average intake of folate was about *one-fifth* the recommended amount. Over 99 percent of the children consumed less than half of the daily recommended amount *(Journal of the American Dietetic Association)*.

A nutritional survey of 46 elderly long-term surgical patients showed that most of them had inadequate intake of folate *(International Journal of Vitamin and Nutrition Research).*

Dr. Pfeiffer notes that folate intake is "one of the most widespread insufficiences in our diets."

But a folate deficiency can result from more than just not getting the Recommended Dietary Allowance. Vitamin C is necessary for the reduction of folate to the active form the body can use. A deficiency of that vitamin can aggravate the ill effects of a marginal supply of folate.

An unusual property of folate in supplemental amounts is that it can mask some of the effects of vitamin B_{12}-deficiency anemia—pernicious anemia.

Because of this, the FDA continues to put a limit on the amount of folate in over-the-counter supplements, even though new techniques now make it possible to diagnose pernicious anemia even when folate levels are high. Actually, folate deficiency is far more common than B_{12} deficiency. As we suggested in the last chapter, if you want to ensure folate nutrition with a B-complex supplement, make sure it contains 400 micrograms (1.4 milligrams). If you're pregnant, you'll need double that amount (800 micrograms). And if you're a nursing mother, you'll need 500 micrograms.

And just remember that, although folate itself may not sparkle like a diamond, it can sure help *you* to sparkle from head to toe.

CHAPTER
36

PANTOTHENATE—THE ANTI-STRESS VITAMIN

Colitis. It's the disease God forgot to give Job. Even the mild variety comes complete with diarrhea and bloody stools. And severe colitis pulls out all the stops—literally—diarrhea so constant the bathroom seems like a prison cell; stomach cramps; pale, feverish skin blotched with rashes . . . .

If this description is turning your stomach, please *don't* turn the page.

We wanted to give you a really dramatic example of the role of pantothenate (pantothenic acid)—one of the B-complex vitamins. Perhaps the best way to see how a vitamin works to keep you healthy is to see how *un*healthy you can get when it's missing. And while colitis—a disease in which the colon is inflamed—is not caused by an outright deficiency of pantothenate, it may well be the result of the body's failure to efficiently utilize this vitamin.

Normally, your body uses pantothenate by turning it into another substance, coenzyme A (CoA). Put another way, CoA is the metabolically *active* form of pantothenate. But researchers at the University of Manitoba, Winnipeg, Canada, and at the

215

Mayo Clinic in Rochester, Minnesota, found that, although 29 patients with colitis had normal levels of pantothenate in their blood, the level of CoA in their colons was only one-half of that found in the colons of 31 patients who did not have colitis *(American Journal of Clinical Nutrition)*.

The researchers offered *six* possible explanations—all speculations—as to why colitis patients had low levels of CoA in their colons. Why the uncertainty? Because CoA is hard to pin down. It helps the heart beat, the stomach digest, the lungs pump. And more.

CoA is vital in the health of your adrenal glands and in the production of the adrenal gland hormones, the hormones that give you the emotional and physical energy you need to cope with stress—*any* stress. From a bitter argument to a bitter winter. From a traffic jam to jam spilled on your shirt. From a mosquito bite to the seven-year itch. In fact, CoA is so important for healthy adrenal glands that pantothenate (which turns into CoA) has been dubbed an anti-stress vitamin.

Way back in the 30s, researchers had already discovered that rats deprived of pantothenate had severely damaged adrenal glands. They also found that rats fed a pantothenate-deficient diet reacted poorly to stress, while rats given extra pantothenate coped with stress better.

In one study, rats were divided into three groups. One group got a diet deficient in pantothenate. Another group got a diet adequate in pantothenate. The third group got a diet high in this vitamin. Then all the rats were put in cold water and made to swim until they were exhausted. The pantothenate-deficient rats swam an average of 16 minutes. The "adequate" group did better: They swam an average of 29 minutes. But the rats with a diet high in pantothenate swam an average of 62 minutes *(Metabolism)*.

But what's true for rats is not necessarily true for us humans. So in 1952, Elaine Ralli and her co-worker, Mary Dumm, researchers in the department of medicine at the New York University–Bellevue Medical Center in New York City, tested the anti-stress effects of pantothenate on humans.

Standing Up to Stress

The researchers immersed a group of normal men in 48°F water for eight minutes. Precise chemical measurements of the men's blood and urine were taken before and at intervals after the stress. Then, for six weeks, the men received 10 grams of calcium pantothenate (a common form of pantothenate) every day. At the end of six weeks, they were again immersed and the same measurements were taken.

Usually, stress causes a decrease in some of the white blood cells that protect the body against infection. After taking the pantothenate, the men had a "less pronounced" drop in these white blood cells. Also, levels of vitamin C—a nutrient burned up by stress—were "significantly higher." And the men excreted less uric acid, a sign that the body had not undergone as much wear and tear. Importantly, they also had lower cholesterol levels *(Vitamins and Hormones)*.

A stress that's every bit as intense as cold water is the cold steel of a surgeon's knife. Fifty patients undergoing abdominal surgery were given 500 milligrams of panthenol—a substance similar to pantothenate—the day of surgery and for five days afterwards. Another 50 patients were not given panthenol.

The group receiving panthenol had quicker recoveries, with less nausea and vomiting—"a more benign postoperative course," in the words of the researchers conducting the study *(American Journal of Surgery)*.

Armor against X Rays

But perhaps the most severe stress is X-ray radiation. Radiation is like tiny bullets shooting into the body.

In an experimental study, Dr. I. Szórády, of the department of pediatrics, University Medical School, Szeged, Hungary, exposed 200 laboratory mice divided equally into four groups to total body irradiation with X rays.

The rate of survival was highest in the group of mice receiving pantothenate for a week before irradiation. Half were still alive 21 days following the massive stress. But among 50 other mice *not* protected by supplemental pantothenate, half were dead within eight days of X-ray exposure *(Acta Paediatrica Hungaricae)*.

"It follows that, as compared to controls, survival was prolonged by 200 percent," Dr. Szórády concluded. "Due to its metabolic key position, pantothenic acid thus seems to induce slow biochemical processes which ensure enhanced protection against radiation injury."

These "slow biochemical processes" may be one key to how pantothenate shuts the door on stress.

Stress speeds you up. Thoughts flash through the mind. Blood pressure shoots up. The heart races. If you have a hard time steering through the stress in your life, your body may be in chronic fourth gear—but your health will come in last. Pantothenate may help keep your body moving at the speed it was built for.

A Longer Life

Added proof for Dr. Szórády's theory of pantothenate's power to "slow biochemical processes" comes from Roger Williams, Ph.D., the first man to isolate, identify and synthesize pantothenate. Dr. Williams, a research scientist with the Clayton Foundation Biochemical Institute at the University of Texas, believes that pantothenate can actually prolong life.

He conducted an experiment with two groups of mice, feeding both of them an identical and nutritionally complete diet. One group, however, got extra pantothenate in their drinking water.

The animals without extra pantothenate lived an average of 550 days. But those getting the extra pantothenate lived an average of 653 days.

"If the 550 days is regarded as equivalent to 75 years for a human, then the 653 days would be equivalent to 89 years," Dr. Williams wrote in *Nutrition against Disease* (Pitman, 1971).

"On a purely statistical basis," he adds, "I would be willing to wager that if a large number of weaned babies were given 25 milligrams of extra pantothenate daily during their lifetime, their life expectancy would be increased by at least 10 years."

And they might have fewer runny noses, too.

Dr. Szórády conducted a standard allergy skin test on 24 children, injecting them with histamine. "Pantothenic acid reduced the intensity of the skin reaction by 20 to 50 percent in all children," he reported. In his paper on pantothenate, he also cites a study in which a researcher "applied pantothenic acid treatment of allergic adults with satisfactory results."

Raw Foods a Must

You'd assume that Mother Nature would have stocked her pantry with a hefty supply of a vitamin so critical to overall health and well-being. And you'd be right. *Pantos* is the Greek word for *everywhere*, and pantothenate lives up to its name: It's found in almost all foods. But Mother Nature's pantry—brimming with vegetables, lean meats, whole grains, fruits, nuts and seeds—is a far cry from the pantry in most modern households, where canned, frozen and highly processed foods crowd out the real thing. As far as pantothenate goes, these cupboards are just about bare.

That's because processed foods are losers. So concluded Henry Schroeder, M.D., former director of research at Brattleboro Memorial Hospital and professor of physiology at the Dartmouth medical school.

"It is apparent that raw foods supply adequate amounts [of pantothenate] . . . ," wrote Dr. Schroeder. "It is not apparent, however, that persons subsisting on refined, processed and canned foods will be provided with adequate amounts. . . ."

Facts back him up. When fresh vegetables are frozen, pantothenate gets the cold shoulder—the vegetables lose anywhere from 37 to 57 percent of this vitamin. Canned vegetables lose from 46 to 78 percent of their pantothenate. Processed and refined grains—the kind used in baking most of the breads, cakes, cookies and crackers sold in supermarkets—lose 37 to 74 percent of this nutrient. Processed meats do no better, losing one-half to three-quarters *(American Journal of Clinical Nutrition)*.

"These data," believed Dr. Schroeder, "cast doubt on the adequacy of the American diet for . . . pantothenic acid," and "demonstrate the dietary needs for the use of whole grains and unprocessed foods of most varieties."

And that goes double for babies. A Canadian study showed that processed, strained baby foods provide *only 25 percent* of an infant's need for panthothenate *(Nutrition Reports International)*.

Another scientist who doubts whether most people get enough pantothenate is Dr. Klaus Pietrzik of Germany. Speaking to the 1975 annual meeting of the Federation of the American Societies for Experimental Biology, Dr. Pietrzik warned that a diet with a 25 percent deficiency in pantothenate would damage the central nervous system after only six months. "The desirable doses of pantothenic acid possibly should be increased," he asserted. But what are the "desirable doses"?

It depends on whom you ask.

The No-Deficiency Diet

There is no Recommended Dietary Allowance for pantothenate. According to the scientists responsible for setting the RDA, however, "an intake of 4 to 7 milligrams a day would be adequate for adults," and "a higher intake may be needed during pregnancy and lactation."

According to Dr. Williams, a much higher intake would be beneficial for mothers-to-be. "I would be willing to give ten-to-one odds that providing prospective human mothers with 50 milligrams of this vitamin per day would substantially decrease the number and severity of reproductive failures,'' he wrote.

And while Dr. Szórády suggests a daily 15-milligram intake, he adds that "physical work, surgical intervention, injury, burns and grave infections, those of tbe gastrointestinal tract in particular, may double the pantothenic acid requirement of adults.''

So, how do you meet your daily requirement?

Your best bet is not to fool with Mother Nature. Follow Dr. Shroeder's advice and include plenty of whole, unprocessed foods in your diet. Whole grains like brown rice, oats and whole wheat are good sources of pantothenate. A bowl of oatmeal sprinkled with wheat germ or bran is a good source. Eggs, too, supply plenty of pantothenate.

If you ask for dark meat this Thanksgiving, you'll have even more to be thankful for. The dark meat of turkey (and chicken) is an excellent source of pantothenate. Organ meats are also rich in the vitamin—especially liver. B vitamin–packed brewer's yeast is another fine source of pantothenate.

These foods, along with a B-complex supplement with at least 10 milligrams of pantothenate, should supply you with more than enough of this vitamin. (Most B-complex supplements have more than 10 milligrams of pantothenate, some have up to 100 milligrams. It may be listed as pantothenic acid or calcium pantothenate on the label.)

So if the stress in your life is getting you down, it's time you upped your intake of the anti-stress vitamin, pantothenate.

CHAPTER
37

TAN WITHOUT BURNING WITH PABA

An argument could be made that the whole idea of working on a suntan is a little crazy. After all, there was a time when the world's BPs (that's "beautiful people" in affluent-ese) were into ivory and alabaster skin. Anyone with a tan was considered strictly working class, and who wanted to be one of those?

That twisted notion still influences us today, except that a tan no longer provokes the image of a stoop-shouldered peasant working in the fields. People associate tans with sailing, sunning and lounging at pool side. The only time BPs want to appear white is when they're decked out in their tennis togs. People with neither the time nor the money to loaf in the sun are the new working class. The only rays they're soaking up are emanating from their office desk lamps.

The problem with cultivating a tan is that people can overdo it. Getting a bad sunburn is no fun, and too much sun can lead to serious skin problems. We're certainly not suggesting that you devote all of your spare time to exploring caves. You should get out and enjoy the sun, but you also should be sensible about it. Before stepping outside, you might put on a sun screen that will absorb, reflect or scatter the ultraviolet light of the sun—reducing

222

the amount that reaches your skin. The best sun screens will contain one of the B-complex vitamins, para-aminobenzoic acid, or PABA.

People with light skin color and blue or green eyes generally are more inclined to burn. They can exceed their sunburn threshold tolerance in 10 to 20 minutes under a noontime summer sun. Other people, who rarely burn and readily tan, may not even become red after 45 minutes or more in the same setting.

Wrinkles, Aging and Cancer

Since people with fair skin and blue or green eyes are more susceptible to the sun, they also are more vulnerable to skin cancer. Ireland, for example, ranks 10th for women and 20th for men in the incidence of death from skin cancer among 42 countries. The high rate exists despite the fact that Ireland is in a latitude that receives less than half the burn-causing ultraviolet radiation of any of the other countries.

"The most important skin carcinogenic factor in man is sunlight exposure," says Allan L. Lorincz, M.D., professor and chief of dermatology at the University of Chicago. Too much sun also can produce other chronic skin damage like pigment alterations, premalignant lesions and premature wrinkling and aging. That's why you rarely see a fashion model who's keen on tanning rituals.

People who are, however, may think they can splash on anything and be protected from burning. "Suntan lotions are designed to be *not* so absolutely protective," says Dr. Lorincz. "They use weaker sun screens to let modest amounts of the sun through to stimulate new pigment formation in the skin."

PABA, the B vitamin, has stood up as one of the most potent sun screens on the market, he continues, and it has few complications in regard to its use. PABA's screening ability was discovered in the 1920s by Dr. Lorincz's predecessor and former colleague at th University of Chicago, Stephen Rothman, M.D.

PABA protects against the UVB wavelengths of the sun,'' Dr. Lorincz told us. UVB is the form of ultraviolet radiation which causes sunburn and other skin problems to flare. At the same time, PABA permits UVA rays, which are the less dangerous, tanning rays, to travel through to the skin.

The superiority of PABA as a sun screen has been documented in various laboratory tests. Harvard scientists found that, of 24 screening agents tested, a solution of 5 percent PABA in alcohol provided the best protection against ultraviolet radiation *(New England Journal of Medicine).*

At the University of Miami, investigators discovered that putting a 5 percent solution of PABA on hairless mice protected them from later exposure to ultraviolet light. Mice not treated with PABA developed severe skin lesions after they were exposed *(Journal of Investigative Dermatology).*

Which Form of PABA Is Best?

In the past few years, chemical derivatives (esters) of PABA have appeared on the market which outperform the original 5 percent PABA solution. Dr. Lorincz does not favor the esters because ''there is a theoretical reason to believe that the esters can cause a higher risk of allergic sensitization.

''With a 10 percent PABA solution in alcohol, you get up to two hours of midday sun protection,'' he says. ''You can still tan—you'll just tan more slowly.''

The ability of a sun screen to remain effective under the stress of prolonged exercise, sweating and swimming is called its *substantivity.* PABA sun screens in alcohol are considered to be quite substantive, says Dr. Lorincz. Still, when using a sun screen, people are advised to apply it both before they go out and several times during sun exposure, especially after swimming or perspiring.

PABA is not a carte blanche to sunbathe. It allows you to stay out a little longer, but if you overdo it, you'll burn.

CHAPTER

38

BIOTIN—THE LITTLE-KNOWN LIFESAVER

At first, she looked like a perfectly normal baby, so no one suspected a thing. But by three months of age, it was obvious that something was terribly wrong. She began to have seizures—about ten a day—and nothing seemed to help. By 14 months of age, all of her hair had fallen out—even her eyebrows and eyelashes. A red, scaly rash marred her body. Her eyes, once bright and shining, became swollen and painful from severe inflammation.

On top of that, she became increasingly irritable and sleepy. Her muscles grew steadily weaker until she could barely walk. Lab studies of her blood and urine revealed a high level of accumulating poisons, the kind found in severe metabolic disorders. And the levels of lactic acid in her blood rose to over twice that of the normal value, causing it to become dangerously acidic.

The doctors were understandably alarmed by the downward course the child was taking, especially since they didn't really know what was causing it or exactly how to correct it. But they did know that she would surely die if something wasn't done soon.

At that point, they began giving the little girl large doses of biotin, an essential B-complex nutrient.

"The clinical response to 10 milligrams of biotin per day was dramatic," says Jess Thoene, M.D., of the department of pediatrics, University of Michigan at Ann Arbor. "Within 12 hours the plasma [blood] lactic acid concentration had fallen to normal and her state of consciousness had improved. After 48 hours of biotin therapy, all of her blood chemistries had normalized. Over the next four months she reached all the developmental milestones that had been lost during the illness. Her hair, including eyebrows and eyelashes, began to regenerate, and her muscular coordination was regained. Biotin not only saved her life, it allows her to have a normal, healthy childhood without any of the signs of her former illness (*New England Journal of Medicine*, April 2, 1981).

But why biotin? How did the doctors single out this particular, little-known nutrient as the special one to cure this child's ailment?

Actually, it wasn't easy. It took a lot of detective work (and a little luck) to finally fit all the puzzle pieces together.

First, scientists learned that certain enzymes depend on biotin for normal functioning. Without those enzymes, the body can't utilize carbohydrates, proteins and fats. When that happens, specific abnormal metabolites (poisons) build up in the body, creating a whole host of devastating symptoms.

When modern equipment made it possible to identify those abnormal metabolites, it wasn't long before doctors were able to pinpoint exactly which enzyme systems were malfunctioning.

That information, combined with the fact that this patient had symptoms strikingly similar to another child whose enzyme deficiencies were corrected with biotin, decided the course of action here, says Dr. Thoene.

"These defects in the metabolism of biotin may be much more common that we once thought," adds Herman Baker, Ph.D., another doctor actively involved with the case.

"Not long ago, we had no way to test for biotin deficiency, so many cases probably went undetected. Now we have a method which can isolate as little as one part in a trillion of the nutrient,"

Dr. Baker, a professor of preventive medicine at the New Jersey Medical School in Newark, told us. "At present, we are the only ones in the country who have this procedure for detecting low levels of biotin with such extreme accuracy. Ever since this case study became publicized, we've been deluged with requests for biotin levels by doctors whose patients have similar symptoms."

And no wonder. It's rare to be able to cure a potentially fatal disorder with a remedy that, so far, has shown no side effects and is completely safe.

That's how Morton J. Cowan, M.D., an immunologist from the department of pediatrics at the University of California at San Francisco feels about biotin, too. He's seen for himself how biotin works in youngsters with this same genetic defect.

"The children I've seen," says Dr. Cowan, "had defects in their immune systems along with all the other symptoms. In fact, two of the kids died from overwhelming infection in combination with progressive central nervous system deterioration before we knew that biotin could reverse the disorder" (*Lancet*, July 21, 1979).

"We still don't know for sure what's actually happening with these kids," Dr. Cowan told us. "It may be that their bodies can't metabolize biotin normally. But the problem may also be one of absorption. These kids have had a normal exposure to biotin in their diet, yet, in some of the children, the blood and urine levels are low. The body may just not be able to transport the biotin across the cellular membranes. We don't know why this is so. But we do know that flooding the system with 10 to 40 milligrams a day of biotin somehow pushes it across the barrier and into the bloodstream and cells, where it's needed for the metabolism of fats, carbohydrates and proteins.

"With our patient, that's what it took for complete recovery. What's more, she was relieved of the numerous infections that continuously plagued her.

"From what we've seen, immune deficiencies seem to go along with biotin deficiencies whether the problem is genetic [like the cases mentioned so far] or acquired," Dr. Cowan told us.

Less Biotin, Fewer Antibodies

That seems to support the conclusions made by Mahendra Kumar, Ph.D., and A. E. Axelrod, Ph.D., of the biochemistry department at the University of Pittsburgh school of medicine in Pennsylvania.

They found that rats that were made deficient in biotin showed a marked decrease in the number of cells which produce antibodies (the protein which fights off infection).

The antibody-forming cells were reduced by 96 percent in the biotin-deficient rats, report Drs. Kumar and Axelrod, but were partially restored to normal when biotin was administered to the animals (*Proceedings of the Society for Experimental Biology and Medicine*).

Fewer Eggs, Less Biotin

Most researchers and nutritionists have long believed that it is next to impossible to acquire a biotin deficiency. That's because such small amounts are required (about 100 to 300 *micrograms* per day, a mere fraction of what the sick babies were receiving).

And what you don't pick up from the good food sources that you eat (like liver, eggs, peanuts and dried beans), say the scientists, the friendly bacteria that live in your large intestine will manufacture for you.

Between those two sources, how can anyone become deficient?

But apparently it's not that simple. "First of all," says Mary Marshall, research nutritionist with the U.S. Department of Agriculture's human nutrition center, "many people have cut their intake of eggs and liver, the best sources of biotin, because of their high cholesterol content.

"I also think it's a myth that the bacteria in your gut can supply you with the biotin you're not getting in your diet. It's true that they make it, but they do it in the lower part of the large intestine, and absorption does not take place at that location.

"Besides," Mrs. Marshall told us, "we don't even know if we have the same bacteria now as we did long ago, because of all the antibiotics we've consumed over the years."

In fact, every time you take an antibiotic or sulfa drug, you may be killing off the biotin-manufacturing bacteria in your gut. So even if you *could* absorb the biotin they're making, they may not be there to make it.

Elderly People Need More

But even if you haven't taken an antibiotic in years, you still could be low in biotin, that is, if you're physically active or elderly.

A study done in Basel, Switzerland, measured the blood levels of biotin in various populations. The results showed that the elderly and athletes had significantly lower levels than the control group *(International Journal of Vitamin and Nutrition Research)*.

"The elderly may have a problem with absorption," says Mrs. Marshall. "They do with many other nutrients, so it's possible that biotin is among them. We really don't know for sure."

"As for the athletes," speculates Dr. Baker, "exercising causes a buildup of lactic acid in the muscles. Biotin is part of the enzyme system which is needed to break it down again. The more lactic acid that accumulates, the more biotin is needed.

"We will be conducting a study soon on the effect of exercise on biotin levels in humans, so we should have some definite answers."

Meanwhile, increased need is not just limited to the elderly, athletes and people taking antibiotics.

Hospital patients on total intravenous feeding should be aware that biotin deficiency can result. That's what happened recently to one little girl. Unlike the other sick babies, this patient did not have a genetic defect in biotin metabolism. (It was only after three months on intravenous feedings that the familiar biotin deficiency symptoms developed.)

Ten milligrams of biotin per day did the trick for her, too, and after seven weeks of therapy, her dose was reduced to only 100 micrograms daily (*New England Journal of Medicine*, April 2, 1981).

Children recovering from burns and scalds may need a biotin boost, too.

A study of nine children suffering from those injuries was conducted at the Institute of Child Health in London. Plasma biotin levels were significantly below the control values in all the children. "The evidence suggests," write the researchers, "that low plasma biotin levels found in children with burns and scalds are due to the injury either through loss of the vitamin or through increased requirements for tissue repair" (*Journal of Clinical Pathology*).

Sudden Infant Death Syndrome

There's also some impressive evidence that low biotin levels may be involved in cases of sudden infant death syndrome (SIDS), a tragic phenomenon in which babies are found dead in their cribs for no apparent reason. Researchers in Australia and Great Britain say that SIDS closely resembles a disorder in which marginally biotin-deficient chickens die when subjected to even mild stress. None of the classic signs of biotin deficiency are present in the chickens, but there are low levels of biotin in their livers, and supplementation with biotin eliminates the problem.

The researchers speculated that the same thing may be happening in human infants, as well. To test their theory, they examined the livers of infants who had died of various causes and found that those with SIDS had significantly lower levels of biotin, just like the chickens. All of the SIDS victims but one had suffered some mild disease at their deaths, but nothing severe enough to explain why they died.

"We do not suggest," say the researchers, "that SIDS results from biotin deficiency alone, but . . . we postulate that biotin insufficiency may leave the infant in a condition in which SIDS can be triggered by mild stress, for example, infection, a missed meal, excessive heat or cold or a changed environment" (*Nature*, May 15, 1980).

It's been reported that SIDS is more common among bottle-fed babies than breast-fed ones. That may be because a considerable loss of biotin occurs during the manufacture of certain infant formulas. It's been recommended that infant formulas be supplemented with biotin as a precaution against SIDS.

It seems that babies get the brunt of the biotin-deficiency problems. Fortunately, they also reap the benefits of ample supplementation.

For adults, there isn't enough information available yet to determine exactly how much biotin is really needed—that is, unless you're talking about blood lipids (fats). Mary Marshall has conducted a few experiments which show that supplementation with 0.9 milligrams biotin per day can reduce blood lipids. "We tested rats and humans with high lipid levels," Mrs. Marshall told us, "and we found that biotin supplementation caused an initial rise in lipids followed by a drop to below prestudy levels (*Artery*, March, 1980).

"So much work still needs to be done," says Mrs. Marshall, "because right now we have more questions than answers. We think there may be a connection between biotin and diabetes, for example."

Dr. Baker agrees. "Biotin seems to affect glucose (blood sugar) metabolism. There's some evidence of that, and we plan to check out that possibility," he told us.

The role of biotin in immunity is another area ready to be explored. "We have no scientific evidence right now that taking more biotin will help normal people fight off viruses," says Dr. Cowan. "But it did relieve the kid with the genetic biotin deficiency of their multiple infections."

A few years ago, nobody paid any attention to biotin. Now, it looks like biotin may not stay the unknown B vitamin for long. The more we learn about it, the more evident it becomes that it is vital to our total well-being.

39

CHOLINE FOR A SHARPER MEMORY

How good is your memory?

Quickly, now, can you recall what you ate for dinner the night before last? Do you remember the title of that Barbra Streisand movie you saw two years ago? What if you bumped into an old school friend you hadn't seen for many years? Would you remember the name—or even the face?

Clearly, if a lifetime is built of pleasant memories—growing families, graduations, weddings, wonderful vacations—then the quality of your memory becomes the key to a good and satisfying life.

That's not meant to suggest that your brain should be like some vast computer, endlessly spinning a printout of every sight, sound, smell and textbook fact that ever nestled—however briefly—in your consciousness. Many things are meant to be forgotten. But being able to recall *important* events, experiences and information vividly and in fine detail is not too much to ask.

And while nature hasn't skimped in giving us the gray matter to get the memory job done, that hasn't stopped scientists from searching for some agent that would boost our recall capacity even more. They haven't yet found the magic potion or elixir, but investigators at the National Institute of Mental Health (NIMH) have found something that gives forms of recollection a welcome nudge—especially in people whose memories are a bit below par to begin with.

That substance is choline, an essential dietary component found in a wide range of meat and vegetable foods. Choline is thought of as a vitamin by some nutritionists (it's included in many of the more complete B vitamin supplements). What's more, our bodies can manufacture additional choline, provided we eat a healthful diet that supplies the raw materials.

"Our studies show that choline has a weak to moderate memory enhancement effect," research psychiatrist N. Sitaram, M.D., told us. "It's not a robust effect, but it can be measured."

Dr. Sitaram, who is now director of affective disorders at Lafayette Clinic in Detroit, was interested in testing choline because it is a precursor, or forerunner, of acetylcholine, a brain compound that is essential for the smooth flow of nerve impulses. Other studies have shown that extra choline in the diet increases levels of acetylcholine in the brain. Dr. Sitaram and his colleagues, Herbert Weingartner, Ph.D., of the laboratory of clinical psychology, NIMH, and Christian Gillin, M.D., currently at the University of California at San Diego, wanted to find out if this would aid memory.

On two separate days, they gave ten healthy volunteers, ranging in age from 21 to 29, either a supplement of 10 grams of choline chloride or an identical-appearing but worthless substitute. Then after an hour and a half, the people were given two kinds of memory tests.

In the first, a serial learning test, subjects had to memorize *in proper order* a sequence of ten unrelated words. The list was read to each person and repeated as often as necessary until perfect recall was achieved and could be repeated twice in a row.

"Choline significantly enhanced serial recall of unrelated words as measured by the number of trials required," the researchers reported. "Furthermore, the enhancement was more pronounced in 'slower' subjects . . . than in subjects who performed well" *(Life Sciences)*.

In other words, the people most in need of help had their memories prodded the most when they took choline. One individual who normally needed six trial readings to master a ten-word list cut that to four after taking choline. Another dropped from seven to five attempts with the choline supplement.

In the second test, the volunteers were read lists of 12 common words. Half the words were highly imageable, concrete words like *table* and *chair,* which can be easily visualized. The rest were low imagery words like *truth* and *late,* which represent abstract, hard-to-visualize concepts and are more difficult to memorize.

In these trials, subjects didn't have to learn the lists in any particular order, but the words were read to them again and again until all 12 words could be successfully recalled twice in succession.

The results, as the authors describe them, were "extremely interesting." People didn't fare any better overall when they took choline, but when the test was divided into high-imagery and low-imagery words, they registered much better scores in the latter, more difficult category while taking the supplement. In other words, choline seemed to selectively enhance memory to meet the challenge of the tougher learning tasks.

Learning Time Cut in Half

One person who normally required ten trials to master a list of difficult words reduced that to five (a 50 percent improvement!) after taking choline.

And unlike certain drugs which also raise acetylcholine levels in the brain, the authors point out, choline is a natural food component which is usually safe even in large amounts. The doses of choline in these tests were at least ten times as great as the 900 milligrams or less supplied by a typical diet. (These amounts, however, should be taken only under a doctor's supervision.)

As promising as Dr. Sitaram's results were, however, he was quick to point out to us that many questions still remain. For example, these tests measured memory 90 minutes after a single dose of choline. We still don't know how long the effects last or whether they would continue over several weeks or months if extra choline were consumed daily.

And the trials involved only younger, healthy volunteers with a normal range of remembering ability. The real challenge, according to Dr. Sitaram and the other NIMH researchers, will be to determine if choline can help elderly people with serious memory impairments brought on by the brain deterioration of senility.

CHAPTER

40

VITAMIN B$_{15}$— MIRACLE OR HOAX?

The story of this "vitamin that isn't" is a long, complicated and checkered tale of promotional *chutzpah* and scientific skepticism, including among its cast of characters a beleaguered father-and-son research team, chemists from the Soviet Union, and zealous representatives from the U.S. Food and Drug Administration (FDA)—all at odds. It hasn't exactly got the pace and suspense of *Three Days of the Condor;* instead, if most of the evidence is correct, it's more like four decades of the turkey. Here's the condensed version.

Credit for discovering "vitamin B$_{15}$" (we put it in quotes because, by definition, it's not a vitamin—that is, its absence in the body isn't linked to any deficiency disease, the way vitamin C is to scurvy) goes to the Ernest Krebses, father and son, who are also the boys who came up with laetrile and called it vitamin B$_{17}$. Krebs senior and junior christened their crystalline concoction pangamic acid because it was found in all *(pan)* seeds *(gamete)*. Over the years, it has also attracted the labels calcium pangamate, "the famous Russian formula," and a host of brand names that made sure to use the number 15 in them.

236

During these same years, a slew of alleged benefits were attributed to pangamic acid; it was said to positively affect heart disease, diabetes, schizophrenia, alcoholism, asthma, nerve and joint infections, eczema and you name it. *Panacea,* not pangamic, is what the acid should have been called. The Russians, especially, touted the substance and made great claims for its ability to lower the body's oxygen needs, thus helping athletes by transporting oxygen more efficiently to their muscles. Coaches worldwide dropped their whistles and ran for B$_{15}$.

The only problem was, there were problems:

1. The Russian studies were pretty sloppy, without proper controls, loaded with unsubstantiated data and looking about as water tight as a colander.
2. There is no clear chemical identity for pangamic acid, so companies producing it can pretty much put into it whatever they want. The FDA says that it is "not an indentifiable substance."
3. In 30 years at the Bunsen burner, the Krebses were able to isolate pangamic acid from seeds only once. But since naturally occurring substances can't be patented anyway, they redoubled their efforts to find a synthetic counterpart. Both they and the Russians succeeded in doing so. Most companies producing the stuff say they follow the Russian-style directions and call the results calcium pangamate, which is alleged to contain DMG, the essential extract that is supposed to be responsible for all the good deeds. But according to the FDA, it has never analyzed a batch of pangamic acid that contained what the Krebses said they'd been able to isolate from seeds. Furthermore, DMG has been shown in some labora-

tory experiments to be a potential carcinogen, and so has DIPA-DCA, a major component of the second-largest-selling form of calcium pangamate

4. The FDA says DMG is not a natural food substance, but a food additive, and that, until it goes through the usual tests and safety checks, it must be removed from the shelves.

Court cases and shipment seizures have been going on for years, with the FDA ahead in suits won and the companies victorious in the piling up of sales dollars. For even though pangamic acid, by federal regulation, ought to be off the shelves of pharmacies and health foods stores, you can still find it there, either boldly obvious or in various disguises, because there's money to be made from it and the FDA can't be everywhere at once.

And our view? Well, so far, nothing that we've seen or heard about B_{15} has made us feel like dropping *our* whistles and running for it.

CHAPTER

41

BRIMMING WITH HEALTH (AND VITAMIN C!)

What would happen to you if your body tissues were drenched with vitamin C, saturated like the soil after a downpour? And what if this soaking lasted for more than just a few hours, but for days and days, for the rest of your life? What would be the consequences?

The fate that would befall you would likely be better health. That's the opinion of a growing number of researchers looking into the vitamin C requirements of your body. The word is that the right daily intake of C is the one that ensures this maximum permeation of your tissues in what's called a steady state.

It's a condition existing everywhere in the animal world, and that fact set a lot of people thinking about the implications for man. Unlike humans, most animals can synthesize (manufacture) vitamin C internally. Since these C makers have high saturation levels of the vitamin, scientists reasoned, the steady state must be ideal for their health. So the same saturation condition might be optimal for humans, who have to make sure their C intake keeps their tissues loaded.

Emil Ginter, Ph.D., a distinguished vitamin C researcher from Czechoslovakia, was among the first to test these assumptions. Initially, he set out to discover what a maximum saturation would do for a creature that shared man's inability to synthesize vitamin C—the guinea pig. In test after test, he found that guinea pigs on close-to-maximum saturation levels of C fared better than guinea pigs with lower levels. The animals with higher vitamin C levels handled cholesterol better and developed fewer gallstones when placed on a gallstone-producing diet. The saturation animals were not only better off than those guinea pigs on deficiency intakes of C, but they were even healthier than those getting many times the intake needed to prevent scurvy—the vitamin C–deficiency disease (*Nutrition and Health*, vol. 1, no. 2, 1982).

Evidence is accumulating that in humans, too, a state of vitamin C saturation is optimal for health, says Dr. Ginter. Here and abroad, studies have demonstrated that a full store of C can help battle harmful levels of cholesterol and triglycerides, detoxify potentially dangerous histamines (substances produced in the body), neutralize unwholesome chemicals in your diet and more.

Beyond Your RDA

But the question is what daily intake of vitamin C will keep your cache—your body pool—brimming?

Whatever the quantity is, many researchers and doctors are convinced that it has little to do with the Recommended Dietary Allowance (RDA) of 60 milligrams a day. "Sixty milligrams is enough, all right—if you want merely to stay just above scurvy level," says W. M. Ringsdorf, Jr., D.M.D., of the University of Alabama in Birmingham. "But if you want to live a life of reduced infection, if you want to promote healing and sharpen your immune system, if you want optimum triglyceride levels in your blood, you'll want a daily intake of C far above the RDA."

"It is certain," notes Dr. Ginter, "that the officially recommended doses are unable to ensure a maximum body pool, for they do not lead to maximum levels of ascorbate [vitamin C]

. . . in the blood, and much less in tissues." And that's where some major studies come in. They can help you figure out just how far above the RDA you should go.

In one of these experiments, researchers used vitamin C "tagged" with harmless levels of radioactivity to trace vitamin C in the body. Anders Kallner, M.D., Ph.D., of the Huddinge University Hospital in Sweden, and his colleagues chose 14 healthy, nonsmoking males, put them on daily C intakes of 30 to 180 milligrams, and had them drink water containing the tagged vitamin C. After tracking the C in blood plasma and urine, the research team was able to gauge the men's maximum *body pool* and turnover (the amount of vitamin C metabolized or used).

The average stockpile of C was assessed at 1,500 milligrams, with a daily turnover of 60 milligrams. The study concluded that, to maintain such a pool and to compensate for turnover and incomplete absorption of C, healthy, nonsmoking males should ingest about 100 milligrams a day (*American Journal of Clinical Nutrition*, March, 1979).

But that is not the last word on your C requirements. A more recent study recommends an even higher daily intake for men—and a different one for women.

For five years, Philip J. Garry, Ph.D., and his fellow researchers monitored the vitamin C levels of 270 healthy elderly men and women in the Albuquerque area. They checked the subjects' diets, their intakes of vitamin C supplements and the amounts of C in their blood. The picture that emerged was of a health-conscious group of seniors with apparently normal abilities to absorb and store vitamin C. Dr. Garry and his colleagues concluded that, for men to have a full C concentration in their blood (maintaining a body pool of 1,500 milligrams), they need to ingest 150 milligrams of C per day. And for women to get the same concentration, they need to take 75 milligrams a day. Intakes at lower levels simply can't keep our body pools on the "full" mark (*American Journal of Clinical Nutrition*, August, 1982).

Indeed, even dietary intakes *three times* the RDA aren't quite up to snuff, according to Dr. Ginter. He cites some provocative evidence suggesting that your maximum body pool of C is an even mightier flood than some researchers think. "This value [of 1,500 milligrams] appears unduly low," he says. "It is certainly much lower than data on animals capable of synthesizing ascorbate [vitamin C]. In addition, there are large organs in the human body, such as, for instance, the liver, brain and gastrointestinal tract, in which maximum ascorbate concentrations determined by direct analysis are at least 10 times higher."

If you examine the C content of human tissues, explains Dr. Ginter, you discover that the maximum pool is actually about 5,000 milligrams (approximately 32 milligrams of C per pound of body weight). And that's a pool value similar to those found recently in monkeys.

"Vitamin C doses necessary for maintaining such a high body pool in humans have not as yet been experimentally determined," Dr. Ginter points out, "but they may be calculated approximately from available data." Since we know the turnover and absorption rate of C, he says, it's a simple matter to compute the intake that we need to keep our reservoirs topped off at 5,000 milligrams: about 200 milligrams a day.

Vitamin C to the Rescue

Let's say you're flat on your back in the hospital, recovering from abdominal surgery. Or money problems are weighing on your mind. Or you're walking down a city street choking on smog. How much vitamin C does your body need now?

More than you might think. We now know that your countermeasure for these and other traumas should be *extra* vitamin C—above and beyond your saturation intake. When your body is under the gun, it demands additional C to heal itself or fight off enemies within.

"Stress is just one factor that steps up your vitamin C requirements," says Robert Haskell, M.D., of San Francisco. "If anything helps you battle the effects of stress, it's extra vitamin C."

"It appears that all forms of pollution increase the requirements of vitamin C in humans and experimental animals," notes Dr. Ginter. "It has been repeatedly shown that various pesticides, industrial toxins, certain drugs, particularly antipregnancy pills, and smoking decrease blood vitamin C levels."

And if you have a wound that needs healing, you can observe the most dramatic example of extra C power firsthand. For an "excess" of the vitamin not only puts wounds on the mend, but hurries the healing along at record speeds.

That fact was confirmed by Dr. Ringsdorf and an associate when they reviewed a series of clinical studies testing C's healing ability. The subjects were people without C deficiencies who had a variety of wounds—bed sores, leg ulcers, gum damage, even wounds from surgery. When these patients went on daily C intakes of 500 to 3,000 milligrams, fast-paced healing set in. Recovery time from both surgery and injury dropped by as much as 75 percent (*Oral Surgery/Oral Medicine*, March, 1982).

And no wonder. Vitamin C, it seems, is a crucial ingredient in all human wound healing, fast or slow. "This nutrient is unique among vitamins," reports Dr. Ringsdorf, "because it regulates the formation and maintenance of intercellular cement and collagen [a supportive protein that helps bind up wounds]. Thus, the structural integrity of every tissue and organ is dependent on this vitamin."

And you're never more dependent than when you're hit by more than one C-demanding trauma—when you're under stress and you light up a smoke to calm your nerves, for example, or when you're nursing multiple wounds. All the factors that boost your vitamin C needs, says Dr. Ginter, are probably cumulative. And that means your body's C requirements may add up like bills—payable upon demand. "Personally, I believe that in such situations," he says, "the optimum dose is several hundreds of milligrams per day."

That sounds like small payment for some bills your body can't afford to ignore.

CHAPTER

42

VITAMIN C: CHANGING YOUR BODY FOR THE BETTER

"Vitamin C is unique among vitamins because it is the only one that seems to play a role in every bodily function, as it holds the cells together," observes Reginald Passmore, M.D., professor of physiology at Edinburgh University in Scotland. "When it is deficient, furthermore, it wreaks more havoc in more places in the body . . . than any other nutrient" (*Nutrition Today*).

Adds Irwin Stone, one of the early pioneers of vitamin C research: "Ascorbic acid (vitamin C) is involved in so many vital biochemical processes and is so important in daily living that, after forty years of research, we still have no clear idea of all the ways in which it works" (*The Healing Factor,* Grosset and Dunlap, 1972).

It's such a versatile performer, in fact, that vitamin C has been called "an oil for the machinery of life." Yet, your body can't manufacture it or store more than a few grams, so keeping your cells saturated with a rich, daily supply of C is crucial. Just *how* important has been demonstrated in studies showing what happens when you *don't:* Deficiencies interfere with everything from the production of collagen, the protein "cement" that holds your cells together and helps in the healing of wounds, to your ability to digest food and fight the effects of stress.

Researchers at Cornell University have even found that deficiencies of the vitamin impair the body's ability to metabolize drugs, which could have serious implications for the elderly, in particular.

"In guinea pigs, we've found that deficiencies of vitamin C impair the liver's ability to detoxify drugs, which results in more of the drug affecting the body—causing, in effect, an overdose," one researcher told us.

But one of the most important gears the "oil of life" greases is the body's immune system—your defense against infectious disease. In one study at South Africa's University of Pretoria, vitamin C was found to stimulate the immune system.

When a germ, virus or any other microscopic invader penetrates the body, a healthy immune system, like a football team, musters a front line of defenders and hustles them off to the site of the invasion. One unit of this defending team is made up of specialized white blood cells called neutrophils, which simply eat up the enemy—rather like the body's very own mean Joe Greenes. In both human subjects and human cells in test tubes, the South African scientists found that vitamin C increased the mobility of these neutrophils, speeding up their rush to the line of scrimmage. Vitamin C also helped stimulate the immune response by stepping up the body's production of lymphocytes, another kind of white blood cell (*American Journal of Clinical Nutrition,* September, 1981).

How do neutrophils know where the attackers have threatened the body and how to get to the scene of the invasion? They do it by following the "scent" of a chemical distress signal the body produces when it becomes inflamed by injury. The neutrophils' amazing pursuit through the body's byways, hard on the enemy's trail like angry linemen, is called *chemotaxis*—and it doesn't always work. When neutrophils are exposed to a chemotactic signal once, they become deactivated—that is, they fail to respond to a subsequent signal.

Yet, Italian researchers have found that vitamin C "completely prevented the loss of true chemotactic responsiveness by cells." In other words, human neutrophils, exposed to chemical distress signal, responded right on cue to a second signal—*if* they were saturated with vitamin C. Otherwise, they didn't respond at all (*British Journal of Experimental Pathology,* vol. 61, no. 5, 1980).

For a Healthy Pregnancy

Vitamin C may also be needed to ensure a healthy pregnancy, other research suggests. A study conducted at the Methodist Hospital in Brooklyn, New York, by Dr. C. Alan B. Clemetson discovered that, when the levels of vitamin C in the blood fall below a certain level, blood levels of histamine rise significantly. Evidence going back as far as 1926 indicates that histamine might be responsible for a potentially fatal complication of pregnancy called abruptio placentae, in which the placenta separates from the womb prematurely.

Studies of women with that condition have found that they usually have abnormally low levels of vitamin C in their blood. And Dr. Clemetson found that histamine begins to build up in the blood long before vitamin C levels fall to the point where scurvy, the classic C-deficiency disease, begins to develop. The blood levels of C are low, but by no means *deficient* as the term is commonly defined (*Journal of Nutrition,* April, 1980).

So Dr. Clemetson believes that it might be a good idea for pregnant women to supplement their diets with vitamin C. He does not have the final, unshakable proof that C prevents abruptio placentae, any more than we have *unshakable* proof that C prevents the other problems we've been discussing. But Dr. Clemetson thinks taking C might be a good idea all the same.

C Saves Body Tissue

A true believer in vitamin C is former *Saturday Review* editor Norman Cousins. Upon returning from a stressful trip to Russia in 1964, Cousins felt like a grimy passport with every page stamped "pain." He had difficulty moving his neck, arms,

legs and fingers. He was diagnosed as having ankylosing spon-
dylitis, a rare collagen disease affecting the joints of the spine.
But he fought his way back to health with up to 25 grams daily
of vitamin C and mirth sessions of Marx Brothers movies and
"Candid Camera" classics.

Cousins' diagnosis may have been rare, but collagen is not.
It is everywhere in the body, comprising fully 30 percent of all
body protein.

If vitamin C is lacking, the result will be a defective collagen
molecule that means, ultimately, weak tissue. Scurvy (gross vitamin C deficiency) is a hideous culmination of tissue collapse,
wherein old scars break down, new wounds won't heal, blood
vessels hemorrhage and the gums can't even hold their teeth
anymore.

Science is just beginning to scratch the surface of how collagen does its job. An editorial in the British medical journal
Lancet opened: "Long regarded as inert, uninteresting, and purely
mechanical in function, collagen is attracting the close attention
of physicians and biochemists. This reversal in outlook is partly
due to the realization that collagen is involved in many diseases,
from fatal heart and lung diseases to back pain and minor skin
disorders."

The editorial goes on to say: "At present we recognize disorders primarily when mechanical malfunction occurs, but collagen may be involved in other diseases at a more subtle level."

Needs for C May Be Special

How much vitamin C is necessary to maintain healthy collagen production? The amount can vary widely, as revealed in
the case of a young boy studied by two southeastern doctors,
reported in the *Journal of Pediatrics*.

The boy, age eight when first diagnosed, had absurdly
stretchable skin. His muscles were weak; his skin was brimming
with hemorrhages and scars; he was mildly myopic and the diameter of his cornea was unusually small. At first he was diag-

nosed for vitamin C deficiency, but blood and urine tests showed that he was not suffering from any deficiency in the narrow clinical sense that doctors are trained to look for.

What he suffered from was a *vitamin dependency*. His doctor, Louis J. Elsas II, M.D., of the division of medical genetics at Emory University's school of medicine, discovered the boy to be in need of much more vitamin C than most people need for collagen formation because of an inherited disorder that hampered the process.

After 20 months of therapy (4 grams daily of vitamin C taken orally), the boy's wound healing and muscle strength improved and corneal diameter actually grew—something that's not supposed to happen after the age of four.

The case is unique, Dr. Elsas explains, because "this is the first inherited metabolic disorder in which ascorbic acid [vitamin C] has been clearly demonstrated as a requirement in pharmacologic [hefty] doses." Somehow, the genetically impaired protein that's causing the faulty collagen formation works better with a lot more help from vitamin C than is usually necessary.

The boy's collagen disorder is rare, but increased metabolic requirements for vitamin C may not be so unusual. "Conceivably, a vast number of individuals could have a different vitamin requirement," a spokesman for the research project said. "Their genes are different; you can almost state that categorically." And since people's genes are different, "you could expect large variations" among individuals in the shape and effectiveness of the proteins we make to maintain our life processes.

Dr. Elsas' research may be at least as important for the new questions it raises as for the old questions it answers. The spokesman says an increased vitamin requirement might be discovered in some patients with "dislocated limbs, myopia . . . all sorts of clinical manifestations" that could be associated with collagen disorders.

Corneal diameters, rare collagen defects: Is this getting too esoteric?

Then consider bedsores, a common problem among the bedridden.

Faster Healing

At the Human Tissue Reconstruction Institute at Bethany Methodist Hospital in Chicago, Anthony N. Silvetti, M.D., was confronted by about 30 patients with stubborn bedsores, skin ulcers due to varicose veins or diabetes, and burns due to heat or caustic chemicals. These sores had festered for between two months and several *years* with no response to conventional treatments.

Vitamin C helped heal the sores dramatically. Dr. Silvetti prepared a solution of simple and complex sugars along with essential amino acids and vitamin C. He cleared dead tissue from the sores, washed them with a salt solution, then applied his therapeutic poultice to the wound every day, covering it with a sterile nonadhesive dressing.

"Within the first 24 to 73 hours of beginning the nutrient treatment," Dr. Silvetti and his co-workers reported, "the wounds became cleaner. The foul smell disappeared and the wounds exuded less pus. The infected tissue rapidly transformed into healthy growing tissue full of new blood vessels. . . . Small to medium-sized wounds eventually healed completely with little scarring. Larger wounds accepted early, successful skin grafts" (*Federation of American Societies for Experimental Biology*, April 15, 1981, abstract no. 3929).

The sores hadn't healed before, Dr. Silvetti explained, because oxygen and nutrients required for new tissue formation weren't circulating to the site of infection. So he applied those nutrients—vitamin C, amino acids and sugars—directly to the damaged skin.

The treatment even boosted patient morale, Dr. Silvetti noted, because healing began so quickly. There was "daily visible improvement" in the sores.

At the University of Genoa medical school in Italy, researchers treated patients who were unable to resist bacteria infections normally. Their white blood cells couldn't "chase" or kill bacteria, and as a result, they suffered chronically from abscesses and boils. One patient had had 43 abscesses in two years. None had gone infection free for as long as a year.

Again, vitamin C proved effective without causing side effects. Three of the patients took 1 to 2 grams of C a day and improved within a few weeks. After a year, their skin was still clear. It was the longest stretch of skin health they had ever enjoyed.

"The laboratory and clinical results obtained with ascorbic acid in our patients and the safeness of this drug strongly suggest its use for the prevention and treatment of recurrent infections in patients with defective chemotaxis [the ability of white blood cells to chase germs] and/or bacterial killing" (*British Journal of Dermatology*, January, 1980).

But besides these particular infections, vitamin C has also shown that it can hit the target on a lot of other distressing conditions.

Malaria has shown an interesting response to vitamin C.

In malaria, a parasite lives in human red blood cells. Once infected by a mosquito bite, a person carries the parasite permanently, suffering from intermittent attacks of chills and fever. Drug-resistant strains of the parasite breed constantly.

At the University of Lowell in Massachusetts, Nicholas J. Rencricca, Ph.D., was testing the effects of high-pressure oxygen on the red blood cells of malarial mice. He supplemented the mice with vitamin C on the hunch that the vitamin would protect their red blood cells from the "rusting" effect of too much oxygen.

Unexpectedly, the vitamin C helped destroy the blood cells that carried the malaria parasite but didn't harm the healthy unparasitized blood cells, and the mice lived longer than expected. "I believe in it," Dr. Rencricca told us about vitamin C. "Even in large doses. I wasn't out to prove or disprove anything in my experiment. There's definitely something to it."

A nine-year study of Japanese hospital patients who had received blood transfusions revealed that 2 grams of C given daily sharply reduced the number and severity of serum hepatitis cases. A particularly troublesome viral disease, hepatitis often strikes surgical patients who have had blood transfusions. By the seventh year of the study, hospital administrators felt so strongly about the preventative properties of the nutrient that "the decision was made, for ethical reasons, to give vitamin C in large amounts to essentially every patient.

"During the period 1967 to 1973," the report continues, "there were 150 patients who were given blood transfusions and who received little or no vitamin C (less than two grams per day). Of these patients, 11 developed hepatitis (7 percent) . . . . Among 1,100 similarly transfused patients who received two grams or more of vitamin C per day, there were no established cases of hepatitis and only a few questionable cases" (*Journal of the International Academy of Preventive Medicine*).

Rheumatoid arthritis is another baffler that often cripples older people. A Canadian research team took normal and arthritic cells from human joints and cultured them with aspirin, vitamin C, vitamin E and combinations of the three. Aspirin was found slightly effective in inhibiting growth of arthritic cells and reducing their population, but "high and low concentrations of vitamin C had little effect on normal cells, and a low concentration had little effect on [arthritic] cells. *However, a high concentration eradicated these [arthritic] cells*" (emphasis ours) (*Experientia*, vol. 35, no. 2, 1979).

The researchers concluded that an aspirin–vitamin C combination might be the best way to reduce the growth of arthritic cells.

Divided Doses Best

Since vitamin C does so many helpful things, what's the best way to make sure you're getting enough? A diet rich in fresh fruits, vegetables and greens should provide plenty, most researchers say. Yet, many things are known to increase the body's demand for C, notably stress and smoking. In fact, in one Swiss study, it was suggested that the minimum daily requirement for vitamin C be increased from 70 to 100 milligrams for nonsmoking adults and to 140 milligrams for smokers.

Alcohol also appears to interfere with vitamin C absorption. In a study at Deakin University in Victoria, Australia, five healthy volunteers agreed to eat a very odd breakfast: a buttered bun, coffee, 2 grams of vitamin C and 35 grams of ethanol, or ethyl alcohol (roughly equivalent to two martinis or three light beers). Later, they ate a boozeless breakfast for purposes of comparison. Result? "Plasma ascorbic acid concentrations were significantly lower for at least 24 hours" after their alcoholic meal (*American Journal of Clinical Nutrition,* November, 1981).

If you take vitamin C supplements as a sort of nutritional "insurance policy," what's the best time to do so? A trio of researchers from the University of Toronto faculty of pharmacy and the University of Arizona college of pharmacy put that question to the test.

To ensure accurate measurements, the scientists first saturated the tissues of four subjects by giving them a gram of vitamin C a day for two weeks. Then they examined the extent of vitamin C absorption by measuring the amount of C they excreted in urine after taking a gram of C in three different ways: as a single dose in solution, divided into eight equal parts and taken at 15-minute intervals, or a single dose right after eating a meal high in fat.

Dividing the doses, the researchers found, increased vitamin C absorption by 72 percent over taking it in a single dose. Taking it after a meal increased absorption by 69 percent. "From a practical point of view," they concluded, "AA [ascorbic acid, i.e., vitamin C] absorption may be improved by either dividing a daily dose into several smaller doses taken during the day or by ingesting the vitamin after a meal" (*Life Sciences,* vol. 28, no. 22, 1981).

If smaller doses divided through the day are better than a single, larger dose, what about timed-release vitamins, which are supposed to do the dividing for you? The same trio of researchers recently studied that question, too.

Four volunteers were given a gram of vitamin C in several different forms: a powder dissolved in water, a tablet, a chewable tablet and a timed-release capsule.

The researchers found that the solution, tablet and chewable tablet delivered their load of vitamin C to the body with roughly the same effectiveness—for each, about 30 percent of the total was absorbed. But the timed-release capsule was a different story, delivering only about 14 percent of its contents to the body. "The timed release capsule examined here appears to be a more expensive and less reliable means of providing oral vitamin therapy compared with more conventional dosage forms," the scientists remarked (*Journal of Pharmaceutical Sciences,* March, 1982).

Why did the timed-release capsules perform so poorly? Research team member Michael Mayersohn, Ph.D., of the University of Arizona, says that the vitamin may have been incompletely released from the chemical formulation that is designed to release it slowly, or it may still have been bound by the formulation when it passed the body's vitamin C absorption site (believed to be in the upper part of the small intestine).

Dr. Mayersohn added that there was a wide variation in the individual subjects' ability to absorb the vitamin, suggesting that "some people may simply be good absorbers of vitamin C and others may be poor absorbers."

Whether you're a good absorber or a poor one, a steady supply of vitamin C changes your body for the better in a remarkable variety of ways. It may even "oil the engines" of your life.

CHAPTER
43

VITAMIN C,
SUPER HEALER

Whenever Lois Lane heard it said that her pal Clark Kent—wimpy old Clark—might possibly be the champion of good in Metropolis and true hero of her heart, she was aghast: "Clark? *Superman*? You've got to be kidding!"

It was an agonizing spectacle. How could she be so dumb? Case after case, year after year, every time there was a job for Superman, Clark would disappear. Get with it, Lois.

But Lois never did catch on. For her, there couldn't be anything heroic about a mousy guy who hung in there right beside her every day, unobtrusively going about his business.

Now, there's something Lois Lane-ish about the common inability to realize that vitamin C—everyday C—could possibly do so much good in the streets and back alleys of the city inside us.

Funny: Every time there's "a job for Superman," like a heart attack, vitamin C appears on the scene. We need it to rout the foe because C is our natural superhealer.

A bit farfetched? Sure. But the idea of using vitamin C to speed the healing of a chemically burned eye seems just as farfetched—even to the ophthalmologists who are testing the revolutionary treatment.

"What seems interesting to me," says Roswell Pfister, M.D., of his own experiment, "is that we're using a perfectly normal foodstuff to reverse the tissue degeneration" of a severely damaged eye.

Dr. Pfister, former chairman of ophthalmology at the University of Alabama–Eye Foundation hospital in Birmingham, has been working with Christopher Paterson, Ph.D., of the University of Colorado medical center. Together they experimented with the corneas of 18 rabbits that were burned by a particularly nasty alkali, sodium hydroxide. (The cornea is the clear cap that covers the lens and iris—colored portion—of the eye.) Nine of the rabbits received daily injections of 1.5 grams (1,500 milligrams) of vitamin C after being burned. The 9 others went untreated.

Result: In the nine C-treated rabbits, not one cornea degenerated to the point of perforation. But among the nine other rabbits, 11 of the 18 untreated corneas perforated.

Saving Eyes with Vitamin C

Then Drs. Pfister and Paterson tried giving the vitamin in the form of eye drops. Working again with rabbits, nine were given eye drops hourly after being burned, and one cornea developed a superficial ulcer. Of the 19 corneas in the control group, which received no vitamin drops, nine eyes ulcerated or perforated. Significantly, the one C-treated rabbit that developed an ulcerated cornea had the lowest level of vitamin C in its aqueous humor.

No, *aqueous humor* is not a euphemism for off-color Navy jokes. It's the fluid between the cornea and the lens and surrounding the iris. It nourishes those parts of the eye, and the eye's secretion of it maintains a much-needed pressure on the eye as a whole, Dr. Pfister told us. Without it, "the eye would become mushy."

The amount of vitamin C in the aqueous humor is 18 to 20 times greater than the amount of vitamin C in the blood. Drs. Pfister and Paterson knew this but were not paying it any particular attention until "somewhat by accident" they discovered that the amount of vitamin C in the aqueous humor of the cornea-damaged rabbit eyes "was down to a third of its normal level," Dr. Pfister said.

Was this disappearance of vitamin C, like that of Clark Kent, more than coincidence? The doctors (no Lois Lanes) realized a possible connection. Knowing that the formation of collagen—the stuff that binds cells together—would be crucial to corneal healing, and knowing also that vitamin C plays a vital role in the body's formation of collagen, the doctors theorized that vitamin C "would be required at higher concentrations to repair the devastating effects of an alkali burn," as Dr. Pfister put it.

What happens in the damaged corneas is an all-out war between the forces of creation and destruction. The dead corneal cells break up while the healing process races to hold everything together. If there is a lack of vitamin C fueling the formation of new collagen, the eye loses.

"What we're suggesting" as a result of the experiments, says Dr. Pfister, "is that repair processes have to be helped" by super boosts of C. "This is tissue scurvy, as far as I'm concerned." In contrast to the old approach, which was to apply drugs to prevent old collagen from breaking down, "our objective is to get the healing process carried out," Dr. Pfister says.

The next step in their research is to treat corneal burns in humans with oral doses of vitamin C in hospitals across the nation, to see if the treatment works on humans as well as rabbits. This could take a while. "There are not that many people who get alkali burns in the eye," says Dr. Pfister. (Waiting time would have been less in ancient China, where men were blinded by lye as punishment for looking at another man's wife.)

The corneal healing process does not restore sight, by the way. The cornea is no longer transparent after such a severe burn. But it must be kept from perforating; otherwise, the fluids of the eye would escape. With the cornea intact, sight can eventually be restored by a cornea transplant or the implantation of a plastic cornea, Dr. Pfister points out.

Meanwhile, Dr. Pfister is interested "in other types of eye diseases: bacterial, fungal, viral" that might be helped by vitamin C treatment. "We have no knowledge of what effects it might have," he said. "But if you ask me, 'Could it?' I'd have to say, 'Yes, it could.' "

Skin Saver

Another vitamin C superhealing feat involved a foreman at a printing company. The man was so skillful that he could tell if a job was being printed correctly simply by touching the ink on the paper as it came off the press. But that ink was his poison. It contained hexavalent chromium (a type completely different from nutritional chromium), a widely used industrial chemical that causes more dermatitis (skin disease) than any other. And he had dermatitis—bad.

It hadn't always been that way. For seven years he had lived with it, keeping it somewhat under control by taking antihistamines and steroids. But suddenly it flared up. His hands and wrists began to swell and crack, oozing fluid. He took more drugs, but that didn't help much. And he couldn't wear gloves or use a protective hand cream on the job, because he had to touch his work. His only choice was to spend each Friday evening to Monday morning with his hands wrapped in cold, medicine-soaked compresses. And if that wasn't enough, he slept poorly because of the pain, the antihistamines made him drowsy and his face began to swell and discolor—a side effect of taking steroids both orally and by injection.

Needing him at work, the company finally sent him to a doctor who specialized in occupational diseases—a doctor who knew that in 1969 a researcher had discovered that vitamin C could protect skin from hexavalent chromium.

The doctor prepared a solution containing 10 percent vitamin C, and the foreman kept a container of it next to him while he worked. "Each hour during the work day," writes John Milner, M.D., the physician who handled the case, "he dipped his hands in the liquid and blotted them dry."

Within a week, says the doctor, the symptoms dramatically decreased, and he stopped his antihistamines and his injections of steroids. Within a month, he stopped taking steroids altogether. And he no longer stayed at home weekends with his hands wrapped in bandages—he played golf instead!

"He has continued to use the ascorbic acid [vitamin C] solution," writes Dr. Milner, "and the control of symptoms has been sustained over the course of years" (*Journal of Occupational Medicine*, January, 1980).

CHAPTER

44

INSULATE YOUR HEALTH WITH VITAMIN C

Cold weather means more than the sniffles. It means you could be sniffling at someone's grave side. Statistics indicate that thousands more die during the winter months than in summer. During a cold spell, heart attacks, strokes and pneumonia kill people who would have lived longer if the thermometer hadn't dropped.

Cold weather is serious business. But vitamin C doesn't kid around either. There's substantial evidence that this nutrient can prevent a cold, clear up one that's just getting started or shorten one that's hit full force. And vitamin C doesn't stop there. It also tackles heart disease, circulatory problems and serious viral infections—the conditions that can put your health in a deep freeze during winter.

Most people, however, would be content simply to make the common cold less common. Runny nose, sore throat, fatigue—the heavy traffic of infection that stalls you in bed for a day or two (but won't let you sleep)—who needs it? Your body doesn't, and its immune system is set up to resist the viruses that cause colds. Then why do you catch them? Because, new research shows, to *fully* resist those viruses, the immune system may need large amounts of vitamin C, amounts 10 to 20 times higher than the government's Recommended Dietary Allowance.

The research wasn't with humans, but with guinea pigs. Both species have something in common, though. Neither is able to produce vitamin C in its body, as does almost every other mammal, but instead depends entirely on dietary sources. So when it comes to vitamin C, what's true for guinea pigs is more likely to be true for humans, too.

Enhanced Resistance

In the study, researchers kept two groups of guinea pigs on a diet deficient in vitamin C but supplemented the drinking water of one group with the nutrient. Once a week for three weeks, the immune system of both groups was challenged with a potentially deadly substance. More than twice as many of the vitamin-deficient as the vitamin-supplemented animals died.

In the next month, the researchers fed the surviving deficient animals vitamin C. Some received an amount equivalent to 100 milligrams a day for a human while others received an amount equal to 1,000 milligrams. After three to four weeks, the animals in the 1,000-milligrams group were completely healthy and able to resist the challenging substance. But the animals in the 100-milligram group never returned to health. They failed to gain the weight they lost during their deficient period, and their systems were unable to defend them against the immunologic attack (*Federation Proceedings*, May, 1979).

The authors, Gary Thurman, Ph.D., and Allan Goldstein, Ph.D., who ran the study while professors in the biochemistry department at the George Washington University school of medicine, summarize their research: "This study provides the first definitive evidence that ascorbic acid [vitamin C] plays a major role in the maintenance of immunity and provides a rational mechanism for the postulated beneficial effect of this essential vitamin in the treatment of viral diseases."

The mechanism they're talking about works like this: Stress uses up vitamin C, and cold is a potent stress. When icy weather steals the nutrient, you need more to keep your immune system up to par. If you don't get it, you can catch colds more easily. If you do get it, you have better resistance against the viruses that cause colds. That may be a theory, but it's a good one. Study after study shows that people who take vitamin C have fewer and milder colds.

In a study at the University of Toronto, 407 people received 1,000 milligrams of vitamin C a day and an extra 3,000 milligrams a day for the first three days of a cold. Another 411 people received a worthless placebo. Compared to the placebo group, the vitamin C group spent 30 percent fewer days indoors because of illness and missed 33 percent fewer days of work *(Canadian Medical Association Journal)*.

In a study of crew members on a Polaris submarine, 37 sailors who received 2,000 milligrams of vitamin C a day had 66 percent fewer cold symptoms than a placebo group *(International Research Communication System)*.

In another submarine study (they're apparently popular among researchers trying to get to the bottom of the common-cold problem), scientists from the Naval Medical Research Institute, in Bethesda, Maryland, took a look at the relation between plasma vitamin C levels and the general health of 28 crewmen on a submarine before, during and after a 68-day patrol. They noted that the group with the lowest plasma vitamin C levels "did not differ significantly" in health from the group with the highest levels. Yet, they also observed, in passing, that "the results for upper respiratory infections were in the expected direction . . . with twice as many of the low group showing symptoms of the common cold than the high group" *(Journal of Applied Nutrition,* vol. 34, no. 1, 1982).

By maintaining relatively high levels of vitamin C in their bodies during those long, lightless weeks under the sea, some of the submarines were able to fight off respiratory infections considerably better than their shipmates.

In an Australian study, 95 pairs of identical twins—perfectly matched for age, sex and genetic makeup—were used to compare the cold-fighting power of vitamin C with that of a placebo (in this case, a pill that looked just like the vitamin but contained only lactose, or milk sugar). For 100 days, one of each pair of twins took a gram (1,000 milligrams) of vitamin C daily while the other took the placebo, though neither knew which was which. They were also asked to make careful note of the duration and severity of colds, should they appear.

When the results were analyzed, the research team concluded that "vitamin C had no significant effect except for shortening the average duration of cold episodes by 19 percent" (*Medical Journal of Australia*, October 17, 1981). If you're interested in knocking one day off a five-day cold, in other words, you might try vitamin C. Interestingly, the Australians also found that "females had significantly longer, more severe and more intense colds than males."

In a study of soldiers undergoing training in northern Canada, those receiving 1,000 milligrams of vitamin C a day had about 68 percent less illness than a placebo group (*Report No. 74-R-1012*, Defense Research Board, Department of National Defense).

And in another study from Toronto, 448 people who took vitamin C had up to 38 percent fewer cold symptoms—runny nose, fever, sore throat, tight chest, aching limbs, depression—than a placebo group (*Canadian Medical Association Journal*).

"There is little doubt," wrote the authors of the Toronto study, "that the intake of additional vitamin C can lead to a reduced burden of winter illness."

CHAPTER

45

KEEP COOL WITH VITAMIN C

It's so muggy even the mosquitoes are taking naps. Sprawled in a hammock, with about as much energy as it takes to sip iced tea, Joe turns on the radio and tunes in to a weatherman sizing up the sizzler.

"Well, folks, good news. The temperature's just dropped to 32 degrees in the shade. Thirty-two degrees Celsius, that is."

Joe's not laughing. As far as he's concerned, this is no joke.

He's tired, irritable, and his body feels like a crumpled-up dishrag in a sinkful of dirty dishes.

And have you been feeling like Joe lately? If so, take heart—and take a good bit of vitamin C.

Just about everybody knows that vitamin C has been suggested as a means to prevent the common cold. Well, recent research has also suggested that vitamin C may help prevent the "common hot," that run-down dragged-out feeling that gets washed up on the shore of your life by a summer heat wave.

The research we're talking about wasn't conducted where you might expect: outside, underneath a glaring sun. It was conducted inside, in climate chambers where heat, humidity and wind velocity were controlled not by the whim of Mother Nature, but by the careful design of scientists.

These climate chambers are used in South Africa to acclimate new mine workers to the hot, humid air of the mines. In the chambers, the workers perform a simple exercise called the step test—repeatedly stepping onto and off a step—for hours at a time. By performing this exercise day after day, in progressively hotter and more humid air, they gradually accustom themselves to the same type of conditions they will encounter in the mines.

In 1974, however, researchers found that, despite this preparation, mine workers had a rapid decrease in blood levels of vitamin C during their first three months of employment—even though their vitamin C intake was adequate *(South African Medical Journal).*

Heat Stress Burns Up Vitamin C

That's no surprise, really, because scientists have long known that stress of any kind—from a snakebite to the biting cold of winter—depletes the body of vitamin C. And even if your air conditioner has never broken down, we don't have to tell you that heat is a stress.

When the mercury's on the rise, your body moves quickly to cool itself: Blood vessels expand; the heart pumps rapidly to provide the energy needed to release excess heat; sweat pours off the skin. One theory says that these reactions are sparked by hormones from the adrenal gland, which contains a higher amount of vitamin C than any other body tissue and needs vitamin C to do its job. But if the hot weather just won't quit and your vitamin C is depleted, then the body's temperature *stays* high, and you've got a case of the hot-weather blahs: heat exhaustion, heat prostration—maybe even heatstroke.

To translate this scientific theory into scientific fact, N. B. Strydom and his co-workers in the industrial hygiene division of the Chamber of Mines of South Africa divided 60 miners, who were not exposed to heat for six months prior to the study, into three groups. They asked one group to take 250 milligrams of vitamin C a day and another to take 500. To the third group they gave a placebo—a medically useless pill. The workers were then asked to perform the step exercise for four hours in a comfortable environment, during which time their temperatures, heart rates and sweat rates were measured. On the next ten days, they performed the same exercise, but this time in a hot, humid climate chamber (*Journal of Applied Physiology*).

Although there was no measurable difference in heart and sweat rates, the average body temperatures of the vitamin C–supplemented groups were lower on every single day after the first. Not only that, 35 percent of the workers who took vitamin C were fully acclimated to the heat by the fourth day of the test, while only one person from the placebo group acclimated that quickly.

You probably don't work in an overheated mine. At least, we hope not. But when vitamin C helps those in such an extreme situation to keep their cool, it's a good bet that it'll do the same for you.

Closer to home, Irwin Stone, Ph.D., a noted biochemist, reviews in his book *The Healing Factor: Vitamin C against Disease* (Grosset and Dunlap, 1972) a number of studies in which vitamin C was used to treat heat stress.

One such study describes long-term tests on workers in a Virginia rayon plant who had been exposed to high temperatures and humidities. The study found that heat prostration in the employees was eliminated by the daily administration of 100 milligrams of vitamin C. Before this regimen was instituted, there had been 27 cases of heat prostration; in the following nine years, not a single case was reported in the group taking the daily supplements.

Heat Rash Quickly Cured

Vitamin C may also help eliminate another heat-wave worry: heat rash, or prickly heat.

When heat rash strikes, the pores in the area of the rash shut down and sweating stops. In severe cases, with a large area of the body surface involved, body temperature may shoot up; someone with prickly heat can be a good candidate for heat exhaustion.

Dr. T. C. Hindson, a British dermatologist in Singapore, had been treating an Australian Air Force officer who had an acute case of prickly heat. Nothing that the doctor gave him seemed to help. But one day, the officer felt himself coming down with a cold and began taking 1 gram (1,000 milligrams) of vitamin C. In the course of one week, the prickly heat vanished— after having afflicted him for more than a year *(Lancet)*.

Dr. Hindson immediately began giving vitamin C to five children whose heat rashes he had been treating for some time without success. All of the children threw off the rash, and their skin remained clear as long as they continued taking vitamin C.

To give further weight to his findings, Dr. Hindson conducted a carefully structured study on 30 children with prickly heat, in which 15 children were given vitamin C and another 15 placebos.

At the end of two weeks, the doctor discovered that, of those taking the placebo, 4 showed some improvement, 9 stayed the same, and 2 had worse prickly heat than before. But of those taking vitamin C, 10 were completely rash free, 4 improved, 1 was the same and none worse. Dr. Hindson then gave vitamin C to the children who had been getting the placebo. In future examinations one and two months later, not one rash was seen on any of the 30 children. And *all* of these children had been suffering from severe prickly heat for at least eight weeks before the beginning of the experiment.

The youngsters in this experiment were given vitamin C in dosages based on their weight: A child of 38 pounds was given about 250 milligrams daily, a 19-pounder 125 milligrams, and so forth. In cases where children were too young to take pills, mothers were instructed to crush the tablets in their food. This dose proved virtually 100 percent effective in curing and preventing heat rash.

CHAPTER
46

MAKE VITAMIN C YOUR SHIELD AGAINST POLLUTION

Some people have all the luck. You know the ones we mean. They never gain a pound, never get a blemish, always have the right clothes, their money earns the highest interest . . . and they've never been sick a day in their lives—or so it seems.

Even though they walk through the same environmental traps as the rest of us, they don't get caught. Somehow smog doesn't affect their lungs, and pollutants and poisons seem to bounce off of them as if they were protected by some kind of invisible shield.

Well, maybe they are. There may be a way to protect ourselves from the harmful effects of pollution and other environmental contaminants. And it's not a matter of luck, either. It has to do with our own nutritional status—especially that of vitamin C.

"It is now widely accepted that ascorbic acid [vitamin C] nutritional status markedly affects the toxicity and/or carcinogenicity of greater than 50 pollutants, many of which are ubiquitous in the air, water and food environments," says Edward J. Calabrese, Ph.D., professor of environmental health at the University of Massachusetts, in Amherst.

That's especially true of nitrosamine formation in the stomach. Nitrosamines are carcinogens (cancer-causing agents) that may be formed in the gut when we eat foods treated with sodium nitrate. (Nitrates are added to many processed meats and smoked fish products as food preservatives and as flavoring and coloring agents.)

But now evidence suggests that vitamin C can actually prevent the formation of nitrosamines in your stomach, says Dr. Calabrese, who is the author of *Nutrition and Environmental Health* (John Wiley and Sons, 1980). It's a natural detoxifying agent, but only if the vitamin is in your stomach at the same time as the nitrate-treated foods. So if you take vitamin C only once a day, in the morning, it can't protect you from nitrosamine formation during lunch or dinner, since it would be long gone from your stomach by then. The obvious solution is to take your vitamin C several times during the day with your meals, but for more reasons than one.

First of all, "even if you don't eat foods rich in nitrates, you are still exposed to those chemicals," says Steven R. Tannenbaum, Ph.D., professor of toxicology and food chemistry at Massachusetts Institute of Technology (MIT), in Cambridge. "That's because your body manufactures them automatically. Eating cured foods only adds to the level that's already there."

What's more, if all your vitamin C is combating nitrosamine formation, it will not be available to perform its other vital functions in the body, adds Dr. Calabrese. Consequently, the presence of nitrates in your diet would increase your daily requirement of vitamin C (*Medical Hypotheses*, December, 1979).

That's why it's important to know how nitrates are metabolized and exactly what effect vitamin C has on nitrosamine formation.

To find that out, Dr. Tannenbaum is conducting a study. "Our volunteers are young, healthy MIT students," he told us. "First we put them on a special diet that is completely nitrate free. In that way, we are able to determine how much nitrate is actually produced automatically by the body. After a few days, we add nitrates to the diets and trace the metabolism of the chemical through the body to learn how much of it is converted to nitrosamines.

"In the next part of the experiment, we give each student ascorbic acid to find out whether vitamin intervention affects the amount of nitrosamines formed.

"Right now, we are giving the students 2 grams [2,000 milligrams] of vitamin C per day, and at that level, we have found that nitrosamine formation is blocked nearly completely. We've confirmed that in at least six different people. Less may work also, but 2 grams did the best job.

"When you eat foods rich in nitrates, they are promptly converted to nitrites in the mouth or in the stomach," Dr. Tannenbaum told us. "Vitamin C has the capacity to react with the nitrite form of the chemical faster than nitrogen compounds can. And nitrogen compounds are the substances needed to form the nitrosamines. If the nitrites react to vitamin C and are destroyed, then they can't attach themselves to nitrogen compounds. Hence nitrosamine formation is blocked."

Although there is no absolute guarantee that vitamin C will protect you from the harmful diseases associated with nitrosamines, Dr. Tannenbaum advises people to take it anyway. "It can only help," he says.

Protects against Radiation

That may be good advice for people exposed to X rays as well. And who hasn't been at one time or another? Now doctors are coming to recognize the potential hazards associated with routine irradiation, and many have curtailed their usage. Nevertheless, any form of protection against X rays is valuable, indeed.

That's why the experiment conducted by James A. Scott, M.D., and Gerald M. Kolodny, M.D., is of such interest. In it, they measured the effects of irradiation on normal mouse cells (which had been grown in the laboratory) with varying amounts of vitamin C or with no vitamin C at all.

"We had heard that vitamin C can prevent damage from radiation, and so we decided to give it a try on the mouse cells," said Dr. Scott, assistant radiologist at Massachusetts General Hospital in Boston. "Our experiment showed that it does have this ability, but at relatively high doses—about 10 grams per day for the human equivalent. We're not sure exactly how it exerts its protective effect, but it somehow keeps the radiation from killing the cells.

"We did find one thing that was a real surprise," Dr. Scott told us. "Apparently, the vitamin C slowed down cell division. And since dividing cells are more sensitive to radiation, that may have something to do with the vitamin's ability to protect against damage."

He concludes that "pretreatment with ascorbic acid might alter the cell population such that surviving cells are more resistant to the effects of subsequently administered radiation" (*International Journal for Vitamin and Nutrition Research*, vol. 51, no. 2, 1981).

"So far, we can't say that these results would apply to humans," says Dr. Scott, who is also an instructor at the Harvard medical school. "But if vitamins are necessary for human life in small quantities, maybe some people need more, especially in those situations which stress our bodies—such as exposure to radiation and other environmental pollutants. I take 400 milligrams per day to be on the safe side."

Battling against Ozone

Considering the multitude of pollutants permeating the air we breathe, Dr. Scott may have the right idea—especially when it comes to ozone. Ozone is a highly toxic pollutant gas and is a major component of smog.

But vitamin C may be able to protect us against ozone damage, too. It did just that in an experiment with mice. Researchers at the University of Queensland, in Australia, exposed mice to various concentrations of ozone in the air for 30 minutes. As much as 50 percent of the vitamin C in lung tissue was lost during that time. The vitamin seemed to be used up in its effort to battle the ozone, say the researchers. Scientists had already established that vitamin C could prevent lung damage caused by ozone. This study strongly supported the conclusion that it was the vitamin C *in the lung itself* that was preventing damage by ozone (*Chemico-Biological Interactions*, vol. 30, no. 1, 1980).

Protecting Occupational Health

If you think you have it bad, what about people who must work with toxic chemicals. Now, they really have something to shout about.

Take benzene for example. That's a solvent commonly used in industry. Chronic exposure to benzene has long been known to cause destruction of the bone marrow and perhaps leukemia. The curious thing is that, despite similar levels of exposure to benzene, not all workers become ill. "Given a similar degree of exposure, why do some workers remain apparently unaffected . . . ?" asks Dr. Calabrese.

The answer may lie in the diets of the people involved. "It is hypothesized that inadequate nutritional status of possibly several nutrients including . . . ascorbic acid may enhance susceptibility to adverse effects caused by benzene," says Dr. Calabrese.

At first, the connection between vitamin C nutritional status and benzene toxicity revolved around the recognition of certain similarities between benzene poisoning and scurvy (vitamin C–deficiency disease).

Then a study was done that investigated the effect of chronic benzene poisoning on vitamin C levels in guinea pigs. The researchers found that benzene poisoning diminished vitamin C levels in the blood, adrenals and liver. But the toxic effects were lessened by the administration of vitamin C, and the mortality rate was decreased by 57 percent.

Other researchers have concluded that "exposure to benzene produces an increased requirement of vitamin C and that an extra supply of vitamin C given increases resistance to the effects of benzene vapors" (*Medical Hypotheses*, May, 1980).

If it's insecticides you've been exposed to, vitamin C may be able to come to the rescue again. One in particular, chlordane, acts primarily on the central nervous system leading to symptoms of hyperexcitability, tremors and convulsions. As if that's not enough, it also causes marked degenerative changes in the liver, kidney, spleen and heart.

But now there's a study that shows that vitamin C can counteract some of those adverse effects. In the experiment, the researchers divided rats into three groups. One group acted as the control and was given the regular rat chow. The second group received the same diet plus a dose of chlordane, and the third received the food, chlordane and vitamin C.

As expected, chlordane toxicity drastically altered the tissues of various organs as well as lowering the growth rates of the animals in the second group. Several of the rats' enzyme systems went haywire, too. And the mortality rate was almost 43 percent in the chlordane-treated rats.

The good news here is that the vitamin C–treated rats fared much better. Mortality was nil, and growth retardation was considerably counteracted. Although vitamin C couldn't restore all the damaged parts, it did a good job on the kidneys, where it "could reverse some of these degenerative changes in the kidney tissues" (*International Journal for Vitamin and Nutrition Research*, vol. 51, no. 3, 1981).

As long as we live in a world surrounded by pollution and other poisons, we need all the help we can get. And vitamin C may be one of the best bets around. "It has a lot of properties that haven't even been investigated yet," says Dr. Scott.

"Other areas of research should be directed toward the potential effects of ascorbic acid on the development of silicosis, noise-related adverse health effects, industrial fluoride toxicity and lead intoxication," adds Dr. Calabrese.

But why wait till the research is completed?

The present evidence is already pretty convincing. With vitamin C as our shield against pollutants, who needs luck?

CHAPTER
47

CLEAN CHLORINE FROM YOUR WATER WITH VITAMIN C

It cleans swimming pools, whitens clothes and makes tap water taste like a cross between cod liver oil and Drano. You guessed right—it's chlorine.

Chlorine is added to practically every large urban water supply in the United States. That's not necessarily bad. By killing off waterborne bacteria, chlorine protects us against typhoid fever, dysentery and cholera. But making every glass of water a chlorine cocktail is not necessarily good, either. For chlorinated water not only wipes out *foreign* bodies like germs and microbes, it may also stage an attack on *our* bodies, damaging red blood cells.

John Eaton, Ph.D., associate professor of medicine at the University of Minnesota, told us that chlorinated water has a "deleterious effect" on red blood cells, crippling them so that they can no longer efficiently perform their function of carrying oxygen to every part of the body and causing their premature destruction.

But he also told us what to do to prevent those cells from being lamed by chlorine: "Put vitamin C in your water before you drink it.

"It's odorless and tasteless in the tiny amount needed—just a trace—to neutralize the chlorine," Dr. Eaton said. "And vitamin C works very rapidly," he added.

The research scientist made his two discoveries—that chlorine damages red blood cells and that vitamin C neutralizes it—in the course of finding out why patients at two of three artificial kidney centers in Minneapolis were developing severe anemia.

It turned out that, at those two centers, the water used in the blood-cleansing kidney machines was not chlorine free. In his laboratory, Dr. Eaton found that the chlorine severely damaged the red blood cells of the kidney patients, causing anemia. He also found that, by adding vitamin C to the dialysis water, he could set up a chemical reaction that neutralized the chemical *(Science)*.

But Dr. Eaton is not the first researcher to discover that, while chlorine clears the muck out of stream water, it can also muck up your bloodstream.

In 1972, Russian scientists found that people drinking water with 1.4 milligrams of chlorine in it showed higher blood pressures than those drinking water containing only 0.3 to 0.4 milligrams.

Reading about these studies, we might want to plug up the faucet for good and rely solely on spring or well water. While that might not be a bad idea, it isn't convenient for some of us. Instead, add a little piece of a vitamin C tablet or a scant pinch of the powder to your glass of chlorinated water before you drink it. Not only will chlorine's taste and odor disappear, so will its threat to your good health. Cheers.

CHAPTER
48

C IS FOR CHOLESTEROL— AND ITS CONTROL

Forget Son of Sam, Jack the Ripper and the Boston Strangler: The greatest killer of all time is heart disease. Specifically, it is heart disease caused by atherosclerosis, or hardening of the arteries, and its favorite weapon is cholesterol.

Mention cholesterol, and most people want to do something about it. So they start thinking about breakfast. Now, that's not a bad place to start, but they immediately implicate eggs. And that's a crime. What they should be doing is pouring themselves another glass of orange juice. Vitamin C, researchers have found, is a good defense against cholesterol, hardened arteries and heart disease.

One testimony comes from England, where 11 elderly hospital patients with coronary artery problems took 1 gram (1,000 milligrams) of vitamin C daily—resulting in a decrease of total blood cholesterol levels in only six weeks. That prompted researchers to assert that "atherosclerosis and ischaemic heart disease are not inevitable features of aging" (*Journal of Human Nutrition*, vol. 35, no. 1, 1981). That's not all they found.

As a little background on the case, cholesterol's guilt is

purely by association. Left to itself, cholesterol actually does some good. It helps our digestion by producing bile, without which we can suffer gallstones. Our bodies need cholesterol to manufacture vitamin D, and there is some evidence that it protects us from cancer. Its home turf is the liver, but cholesterol goes out a lot. Its traveling companions are called lipoproteins, and they chauffeur it around the bloodstream.

In the company of high-density lipoproteins (HDLs), cholesterol's joyride is relatively safe. But introduce it to low-density lipoproteins (LDLs), and look out, cholesterol is up to no good. Scientists now believe that lowering total cholesterol is less important than getting most of it on the HDL route. And that, the British research team learned, is another thing vitamin C does.

When they started their gram-a-day supplementation, most of the heart patients had vitamin C deficiencies; the *men* also had correspondingly low levels of HDL cholesterol. "After six weeks' treatment with ascorbic acid [vitamin C], the mean [average] HDL-cholesterol concentration had increased," the study team noted. What's more, that benefit was not restricted to the heart patients; all 7 men in the 14-member healthy control group enjoyed it, as well.

The seven women who acted as controls experienced no significant change in lipoprotein cholesterol, but that doesn't mean vitamin C is guilty of sex discrimination. Women naturally have higher HDL levels, which is one reason they are less prone to heart attacks than men. All the women in the control group had healthier HDL levels.

The evidence that vitamin C can protect as well as defend, that it is as beneficial to high-risk subjects as to those already afflicted with heart disease, may be the most compelling aspect of the British investigation. The research team has entered a plea for higher recommended daily intake of vitamin C because "latent ascorbic acid deficiency may be one of several preventable 'risk' factors contributing to the present epidemic of ischaemic heart disease in the western world."

Deficiencies Are Common

Not only has it been linked to heart disease, but a vitamin C deficiency is more common than you might think.

The heart patients in the British experiment weren't the only ones suffering vitamin C deficiencies at the outset: Some of the 14 "healthy" control subjects were deficient, too. The authors noted that "low blood ascorbic-acid levels are often found in elderly patients."

Nobel Prize–winning vitamin C advocate Linus Pauling, Ph.D., suspects that as much as 99 percent of the world's population suffers from a deficiency of the nutrient. Dr. Pauling, who personally takes 10 grams daily, agrees that the current Recommended Dietary Allowance (about 60 milligrams) is "much too low" and says he would like to see it raised to "at least 150." Dr. Pauling's colleague, scientist Irwin Stone, and British physician Geoffrey Taylor are two other vitamin C champions who go so far as to suggest that today's coronary epidemic may be but a modern version of that ancient sailors' scourge: scurvy.

Like human beings, guinea pigs are one of a handful of species unable to manufacture vitamin C in their own bodies. When the vitamin is withheld from their diets and scurvy is induced in the laboratory, guinea pigs develop weak arteries with interior bruises like those that are symptoms of the beginnings of atherosclerosis. No matter how those bruises are acquired, they become a magnet for wayward LDL cholesterol, which collects there in layers called plaque—perhaps a misguided attempt to shelter the injured area. If such is plaque's intent, it succeeds all too well, eventually narrowing the blood's passageway until it becomes a dead-end road. The body's reaction is a heart attack.

The detour signs start going up in guinea pigs' arteries when their vitamin C reserves are in the range of 15 micrograms per gram of body weight (a microgram is one-millionth of a gram). That's about the level we're at when we have a cold—if we've been getting only the RDA. Taking greater amounts of vitamin C puts us way ahead of the game.

Vitamin C isn't just a policeman directing cholesterol traffic through the bloodstream and forcing loitering platelets to break it up and move on. After a heart attack has occurred, a high level of C can pay off like an insurance policy.

C Repairs Heart Damage

That's what Scottish physicians at Southern General Hospital in Glasgow reported several years ago when they discovered that blood levels of vitamin C drop down to scurvy levels within 6 to 12 hours after a person suffers a heart attack.

They concluded that the vitamin C was diverted to the heart to help rebuild the damaged coronary tissue *(British Heart Journal)*.

Their findings were borne out by a more recent study in which Jairo Ramirez, M.D., and colleagues at the University of Louisville, Kentucky, found that the vitamin C concentrations in the white blood cells of 150 patients with heart disease were "significantly lower" than those of a control group. And they remain dangerously low for several weeks after a heart attack before gradually increasing to a stable level. That phenomenon may occur even when there is no change in daily vitamin C supplementation *(American Journal of Clinical Nutrition*, October, 1980).

Dr. Ramirez, now engaged in private practice in San Antonio, Texas, also noted that cholesterol is higher in patients deprived of vitamin C and that increasing amounts of the vitamin cause an increase in the liver's production of a substance called cytochrome P-450, which speeds up the conversion of cholesterol into bile.

Anthony Verlangieri, Ph.D., associate professor of pharmacology and toxicology at the University of Mississippi, has determined that vitamin C helps the body manufacture another chemical compound with a nifty name: chondroitin sulfate A, alias CSA. Dr. Verlangieri was working in the biochemistry laboratory at Rutgers University when he discovered that CSA acts as a sort of mortar in healthy artery walls and that cholesterol attaches itself only to damaged artery walls that lack this compound.

Preventing One Million Heart Attacks a Year

While Dr. Verlangieri was experimenting with CSA in his New Jersey laboratory, he was unaware that a research team 3,000 miles away, in Culver City, California, had also isolated CSA and was using it to treat heart-attack victims. It worked so well, deaths due to coronary complications dropped by a whopping 80 percent in those patients treated with CSA. Lester M. Morrison, M.D., former director of the Institute for Arteriosclerosis Research at Loma Linda University school of medicine in California, headed the research team. He suggests that CSA can also *prevent* "over one million heart attacks a year."

Dr. Morrison's published findings coincided with those of Dr. Verlangieri, who declared, "My findings show that vitamin C stimulates production of the same compound within the body."

As research continues, scientists are finding that the RDA set for vitamin C is seldom enough and that wholesome foods we've enjoyed for centuries—such as eggs—are rarely to blame for modern diseases.

One of the first to recognize that fact was England's Dr. Constance Spittle Leslie, who put herself on a high-cholesterol diet—but found that her blood cholesterol *dropped* because she also ate lots of fresh fruits and vegetables rich in vitamin C.

If she cooked the fruits and vegetables, however, her blood cholesterol level rose, because heat destroys vitamin C. Results were the same when Dr. Leslie carried out the experiment on 58 human volunteers.

She also found that, when they were given 1-gram supplements of vitamin C every day, the volunteers enjoyed the drop in cholesterol levels even if they cooked their fruits and vegetables (*Medical World News*).

So you don't necessarily have to give up eggs, cheese and the finer things in life out of fear of heart disease. There's ample evidence that vitamin C can safeguard your arteries and your general well-being as it also protects against colds and cancer. There are many stories of the benefits of vitamin C. Neutralizing cholesterol is only one of them.

VITAMIN C, PECTIN AND HEART DISEASE

by Emil Ginter, Ph.D.

The search for substances capable of depressing cholesterol levels in the blood is one of the most pressing in ongoing medical research. Cholesterol concentration (or to be more precise, the level of low-density lipoproteins, or LDL, cholesterol) constitutes an important risk factor for atherosclerotic damage of blood vessel walls that may bring about a heart attack or stroke.

Pharmaceutical companies have developed several drugs that depress blood cholesterol levels in experimental animals and also in humans. The substance most employed has been ethylester of chlorphenoxyisobutyric acid (clofibrate, Atromid) because short-term tests revealed no serious adverse side effects from its use. However, to be effective, this drug must be taken in rather high doses and permanently.

Two extensive surveys lasting several years, carried out in both the United States and Europe and involving several thousand persons, have shown clofibrate to be less effective in de-

Dr. Ginter, who has done extensive research with vitamin C, is associated with the Institute of Human Nutrition in Bratislava, Czechoslovakia.

pressing blood cholesterol than had originally been claimed. In addition, when used continually, this drug has several negative side effects, the most evident of which is the formation of gallstones. The European study even showed the overall death rate in persons on a long-term clofibrate regimen to be significantly higher than for those not taking the drug. And the chemical structure of the majority of other drugs with a cholesterol-depressing action indicates that their regular use also raises the possibility of adverse side effects.

Fortunately, there may be other, safer alternatives. For centuries, men have suspected that fruits and vegetables contain certain natural substances which exert a protective action in circulatory disorders. Physicians in ancient India, for example, used concentrates of certain fruits to treat vascular diseases, and old textbooks of dietetics recommended days of fruit-vegetable diet for cardiovascular patients.

But to come to the present time: Dr. Frank M. Sacks and his team from Harvard compared two groups of people of about the same age consuming either the current North American diet or an essentially vegetarian diet. They found the blood cholesterol levels in those with a high consumption of vegetables and fruits to be substantially lower than in the normal American population. Of particular importance, they found that the low cholesterol levels reflected a reduction of the LDL cholesterol fraction, which is suspected to be the real troublemaker in heart disease. On the other hand, the level of high-density lipoprotein (HDL) cholesterol, which exerts a protective action, was not decreased.

Another group of U.S. researchers in California have noted a substantially lower mortality rate from heart attacks in Seventh-day Adventists, who are predominantly vegetarians. For instance, coronary mortality in Seventh-day Adventist men of a younger age group was only one-quarter of that in a matched sample of the standard California population. The majority of researchers attribute these differences primarily to the fact that vegetarians have a substantially lower intake of cholesterol and saturated animal fat than the average person. Although, of course, that factor plays a considerable role, such an explanation is still incomplete, for it leaves out of account the protective role of certain specific components of vegetables and fruits, namely vitamin C and dietary fiber.

How Vitamin C Protects

Over the past 30 years, several teams of investigators in various parts of the world have pointed out that vitamin C lowers cholesterol levels in humans and exerts a protective action by promoting the transformation of cholesterol to bile acids, which can then be excreted from the body. During a long-term marginal vitamin C deficiency, such as people in many countries experience during the winter and spring months, when fresh fruits and vegetables are less plentiful, cholesterol transformation to bile acids is slowed down, resulting in an accumulation of cholesterol in the liver and the blood.

In animals, if vitamin C deficiency persists for a considerable length of time, cholesterol also accumulates on the vessel walls, and pathological changes take place in arteries reminiscent of human atherosclerosis. On the other hand, high doses of vitamin C accelerate cholesterol transformation to bile acids and prevent such changes from taking place.

If vitamin C is given to people with high cholesterol levels, a decline of cholesterol concentration in their blood is often observed. However, after about six months, when a maximum drop is usually achieved, there is a tendency in some of the patients for cholesterol levels to rise again toward higher values. That is likely caused by a sensitive feedback system. As vitamin C accelerates the conversion of cholesterol to bile acids, some of these bile acid molecules find their way back to the liver and signal a slowing down of the initial reaction. At that point, the cholesterol-lowering effect of vitamin C becomes weakened.

However, if the drug cholestyramine is given with the vitamin C, there is a striking and sustained decline of blood cholesterol level, at least in experimental animals. That is because cholestyramine binds the bile acids in the digestive tract.

So it is evident that a mutual reinforcement of the effect on blood cholesterol level exists between vitamin C and substances capable of binding bile acids in the intestine. Evidence has accumulated in recent years that several naturally occurring substances in plants, designated by the general term *dietary fiber,* exert an effect similar to that of cholestyramine.

Pectin's Vital Role

One such natural fiber is *pectin*, long used in the making of jams because of its ability to form gels. Gel derived from pectin has the ability to bind bile acids in the human digestive tract, thus increasing fecal excretion of bile acids.

Our own studies on experimental animals have produced conclusive evidence that simultaneous administration of vitamin C and pectin significantly decreases cholesterol concentration not only in blood, but likewise in the liver. When taken daily, a test preparation containing 450 milligrams of vitamin C and 15 grams of citrus pectin lowered total blood cholesterol in humans after six weeks. This decline was characterized by a decrease of the dangerous LDL cholesterol, while the concentration of the protective HDL cholesterol remained unchanged.

To sum up, a high vitamin C intake causes cholesterol transformation to bile acids to proceed at a faster rate in the liver. Bile acids from the liver pass into the intestine, where they are then bound to pectin gel and leave the body in the stools. The ultimate result of this interplay of two natural substances is a low cholesterol level in the blood and a diminished risk of atherosclerosis.

Pectin has a number of additional positive effects. It improves stool consistency, acts as a detoxifier by binding heavy metals and carrying them out of the body, and also slows down the absorption of sugar. This last effect may be useful for diabetics.

It should be stressed that this approach to cholesterol control is especially promising because pectin and vitamin C are naturally occurring substances. It seems extremely unlikely that even permanent consumption would result in undesirable side effects. For this reason, persons concerned about high cholesterol levels should substantially increase their consumption of fruits and vegetables. Black currants, for example, are a concentrated source of both vitamin C and pectin. But other abundant sources include citrus fruits, strawberries, tomatoes, raspberries and blackberries. Perhaps some day supplements of vitamin C and pectin in combination will be routinely prescribed to both treat and prevent dangerously increased cholesterol levels.

CHAPTER
50

CAN VITAMIN C PREVENT THE COMMON CANCER?

It's one thing to think of vitamin C in terms of preventing the common cold—but cancer? That's a bit much. After all, there's quite a difference between a case of the sniffles and the second leading cause of death from disease in the country. Nonetheless, some researchers believe that the best way to deal with cancer is to prevent it. And preliminary data indicate that vitamin C may help do just that.

First of all, it's no secret that researchers have been examining vitamin C's effects on already existing cancer cells very closely. In a study at the University of Kansas medical center, researchers found that vitamin C suppressed the growth of certain leukemia cells.

The scientists took bone marrow cells from 28 leukemia patients and placed them in 28 special containers (cultures). In 7 of the 28 cultures (25 percent), the numbers of leukemic cell colonies were reduced markedly when vitamin C was added (*Cancer Research,* April, 1980).

The investigators discovered that lower concentrations of vitamin C worked as well as extremely high levels of the vitamin in that particular instance. They suggested that a study using vitamin C might be conducted on certain types of leukemia patients. But the patients would have to be carefully screened before they could take part in a controlled experiment, the researchers warned. They found that vitamin C will make leukemic cell colonies grow in a few instances.

Apparently, vitamin C also lashes out at certain bad cells while leaving good cells unharmed. A group of researchers from France and Texas found that vitamin C is selectively toxic to at least one type of malignant cell—a melanoma. They also observed that the vitamin C levels needed were at concentrations that might be attained in future studies with humans (*Nature,* April, 1980).

The researchers extracted both cancerous and noncancerous cells from mice. Then they placed the cells in two separate cultures and added vitamin C. The malignant, or melanotic, cells showed a 50 percent decrease in colony formation, cell number and their ability to stay alive.

"Vitamin C may directly inhibit the growth of proliferating cells, and this might explain some of the reported carcinostatic [cancer suppressing] effects," the researchers write. They also note that the preferential toxicity of vitamin C for melanoma cells was greatly increased when small amounts of copper were added.

Cancer Patients Helped

That's great for mouse cells in a dish, but what about vitamin C's effect on cancer patients? Well, a Japanese hospital has been giving cancer patients the vitamin since 1968. Until 1977, they had given smaller doses to some patients, but they found such positive results that they decided to give large doses (5 grams or more per day) to all.

Of patients in the early stages of the disease, 69 percent receiving large doses were still alive at the time of the report, while only 29 percent of those receiving small doses survived. Most striking was the fate of those patients who had been declared terminal: "The average survival time after being pronounced terminal was 43 days for the low-ascorbate [vitamin C] patients and 201 days for the high-ascorbate patients." And further: "None of the low-ascorbate patients survived more than 174 days, whereas 18 (33 percent) of the high-ascorbate group survived longer than 174 days, their average being 483 days (886 days for the 6 still living).

"In many patients, the administration of vitamin C seems to improve the state of well-being, as indicated by better appetite, increased mental alertness, and a desire to return to ordinary life" *(Journal of the International Academy of Preventive Medicine)*.

In light of the Japanese results, a study of 150 advanced cancer patients at the Mayo Clinic needs a closer look. Researchers there found no statistically significant difference in the survival rate, symptoms or apparent well-being of two groups of patients, one of which received 10 grams of vitamin C daily, the other a placebo. They were therefore unable to show evidence of the therapeutic value of high doses of C.

The problem with the Mayo Clinic study was that the patients had already run the gamut of conventional therapy such as chemotherapy and radiation therapy. Their immune systems were wrecked by the toxic effects of the previous therapies, a possibility admitted to by the researchers: "We recognize," they write, "that earlier immunosuppressive treatment might have obscured any benefit provided by [vitamin C]" *(New England Journal of Medicine,* September 27, 1979).

Previous research on cancer victims had far better results. The link between C and the body's immune system is well documented, particularly in cancer victims, who, according to Linus Pauling and other researchers, "generally exhibit diminished immunocompetence and almost invariably have low [white blood cell] ascorbate content.

"The simplest and safest way to enhance immunocompetence in such patients and to ensure that their . . . defense systems are working at maximum efficiency is to increase their ascorbate intake.

"In our view, ascorbate is essential to ensure the working of the immune system" (*Cancer Research,* March, 1979).

Pain Relief

A study of 30 terminal cancer patients given vitamin C by M. L. Riccitelli, M.D., and Edward Elkowitz, D.O., showed "there was no tumor regression," says Dr. Elkowitz, professor at Downstate Medical Center in Brooklyn, New York.

However, Dr. Elkowitz told us, "The patients had less pain, improvement of appetite and improved well-being." And, he notes, the patients taking vitamin C were in far less toxic a state than those patients treated with chemotherapy (anti-cancer chemicals).

The two doctors gave their patients up to 50 grams of vitamin C a day.

"It's probably impossible to give too much because it's harmless," says Dr. Riccitelli, former assistant clinical professor of medicine at the Yale University school of medicine. "After the body is saturated with vitamin C, the rest is metabolized by the liver and excreted."

Dr. Riccitelli himself takes 4 grams a day and believes doing so may help *prevent* cancer. "I'm sure vitamin C works to help prevent cancer," he told us. "Of course, all the evidence is presumptive—you can't *prove* how it works. But that doesn't matter. You can't prove how aspirin works either."

A physician who agrees with him is Ewan Cameron, M.B., Ch.B., a Scottish surgeon who has conducted much of the research on vitamin C and cancer, particularly on patients with advanced cancer.

"I'm pretty convinced that if people maintained a reasonable . . . intake [of vitamin C], that we would see a diminished incidence of cancer," Dr. Cameron told us.

"If you can alter, even a little, the very, very advanced cancer patients, then all logic suggests you should be able to alter the very early stages of the illness," he told us. "And, of course, the earliest stage of the illness is before the person has cancer at all.''

Tumor Growth Reversed

And in Dr. Cameron's studies on advanced cancer patients, the disease was sometimes altered more than a little.

"We published a paper reporting dramatic relief of bone pain in four out of five patients with skeletal cancer," he says. "Bone cancer is usually a pretty painful situation . . . . Vitamin C, however, relieves the pain. And this is not because vitamin C is, itself, a pain reliever or a narcotic. It's because the pain is due to the steady expansion of the tumor against the inelastic bone. Vitamin C slows down the expansion and thus relieves the pain.''

Dr. Cameron has seen cases in which vitamin C not only slowed down tumor growth, but reversed it.

"One old man, a stationmaster, came in with cancer of the pancreas. I operated on him and he went home. He wasn't given vitamin C yet. Four or five months later, he came back with a big, malignant liver. He wasn't going to die that week, but he was a very sick man. Very definitely on a downhill slope. We started him off on vitamin C and his liver shrank back in size and, contrary to many expectations, he went home.''

Over the past eight years, Dr. Cameron has compared the survival time of terminal cancer patients who receive vitamin C to similar patients who don't. He has found that vitamin C increases survival time by an average of 330 or more days (some of the patients are still alive)—*to 6.6 times longer than patients who don't get vitamin C.*

Cancer Prevention

But the studies mentioned so far are of ways in which vitamin C is used to tackle cancer cells which already exist. Other researchers are taking a different approach. They're trying to find out if vitamin C intake can *prevent* cancer cells from developing in the first place, as Drs. Riccitelli and Cameron believe.

According to the National Cancer Institute, about 77,000 Americans develop colon cancer annually, and 42,800 die from it. But there is a lower incidence of colon and rectal cancer in Florida and the southeastern United States, as well as in California and Arizona. The incidence of large-bowel cancer is one-half the national average in those regions, note Henry C. Lyko and James X. Hartmann, Ph.D., who conducted their research at Florida Atlantic University. They suggest that the increased consumption of citrus fruit, which is high in vitamin C, may be the reason. Regular citrus consumption is part of the southeastern Florida lifestyle, they report, and two-thirds of the families there have an average of three citrus trees per household.

The scientists say that people who consume diets high in beef, fats and proteins are at a higher risk of developing large-bowel cancer. But ". . . there is increasing evidence that vitamin C may prevent the development of large-bowel cancer," says Lyko, "and the most encouraging aspect of these findings is that it may be easier to get Americans to supplement their diets with citrus or vitamin C than persuade them to change their dietary habits appreciably."

At Children's Hospital in Los Angeles, researchers have scrutinized vitamin C from another angle. What happens when normal cells are exposed to a carcinogen, and vitamin C is added afterward? Can vitamin C keep tumors from forming? William F. Benedict, M.D., and Peter A. Jones, Ph.D., are only at the earliest stages of working out those questions, but preliminary results are encouraging.

Vitamin C Inhibits Cell Transformation

The researchers took mouse embryo cells and exposed them to a carcinogen for 24 hours. Then they removed the carcinogen and immediately added vitamin C to some of the exposed cells. They found that vitamin C completely prevented cell transformation that normally occurs after exposure to cancer-causing agents.

In a second experiment, the researchers found they could wait as long as 23 days before adding vitamin C to the exposed cells and still get the same results. The vitamin C completely inhibited the cell transformation.

Then the researchers took cells that had already transformed and never before been in contact with vitamin C. They divided the transformed cells into two groups. Vitamin C was added to one group of transformed cells. The second group was left alone. "The dish of transformed cells that got the vitamin C changed back into normal-appearing cells," Dr. Benedict told us. That doesn't happen in every instance, however.

If you took transformed cells and added vitamin C to them, 75 percent of the cells would go back to normal, Dr. Benedict explains. The remaining 25 percent would still be in the transformed state. They would not change back, despite the addition of vitamin C.

"We think the transformation process of a cell is a progression," says Dr. Benedict. "Vitamin C may revert a cell back to normal if the transformation process has only gone so far."

Is there any difference between normal cells and the transformed cells that suddenly appear normal after getting vitamin C? "We don't think there is," says Dr. Benedict.

The doses of vitamin C used were much smaller than those used in other studies, and once the transformed cells had reverted to normal, the researchers discovered the vitamin was no longer needed.

"When we took the vitamin C away, the cells did not transform again," says Dr. Benedict. The vitamin C apparently made an irreversible change in the cells, and they remained normal in appearance. "Usually, when you take other cancer-blocking agents away, within three or four days you have transformed cells appearing in the dish again."

He emphasizes that their research does not address the question of vitamin C's effects on cells *after* they have become a tumor. The relevancy of their findings ties in with blocking a tumor from forming. Vitamin C may change transformed cells back into their normal state before they grow into a tumor, he says.

The researchers hope their results can be duplicated in whole-animal studies, such as those with guinea pigs.

Like humans, guinea pigs are unable to produce vitamin C inside their bodies. The scientists are interested also in learning if vitamin C can prevent cell transformations in the same manner after X rays.

They are cautious about their findings, but they also are excited about them. "We were quite surprised by the results," admits Dr. Benedict, "and as we go along, we get more and more surprised."

CHAPTER
51

USING CORTISONE DRUGS? BETTER CHECK YOUR VITAMIN C!

In our overmedicated society, where doctors write prescriptions as automatically as politicians offer handshakes, you don't have to look very far to find someone who is taking one of the steroid drugs—cortisone, hydrocortisone, prednisone or a related compound. In fact, chances are good that anyone who's ever experienced even a moderate bout of arthritis or any other form of painful inflammation or swelling has taken a steroid or corticosteroid at least for a short time—perhaps you included.

Despite the frequency with which they are prescribed, however, steroids are far from harmless medications. Some of their undesirable side effects are so predictable and so severe that people forced to take them over long periods eventually run into health complications that can overshadow their *original* problems. That's why it's encouraging to learn of growing indications that a stepped-up intake of nutrients, especially vitamin C, can counteract some of the nastiest side effects.

One of the most dangerous and widely recognized consequences of prescribed steroids is reduced resistance to infection. A report by Ellen Ginzler, M.D., assistant professor of medicine at Downstate Medical Center in Brooklyn, New York, gives a new insight into the magnitude of the problem. Dr. Ginzler noted that, among 223 patients with systemic lupus erythematosus—an inflammatory disease that causes a breakdown of connective tissue—high doses of prednisone were directly tied to increased bacterial and fungal infections *(Medical Tribune)*.

Drug-related infection was the cause or major contributing factor in 30 of 55 deaths among patients in the study group. And there were 354 nonfatal infections. Such infections tended to rise as steroid dosage went up.

"No one is particularly surprised. Other studies have suggested the same relationship of steroids to infection," Dr. Ginzler said, "but this is the first study that has specifically looked at the question, trying to separate out the potential risk factors." The results, she added, "strengthen our resolve to minimize steroid therapy" in treating lupus.

But drug-prescribing habits aren't changed overnight, even in the face of hard evidence. What about the hundreds of thousands of Americans who are taking cortisone and other steroids now, and for whom doctors will continue to prescribe those drugs? Here's where new evidence suggests that supplementary vitamin C may be valuable.

Steroids increase the risk of infection by interfering with the ability of tiny colorless corpuscles in the blood, called neutrophils, to engulf and destroy invading bacteria. But extra vitamin C, taken at the same time as the drug, can restore the body's natural defense mechanism and get the neutrophils back on the attack. That's the thrust of recent findings reported by researchers Grant E. Olson and Hiram C. Polk, Jr., M.D., professor and chairman of the department of surgery at the University of Louisville school of medicine.

The Kentucky researchers describe their study in the *Journal of Surgical Research*. Using blood samples collected from normal people, the pair created test-tube mixtures of neutrophils, *Staphylococcus* bacteria and the equivalent of a therapeutic dosage of the steroid drug hydrocortisone. In some samples, vitamin C was added—the equivalent of 2 grams (2,000 milligrams) for a 150-pound man. Other mixtures received no supplementary vitamin C.

Testing revealed that, in the latter samples, the bacteria-killing process was significantly depressed within one hour after the addition of hydrocortisone. But the neutrophil mixtures fortified with vitamin C had a near-normal ability to destroy the staph germs.

The authors concluded that, in patients receiving certain steroids, "ascorbic acid [vitamin C] may be beneficial in reducing the high incidence of infection in this group."

Their findings—and conclusion—parallel a similar study performed by researchers at the Georgetown University hospital, Washington, D.C. In that study, reported in the *Journal of the Reticuloendothelial Society*, blood samples from six patients receiving steroid treatment were exposed to latex particles, meant to simulate a bacterial invasion.

As expected, measurements indicated that among these subjects—who had been taking steroids for from one day to more than five years—neutrophil function was significantly impaired.

But when the same patients were given 2 grams of vitamin C—two 1-gram doses over a 12-hour period—on the very next day it was found that their natural bacteria-fighting mechanisms had returned to normal. And the improvement was rapid, occurring wihin one hour of receiving the second dose of vitamin C.

Steroids Widely Used

If vitamin C can help curb even one of the dangerous adverse effects of steroid drugs, it promises to be of potential value to a large cross section of the American population. For those medications are now being prescribed for a whole host of conditions ranging from treatment of menopause, arthritis, bursitis, asthma, psoriasis and enteritis to kidney disease, eye inflammation and leukemia.

Simply recognizing a particular prescribed drug as a steroid isn't always easy, as they are under a bewildering variety of brand names. For example, Allersone, Cort-Dome, Cortenema, Cortril, Dermacort and Hytone are just some of the brands of hydrocortisone. And prednisone, one of the most popular of the steroids, is marketed by many different companies.

Side effects, as listed in standard prescribing volumes such as the *Physicians' Desk Reference*, are numerous and alarming. In addition to lowered defense against infection, they include peptic ulcers, cataracts, glaucoma, diabetes, heart problems, high blood pressure, delayed wound healing and bone and muscle breakdown.

In addition, people who take steroids continuously for several years to treat a chronic illness often develop a distressing condition known as Cushing's syndrome. Symptoms include painful, fatty swellings on the body, a moon-shaped face, distended abdomen and reduced sexual ability.

Still another side effect, suppressed growth in childhood, also appears to respond favorably to vitamin C. A team of doctors at two hospitals in Athens, Greece, discovered that supplements of 500 milligrams of vitamin C every eight hours helped restore new collagen formation in youngsters taking steroid drugs. Collagen is essential for normal growth, but steroids interfere with its formation. The Greek researchers found that new collagen production was boosted by 52 percent after four days of vitamin C supplementation *(Archives of Disease in Childhood)*.

Given the facts of modern life, cortisone and other steroid drugs are an almost unavoidable part of medical treatment for many people. But we must never forget that they are two-edged swords. Hopefully, as more doctors and patients find out about the counteracting effects of vitamin C, at least some of the terrible consequences of the steroids can be avoided.

52

VITAMIN C AND HEROIN ADDICTION

The heroin addict: His life turned into a hell, the heroin he craves shuts off emotion and sexual desire, warps sleep and, if the needles are dirty, infects the liver and heart.

He has a problem that society, in spite of spending hundreds of millions of dollars, has been largely unable to solve. But he may be helped—perhaps even cured—by a simple substance: vitamin C.

One reason heroin addicts *stay* heroin addicts is that it's physically grueling to go off the drug. Withdrawal symptoms last for days and include runny eyes and nose, sweating, chills, muscle aches and pains, abdominal cramps, diarrhea, loss of appetite and insomnia. Most withdrawal programs deal with those symptoms by treating them with specific drugs: Valium for the insomnia, for instance, or Darvon for the pain. The problem with that approach, however, is that the treatment medications have side effects sometimes as debilitating as the withdrawal symptoms themselves. Also, the medication may itself be addictive! In fact, the most widely accepted treatment for "curing" a heroin addict is giving him methadone—another addictive drug.

What heroin addicts really need is a way to detoxify their

bodies without suffering prolonged withdrawal symptoms. Sound impossible? Not if they take vitamin C.

"Sodium ascorbate [vitamin C] . . . was seen as a cost-effective, convenient, *safe* way to detoxify narcotic addicts," write Valentine Free and Pat Sanders, R.N., former researchers at the San Francisco Drug Treatment Program, who gave large amounts of vitamin C to heroin addicts during their withdrawal (*Journal of Psychedelic Drugs,* July-September, 1979).

The researchers asked 227 addicts—all of whom had used heroin for at least seven years and spent $70 to $100 a day on the drug—to join one of three groups. Group 1 received vitamin C—24 to 48 grams for the first week of withdrawal, then 8 to 12 grams for the next two weeks. Group 2 received "symptomatic relief medications" such as Librium, a tranquilizer. Group 3 also received those medications, but only for three days—for the last 18 days of the detoxification period they received vitamin C. During the entire three weeks of the pilot study, the researchers measured the average number of withdrawal symptoms in each group.

After the first day of the study, the number of withdrawal symptoms in group 1 (vitamin C) was 6.5 while group 2 (medications) had 8 and group 3 (medications–vitamin C) had 9. By the end of the first week, however, group 1 had dropped to 3 symptoms, group 3 had 1.1—and group 2 had 8.

By the end of the second week, the vitamin C group had *no* symptoms, the medication–vitamin C group had 1 symptom and the medication group had 7.5. At the end of the third week, the situation was much the same, with the medicated group dropping to 6.5 symptoms.

They Lost Their Craving for Drugs

And vitamin C helped the addicts in other ways.

The researchers point out that four of the addicts taking vitamin C "reported a loss of 'craving' for drugs." None of the addicts in group 2 noted any change in their desire for drugs.

And, say the authors, the "majority of subjects" in the vitamin C groups "reported the feeling of having increased energy while large amounts of ascorbic acid [vitamin C] were used."

The researchers believe that this increased energy, along with improvements in psychological health caused by vitamin C, should make it easier for detoxified addicts to become responsible citizens: "Patient reports of . . . a sense of well-being add to a greater self-esteem in newly detoxified individuals—a factor which outpatient treatment can build on by encouraging the patient to deal more effectively with the home and community environments."

And, they say, the vitamin C program (which also includes mineral supplements) may help ex-addicts form a new habit— health. "Ascorbic acid and mineral supplements applied to narcotic withdrawal symptoms . . . can easily lead into nutritional counseling and other health perspectives once the detoxification phase has been successfully completed."

This research project was not the first time heroin addicts received large amounts of vitamin C during withdrawal. Irwin Stone, a biochemist who has spent years investigating vitamin C, and an associate conducted a study in which addicts took the nutrient. The results are impressive (*Journal of Orthomolecular Psychiatry*).

"The general improvement in the well-being of the addicts within 12 to 24 hours after beginning sodium ascorbate detoxification is striking," they write. "It is demonstrated by improved mental alertness and visual acuity; appetite is returning, and the addict is amazed that treatment is working without the use of another narcotic."

The scientists also point out a rather incredible observation: If an addict receiving vitamin C uses heroin during the withdrawal period, "it is immediately detoxified and no 'high' is produced. It is like injecting plain water."

Stone and his colleague describe the case of one addict, a 23-year-old who had used heroin since he was 15 and had been through several medication-oriented detoxification programs. "After three days on the regimen," they write, "he began eating and feeling so much better and thinking more clearly . . . and he began to have restful sleep.'' After three months, he was still drug free and had lost his desire for heroin.

In all, the researchers gave vitamin C to 30 addicts. The success rate? "Thirty out of 30 patients were successfully treated.''

CHAPTER
53

BIOFLAVONOIDS FOR HEALTHY CAPILLARIES

Bioflavonoid—the word has a kind of ominous ring to it. You can almost see the movie poster with its garish artwork, the faces of the terrified townspeople, the lurid prose: "What was this strange menace that stalked the city? What did these *things* want? For 24 hours they held an entire community paralyzed with terror! It was—*The Day of the Bioflavonoids!*"

What we're dealing with here is fear of the unknown. The only reason this family of nutrients comes off sounding like some monstrous salad, run amok, is that many of us have never heard of them. The bioflavonoids are often overlooked by nutritional experts, but they have widespread beneficial effects. These "things" are not out to terrorize your town, drain your bodily juices or turn you into a soulless zombi. They come in peace, to help make us all healthier people.

The effects of the bioflavonoids were first observed in 1936 by scientists led by Albert Szent-Györgyi. Dr. Szent-Györgyi, who also discovered vitamin C and was awarded the Nobel Prize for his efforts, noted that, when animals with scurvy were given crude preparations of vitamin C derived from natural sources, they lived longer than animals given pure vitamin C. The impure vitamin C was more effective in healing the capillary (tiny blood vessel) damage that is characteristic of scurvy. Dr. Szent-Györgyi reasoned that there must have been some additional substance present in the impure vitamin C that boosted its healing effects.

That substance was actually a group of compounds, the bioflavonoids. Dr. Szent-Györgyi and his colleagues found that these compounds act to strengthen the capillaries and stop capillary bleeding by lowering the permeability of the capillary walls. Because of this action, he called the compounds vitamin P, for permeability.

Ralph C. Robbins, Ph.D.—a leading expert on the bioflavonoids and a researcher at the food science and human nutrition department, institute of food and agricultural sciences at the University of Florida, in Gainesville—told us that the scientific world reacted quickly to the discovery. "Soon after Dr. Szent-Györgyi discovered the activity of bioflavonoids in animals, a great number of people studied the compounds and found that the biolfavonoids seemed to produce beneficial effects in some 50 diseases."

In most cases, the effects of the bioflavonoids could be traced to their action in the capillaries. These miniscule blood vessels are the link in the circulatory system joining the arteries and the veins. There are some 3.6 billion capillaries, located in virtually every part of the body. The capillaries, and the capillaries alone, carry out the chief purpose of the circulatory system—they deliver oxygen and nutrients to the body's tissues and remove poisonous wastes.

"The important role which capillary dysfunction plays in many diseases is fully recognized by the medical profession, for it is in the capillary system that the essential exchange of body fluids takes place," a team of American scientists told the 20th International Congress of Physiology (*Journal of the American Geriatrics Society*).

Boris Sokoloff, M.D., William Coda Martin, M.D., and Clarence Saelhof, M.D., in a paper delivered to the congress in Brussels, Belgium, listed a variety of diseases in which failure of the capillaries to function properly was a problem. "In viral hepatitis, poliomyelitis, smallpox, measles, primary atypical pneumonia, mumps, virus A influenza, St. Louis encephalitis and other viral infections, capillary fragility and hemorrhage have been observed." The scientists also reported that capillary problems were a factor in arteriosclerosis, hypertension, rheumatoid arthritis, diabetes and bleeding ulcers.

The paper described the researchers' use of bioflavonoids to treat a number of these disorders, particularly those which are likely to strike older people. Age itself tends to produce capillary problems. Tests of 189 patients, age 53 to 88, found that 124 of them, about 64 percent, suffered from capillary fragility. Patients in the group who had high blood pressure were more likely to have capillary problems than those who did not.

The researchers treated 30 of these patients, including 19 suffering from high blood pressure, with bioflavonoids for a period of four weeks. In only one instance was there no change in the patient's condition. In two cases, there was some improvement, and in the remaining 27, the functioning of the capillaries was either completely, or very nearly, restored to normal.

Dr. Sokoloff and his colleagues followed the case histories of 13 patients who had suffered "little strokes"—recurring, relatively minor episodes of bleeding in the brain that, over the course of time, can produce paralysis, palsy, failing intellectual power and personality changes. The problem occurs mostly in older people. The scientists administered 600 milligrams of bioflavonoids daily to the 13 patients. One patient died of a stroke two weeks after his treatment began, and 2 others moved to another city and left the study after a short period of time. The condition of the remaining patients, observed for periods ranging from 12 to 32 months, either improved or remained satisfactory. None of them suffered further strokes.

Because of evidence that capillary fragility was a problem in arthritis, the scientists examined the case histories of 45 arthritis patients treated with bioflavonoids. While the changes were not dramatic, significant improvement was noted in 20 patients, and only 10 patients showed no improvement at all. Patients who had had arthritis for the shortest time responded best to the treatment. The bioflavonoids are hardly a miracle cure for arthritis, the doctors concluded, but "they can be recommended as a supplement to other methods of treatment."

Bioflavonoids have been found effective in countering several of the complications of diabetes. In diabetes, and also in cases of high blood pressure, inflammation of the retina is a frequent problem. The retina is located at the back of the eyeball, where the images we see are received and carried to the brain by the optic nerve. Inflammation of the retina results in impaired vision and is accompanied by the buildup of waxy excretions from the blood vessels. One-sixth of all cases of acquired blindness are the result of retinal disease in diabetics.

Dr. Sokoloff and his colleagues found that, in 85 percent of 198 cases of retinal inflammation treated with bioflavonoids, the bleeding in the retina was promptly controlled.

Cataracts Prevented

Cataract formation, a clouding over of the lens of the eye that can produce blindness, is another possible complication of diabetes. Scientists at the National Eye Institute in Bethesda, Maryland, have found that one of the bioflavonoids, quercitrin, is capable of holding off the development of cataracts in diabetic laboratory animals (*Science*).

In this case, the action of the bioflavonoids has nothing to do with their effects on the capillaries. In 1975, the same team of scientists at the institute reported that several of the bioflavonoids inhibited the action of an enzyme, called aldose reductase, that had been found to play an important part in the formation of diabetic cataracts (*Science*). Three of the bioflavonoids— quercetin, quercitrin and myricitrin—were more powerful inhibitors of the enzyme than anything previously tested.

The researchers decided to test the effects of quercitrin, the most potent of the three, in diabetic animals. They used a South American rodent called the degu, which, because of its particular susceptibility to the action of aldose reductase, invariably develops cataracts 10 to 12 days after the onset of diabetes. The diabetic degus that were not fed quercitrin developed cataracts right on schedule, after about 10 days. The degus receiving the bioflavonoid, however, were free of cataracts 25 days after the onset of the diabetes, even though the levels of sugar in their blood were roughly the same as the levels in the other animals.

Treating Bleeding Disorders

We could go on at great length here about the action of the bioflavonoids in various diseases. Almost any problem that involves bleeding seems to have been alleviated at one time or another by bioflavonoids.

Scientists in France found that the bioflavonoids were a highly effective alternative to hormone therapy in the treatment of abnormal uterine bleeding in women *(Family Practice News)*. The French doctors also reported that the bioflavonoid treatment corrected abnormal menstrual bleeding in 39 of 40 women who had problems following the insertion of an intrauterine contraceptive devide (IUD).

These researchers found that the treatment provided relief for pregnant women suffering from varicose veins, and other studies have shown that a bioflavonoid–vitamin C complex relieves the hot flashes which occur in menopause *(Chicago Medicine)*.

Bioflavonoids have been shown to reduce inflammation in bacterial and viral infections. That is important because of the side effects associated with the use of steroids, the standard anti-inflammatory agents. Scientists in Europe have demonstrated that a complex of bioflavonoids, vitamin C and two anti-inflammatory enzymes acts against a wider variety of inflammations than seven other nonsteroid anti-inflammatory substances and produces no side effects whatsoever *(Arzneimittel-Forschung/Drug Research)*.

Less Blood Cell Clumping

So the bioflavonoids are active against a hodge-podge of many disorders. Coming up with one neat explanation for all these effects is probably impossible, but the bioflavonoids' action in the capillaries is certainly of major importance. Dr. Robbins has done extensive work in this area and believes that the bioflavonoids' effects on capillary permeability may be linked to their regulation of a tendency of blood cells to clump together.

In 1971, Dr. Robbins established that the bioflavonoids have a direct effect on blood cell aggregation, the clumping together of blood cells which often occurs in states of illness *(Clinical Chemistry)*. "Decreased blood cell aggregation," he wrote, "may explain the reported beneficial effects of flavonoids on abnormal capillary permeability and fragility, the decreased symptoms in many diseases, and the protective effect against various traumas and stresses.

"An effect of aggregation is decreased capillary blood flow . . . . Decreased blood flow may be reflected in changes in capillary permeability and resistance to rupture."

Dr. Robbins reported that research had demonstrated a close relationship between blood flow and capillary permeability. When blood flow through the capillaries is blocked, the capillaries become more permeable and components of the blood are lost; when the blood flow is restored, the capillaries return to normal. What happens, then, is that bioflavonoids decrease blood cell clumping, which increases blood flow and results in less permeable, healthier capillaries.

"There are several hundred different bioflavonoid compounds in patients," Dr. Robbins told us. "The ones in citrus fruits are the most active in the body." Because their formation depends on the action of sunlight, bioflavonoids are usually concentrated in the outer tissues of plants, for example, in the rind and peels of oranges.

The bioflavonoids act in plants as natural preservatives, retarding the growth of bacteria and working to prevent the destruction of vitamin C by oxidation. This preservative action is so strong that bioflavonoid-rich onions and garlic, and juices prepared from green pepper, celery, potato peels and tomatoes, have all been shown to preserve the quality of meats.

These things are not visitors from a distant galaxy, after all. The bioflavonoids are an important part of a natural, nutritious diet. They can, and should, become as familiar to you as your own back-yard garden.

CHAPTER
54

HEALING WITH BIOFLAVONOIDS

Mike is prone to colds. So he takes vitamin C. Still, he sniffles and sneezes.

Mary is anemic. So she takes iron supplements until she worries she'll rust in the rain. But still, she feels tired at the end of the day.

John's nose is apt to bleed for no apparent reason. So he eats more vitamin K–rich leafy vegetables to enhance blood clotting. And still, his nosebleeds persist.

Although their symptoms may be different, the solutions to their problems may be the same: All three may be helped by taking bioflavonoids.

Unfortunately, most of us don't eat as many fresh fruits and vegetables as we should, and very few of us eat the skins, membranes and rinds of citrus fruits, which are among the richest sources of bioflavonoids. But increasing our intake of these important nutrients may help clear up a host of nagging health problems we often mistake for symptoms of something else.

The major trauma of a miscarriage, the minor annoyance of a nosebleed and assorted ailments in between may respond well to bioflavonoid therapy because bioflavonoids are particularly adept at strengthening capillary walls.

Babies Carried to Term

As a result, certain young women would do well to baby themselves with bioflavonoid supplements.

"I believe some miscarriages occur because of increased fragility of placental capillaries, and bioflavonoid supplements seem to help toughen those capillaries," says Jack C. Redman, M.D., a family practitioner in Albuquerque, New Mexico. He prescribes citrus bioflavonoids for his patients who suffer from chronic miscarriages. Dr. Redman, who is also a diplomate of the American Board of Family Practice, told us his results with the bioflavonoid therapy have been excellent.

"I've had success giving bioflavonoids to women who have had two, three, even four miscarriages," Dr. Redman explains. "I tell them to begin taking the supplements immediately the next time they become pregnant, and it almost always works. My results have been very encouraging."

Dr. Redman usually prescribes 200 milligrams taken three times a day, for a total of 600 milligrams daily. He tells of one patient who miscarried her first pregnancy but took the bioflavonoids for the duration of the second. "Although she experienced some spotty bleeding during her third month, she carried a beautiful baby girl to term," Dr. Redman recalls. "In that case, as in several others, I found evidence of an old blood clot after I delivered the placenta."

Bioflavonoids Regulate Blood Cells

Another bioflavonoid researcher has found that the bioflavonoids from a grapefruit a day may keep heart problems at bay.

Oranges, lemons, tangerines and grapefruits are good sources of citrus bioflavonoids. Various components present in all of them make up the bioflavonoid complex, but individual constituents of the bioflavonoid-complex family may vary slightly among the different fruits. Their duties vary slightly, too. For instance, bioflavonoids derived from grapefruit help regulate hematocrit levels, which reflect the ratio of red blood cells to whole blood, according to Dr. Ralph C. Robbins, Ph.D., of the food science and human nutrition department, institute of food and agricultural sciences at the University of Florida, in Gainesville. Dr. Robbins is one of the foremost scientists in bioflavonoid research today, and he and others have found that high hematocrit levels are a constant finding in people who are subject to heart attacks.

"In fact, a high hematocrit appears to be a risk factor for heart attacks and strokes," says Dr. Robbins, adding that "high hematocrits were a constant finding with heart attack victims in the famous 'Framingham study,' which established the link between life style and heart disease."

In one of his own studies, Dr. Robbins took 40 people who had a wide range of hematocrit levels and placed them on a diet that included a grapefruit a day—no other restrictions were applied. After 12 weeks, there was a significant drop in the hematocrit levels in the high-hematocrit group (including several heart attack patients) but no significant drop in the hematocrits of individuals already in the ideal range. In addition, those with low hematocrit levels rose to the normal range.

That's important, Dr. Robbins points out, because low hematocrit levels are indicative of anemia. "Hematocrit levels too high and too low are both unhealthy. What we are finding out is that grapefruit helps to stabilize hematocrit levels. Evidence indicates the effect is due to the bioflavonoid naringin."

Some of the other bioflavonoids that have been isolated include rutin, from buckwheat and other natural sources, hesperidin, from oranges and lemons, and tangeretin, from tangerines.

"There are so many bioflavonoids, and their activity varies according to a number of factors, including a person's blood type," notes Dr. Robbins. Most fruits and vegetables contain dozens of different ones, and most bioflavonoid supplements are available in complex form.

"Citrus is a regular cornucopia of flavonoids," says Russel Rouseff, Ph.D., of the Florida Department of Citrus at the University of Florida agricultural research center in Lake Alfred, Florida. "There are at least 40 individual flavonoids that have been identified in citrus. Most of them have been reported to have biological activity. Those are the ones we call *bio*flavonoids."

If you get all your citrus in the form of juice, you may be missing out on many of the most active bioflavonoids, which are found in the rind, the membranes between the fruit segments and in the white, spongy layer called the albedo, just under the rind. Many of the citrus fruits sold in supermarkets have been artificially colored. Powdered citrus peel sold to flavor baked goods, however, has usually not been dyed. Dr. Rouseff believes such products may be good sources of bioflavonoids.

Protection from Cancer

Many bioflavonoids seem to help protect our bodies from the cancer-causing effects of pollutants such as benzpyrene, which is released into the air when some synthetic compounds are burned. Bioflavonoids increase the anti-cancer activity of certain enzymes found in our skin, lungs, gastrointestinal tract and liver. These enzymes metabolize foreign compounds, according to Dr. Robbins, and help convert fat-soluble carcinogens (cancer-causing agents) to water-soluble form so they may be safely excreted from the body. Citrus bioflavonoids are particularly potent in this regard, he notes.

Other researchers have reported on some of the anti-cancer effects of vitamin C. Bioflavonoids may lend a helping hand here, too, because bioflavonoids have been shown to increase the body's absorption of vitamin C. In one Czechoslovakian study, researchers found that guinea pigs absorbed twice as much vitamin C if they were given supplements of rutin and another bioflavonoid at the same time they were given the vitamin C supplement (*Physiologia Bohemoslovaca,* vol. 28, 1979). Like people, guinea pigs are unable to manufacture their own vitamin C within their bodies and must rely on outside sources to get it.

Natural Antihistamines

Neutralizing the cancer-causing agents in air pollution and enhancing the absorption of vitamin C, known for its benefits as an antihistamine, aren't the only ways bioflavonoids may keep us breathing easily. Bioflavonoids are pretty good antihistamines themselves.

According to Elliott Middleton, Jr., M.D., director of the allergy division in the departments of medicine and pediatrics, school of medicine, State University of New York in Buffalo, the bioflavonoid quercetin will inhibit the release of histamine from white blood cells. During a typical allergy attack, histamine is released, causing red, watery eyes, stuffy nose, sneezing, itching and impaired breathing.

Dr. Middleton found that quercetin will also inactivate certain viruses, including herpes type 1 (cold sores) virus, polio virus, parainfluenza virus and a particular respiratory virus that afflicts young children and may be a forerunner of asthma. Although the effectiveness of quercetin under normal dietary conditions has not been established, Dr. Middleton speculates that "certain naturally occurring flavonoids may have a role in antiviral therapy" (*Journal of Allergy and Clinical Immunology,* January, 1982).

Across the country, in Portland, Oregon, nutritional consultant Brian Leibovitz relies on bioflavonoids to keep his allergic patients comfortable throughout the hay fever season. "But bioflavonoids work even better on asthma," Leibovitz told us. "In fact, a standard treatment for asthma, a drug called cromolyn sodium, is nothing more than a synthetic bioflavonoidlike molecule."

For those people bedeviled by another nose problem—frequent nosebleeds—bioflavonoids may offer some hope, also.

In his extensive research, Boris Sokoloff, M.D., successfully used bioflavonoids to treat chronic nosebleeds in 45 people. All of them took 300 milligrams at four-hour intervals for a total of 1,500 milligrams of bioflavonoids a day, and all of them were cured—in some cases in as little as 36 hours!

Help for Cold Sores

Bioflavonoids and vitamin C can help your body heal cold sores in half the time usually required, according to Geza T. Terezhalmy, D.D.S., and other researchers at the National Naval Dental Center in Bethesda, Maryland. The painful blisters that erupt in the mouth and around the lips are the result of infection by the herpes simplex virus (type 1). Fever or exposure to cold, heat, sun, wind or rain often bring about this disfiguring nuisance in susceptible people. Between 80 and 90 percent of us get them at some time in our lives, and about 40 percent have the problem over and over again.

But Dr. Terezhalmy and his colleagues found a way to significantly reduce the time it takes for these annoying sores to heal: supplements of bioflavonoids and vitamin C. Dr. Terezhalmy decided to use water-soluble bioflavonoids and vitamin C because of the many reports that these two substances can be an aid in healing. Vitamin C, he said, appears to play an important role in maintaining the strength of the blood vessels and forming the substances that hold the cells together. Bioflavonoids, he said, have been reported to strengthen the walls of the blood vessels. He told us that a combination of bioflavonoids and vitamin C has been used to successfully treat bleeding gums and viral infections characterized by fragile blood vessels.

Applying this to the problem of herpes simplex infections of the lips and mouth, Dr. Terezhalmy believes that the progression of the inflammation requires weakening of the tiny blood vessels in the tissue and damage to the cement holding the cells together. Dr. Terezhalmy wanted to find out, then, if the tissue-strengthening ability of bioflavonoids would help protect the lips and mouth from the herpes infection.

So he assembled 50 volunteers with recurrent herpes infections on the lips and mouth. Twenty were treated with 600 milligrams each of bioflavonoids and vitamin C divided into three daily doses. Twenty were treated with 1,000 milligrams each of bioflavonoids and vitamin C divided into five daily doses. The other 10 were treated with a lactose dummy pill. Neither the patients nor the examining doctors knew which patients were getting which treatments until the end of the experiment. The standards used to judge the effects of the treatment were the visible signs and symptoms of the infection: itching and feeling of fullness in the affected area, pain, formation of blisters, crusting and disappearance of the blisters.

Before the treatment was begun, there was no significant difference between those who received dummy pills and those who received bioflavonoids and vitamin C. But after the treatment began, the differences were remarkable.

The most remarkable difference, Dr. Terezhalmy told us, was in the duration of symptoms. People treated with the dummy pills were symptom free after an average of 9.7 days. But those treated with 600 milligrams of bioflavonoids and 600 milligrams of vitamin C were completely symptom free after only 4.2 days. There was no significant difference in healing time between those given 600 milligrams of bioflavonoids and those given 1,000 milligrams.

Another interesting result Dr. Terezhalmy mentioned was that all 10 of the placebo-treated people developed multiple blisters, which broke during the course of the infection. But only 36 percent of the bioflavonoid-treated group developed blisters. Giving the treatment early in the course of the infection seemed to make a difference. When bioflavonoids and vitamin C were given at the first sign of symptoms, only 6 out of 26 developed blisters. But when it was given 12 hours or more after the first symptoms, 8 out of 12 developed blisters.

Dr. Terezhalmy told us, "There really hasn't been any adequate treatment for this disease until now, nothing that will actually abort the process of blister formation and minimize the other clinical manifestations.''

"The beauty of all this is that these compounds are in our food,'' muses Dr. Robbins, and Dr. Redman agrees. "Today, bioflavonoids are a by-product of the orange-juice industry,'' Dr. Redman notes, "but I've heard that someday orange juice will be a by-product of the bioflavonoid industry.''

VITAMIN D

CHAPTER

55

DON'T LET THIN BONES LET YOU DOWN

One reason why falls of any kind are more likely to result in fractures for people over 50 is the prevalence of a bone-thinning condition called osteoporosis. As the bones gradually become demineralized, mishaps that once caused bruises are more likely to result in breaks. However, new evidence suggests you can fight back, because osteoporosis, once thought to be an unavoidable consequence of aging, may be preventable. The secret is no fancy trick, either: simply a combination of measures including early diagnosis, calcium supplements, vigorous exercise and vitamin D.

"Osteoporosis in the elderly is an epidemic that's received far too little attention," contends Robert Recker, M.D., chief of endocrinology at Creighton University in Omaha, Nebraska. Indeed, of the six million Americans affected each year, most will be postmenopausal women over 45. And the annual cost of treating fractured hips exceeds $1 billion.

Everyone begins losing bone mineral at around 40 years of age, but women who've had few or no pregnancies are at greatest risk of suffering the fractures that are the major clinical feature of osteoporosis. And except for the use of the hormone estrogen, which has been suspect because of its link to uterine cancer, most therapies for this bone disease are still in the early investigative stages.

For these reasons, "prevention is more important than treatment," declares Harold Draper, Ph.D., chairman of the nutrition department at Guelph University in Ontario. But how do you guard your bones from becoming riddled with holes like Swiss cheese?

Essential to the health of strong bones is vitamin D, the "sunshine vitamin." For most people, the main input is via the skin, where ultraviolet light from the sun converts a form of cholesterol into vitamin D. Vitamin D can also be obtained directly from the diet, in fish liver oils, egg yolks and fortified milk. However, if you're swaddled in heavy clothes all winter, barely touch milk and live in the North, you may have decreased levels of vitamin D in your blood by springtime.

That's cause for concern because, without vitamin D, the body cannot properly utilize calcium. Consequently, bone health suffers and the bones deteriorate, lose calcium and are more susceptible to fractures. Thus, bones are most likely to break in winter and early spring, when the days are short, sunlight (and hence vitamin D) is scarce and calcium availability in the body is low.

D Deters Bone Deterioration

And many studies demonstrate vitamin D's practical benefits. During one investigation, researchers gave a concentrated form of vitamin D to seven women with osteoporosis, all of whom had suffered at least one fractured vertebra. During the year of treatment, the women had an improvement in their calcium balance so that "no further vertebral compression fractures were sustained during the treatment period" (*Clinical Research*).

In a similar study, researchers gave patients with osteoporosis a concentrated form of vitamin D and either 1 or 2 grams of calcium a day (*Clinical Endocrinology*).

The first part of the study lasted a week. Seventeen people received the nutrients. Six had senile osteoporosis, which is "caused" by old age. Five had postmenopausal osteoporosis, which is caused by the postmenopausal decrease in the production of estrogen, a female hormone that plays a role in regulating bone mass. (Almost *every* woman suffers from some degree of osteoporosis within ten years of her menopause.) Six had corticosteroid-induced osteoporosis, which is caused by long, constant use of corticosteroids, anti-inflammatory drugs. A diverse group. But in just one week, every single person had "a significant increase in calcium absorption rate"—a sign that the disease was improving.

Physical Activity Improved

The patients with postmenopausal osteoporosis continued into the second part of the study, which lasted over a year, and were joined by five new patients with senile osteoporosis.

By the end of the study, nine of the ten patients had "greatly improved" physical activity. All but one "became more mobile." And of the five patients who had needed a cane, three no longer did.

The slow, shuffling walk and limited physical activity of those with osteoporosis and osteomalacia may be caused not only by *bone* loss, but by *muscle* loss.

In 1965, researchers discovered that osteoporotic women lost muscle as well as bone. Research has also shown that vitamin D has a direct effect on muscular health. In a study focusing on that link, researchers gave a concentrated form of vitamin D and 1 gram of calcium a day to 11 osteoporotic women for three to six months. At the beginning and end of the study, they measured the women's muscular health (*Clinical Science*, vol. 56, no. 2, 1979).

One of the measurements was a "time dressing test," in which the researchers measured the women's muscular mobility by timing how long it took them to put on stockings, vest, underpants, shirt and a frock. Before the women began taking the nutrients, they needed an average of 3 minutes and 30 seconds to dress. At the end of the study, they needed only 2 minutes and 52 seconds. One woman, who took over 5 minutes to dress at the start of the study, needed just over 2 minutes at the end.

The researchers also measured favorable biochemical changes in the muscle itself. "We suggest," the researchers write, that the patients "had some kind of myopathy [muscle disease] induced by an insufficient production . . . of vitamin D."

CHAPTER

56

THE SUNSHINE VITAMIN CAN BRIGHTEN YOUR HEALTH

You might be a little skeptical of those people who loudly announce their plans to leave the 20th century behind—just deposit their credit cards, mortgage payments and pocket calculators at the edge of the woods and "return to nature." But the truth is, no matter how "civilized" your style of life may be, your body never *left* nature; it's still intimately attuned to the grand procession of natural cycles. And that's something you can ignore only at your peril.

During the winter months, for example, your body responds to the low-lying winter sun with an ebb in the chemical tides that transform calcium and phosphorus into bone. How can the sun's angle affect bone growth? Through vitamin D, a remarkable substance that is synthesized in your skin when it's struck by ultraviolet light and which goes on to play a key role in your body's calcium metabolism.

During the short, dim days of winter, when you're either indoors or bundled up much of the time, lack of sunshine on your skin can result in a steady drain on your vitamin D supply until, by late winter or early spring, your bones may actually begin to ache. Worse, if this shortage is allowed to continue, newly formed bone can become soft and misshapen—a condition known as osteomalacia, or adult rickets.

Fortunately, there's a way around this problem short of waltzing around the back yard in the buff. Ordinarily, you manufacture most of the vitamin D you use through this magical meeting of the skin and sun (hence its nickname, "the sunshine vitamin"), but vitamin D is also available, though not plentiful, in the natural food supply. By making sure your diet is adequate in vitamin D—and seeking out the sun during the darkest months—you can make it through winter without the dull aches and pains of a deficiency. Unfortunately, studies show many people experience a sharp decline in their vitamin D supply during the winter.

One such study was conducted by doctors at the University of Dundee, in Dundee, Scotland, where levels of ultraviolet light in sunshine are "very low or negligible" from November through February. Over a period of a year, the researchers studied the vitamin D status of three groups of people by measuring their serum levels of the major circulating form of vitamin D, 25-hydroxy-vitamin D, or 25-OHD for short.

The groups were divided according to occupation and amount of exposure to sunlight: Gardeners in the local parks department worked outdoors all day, winter and summer; hospital staffers got their sunshine mostly on weekends or after work; and a group of elderly inpatients, who were confined indoors, received virtually no natural or artificial sunlight at all.

The results showed that "in each group the seasonal changes were highly significant," with the highest 25-OHD levels recorded during the late summer and autumn and the lowest during the late winter or early spring. And "25-OHD levels were higher in the outdoor workers than in the indoor workers, who in turn had higher values than did the elderly inpatients" (*American Journal of Clinical Nutrition*, August, 1981).

The researchers noted something else of interest: The more sunshine the subjects got, the later in the season their 25-OHD levels peaked. While ultraviolet light was strongest in July, for example, the gardeners reached their highest levels in November; the inpatients peaked in August.

Perhaps, the researchers suggested, "in the outdoor workers, vitamin D synthesis continues well into the autumn with continued exposure and so vitamin D stores continue to increase."

What all this means to your health was demonstrated in another study conducted by a trio of doctors in Leeds, England. The doctors examined biopsies from hip bones of 134 patients who had suffered suspicious fractures of the femur, or thigh bone, over a period of five years. They concluded that 37 percent of the patients were suffering from osteomalacia. But what was most disturbing was the fact that by far the largest number of fractures occurred in a period stretching from February through June *(Lancet)*.

"As would be expected if this seasonal variation was attributable to variation in the supply of vitamin D dependent on sunlight, the proportion of cases with osteomalacia is highest in the spring and lowest in the autumn," they noted.

Why is there a two-month to six-month time lag between the shortest days of the year (the third week in December) and the appearance of fractures caused by weakened bones? Well, vitamin D is fat-soluble and thus easily stored by the body. Your cupboards may be full to overflowing by the end of the summer and not run out until late winter or even early summer. So it's important to take advantage of sunny weather whenever you can.

Elderly at Risk

That reminder is something older people should make special note of. Because, according to a study at Ichilov Hospital in Tel Aviv, the elderly may have trouble making use of vitamin D even if they live in a sunny climate and get plenty of D in the foods they eat.

The Israeli doctors compared serum 25-OHD levels of 82 elderly people and 30 young control subjects. They discovered that 15 of the elderly subjects—nearly 20 percent—had outright vitamin D deficiencies, and 28 more had borderline levels. Even elderly farm workers, who got plenty of sunshine—while their vitamin D status was considerably better than those older people who were confined indoors—were still significantly lower than the youthful control group (*Israeli Journal of Medical Sciences,* January, 1981).

"It seems likely that impairment of vitamin D metabolism at several points in the metabolic pathway, rather than simple underexposure to sunlight, is a major factor in vitamin D deficiency in the elderly," the doctors concluded. They suggested that perhaps aging impairs the body's ability to produce certain active forms of vitamin D, which in turn slows down the absorption of calcium through the intestine. Result: an increased risk of faulty bone mineralization.

There may be other factors working against vitamin D nutrition in older people, according to Michael F. Holick, M.D., Ph.D., of the department of medicine at the Harvard medical school. "Aging significantly reduces the skin's capacity to produce vitamin D_3," Dr. Holick explains. "The skin of a 70-year-old can make about half of the vitamin D_3 precursor produced by a 20-year-old."

Normally, he explains, ultraviolet wavelengths in sunshine, striking your bare skin, convert a lipid substance called 7-dehydrocholesterol into previtamin D_3. Previtamin D_3 is unstable when heated and slowly converts to vitamin D_3 (an active form) in the deeper layers of your skin. You don't actually make vitamin D_3 during sunlight exposure, Dr. Holick told us; it takes three or four days for the whole manufacturing process to run its course, so your body is busy producing vitamin D_3 long after you come in out of the sun.

In the elderly, however, this marvelous machinery has begun to lose its efficiency. "It's not too surprising, really, because age decreases *all* metabolic functions," Dr. Holick says. Also, the skin actually thins with age, so there are fewer cells to synthesize the vitamin.

What's to stop your skin from producing too *much* vitamin D? (Being fat-soluble and thus easily stored, the nutrient can be toxic in high doses.) It's widely believed that tanning is the answer: In response to extended exposure to sunlight, the skin produced melanin, or pigmentation, to shield its deeper vitamin D–producing layers from ultraviolet light. But Dr. Holick contends that, while this may be a factor, it isn't the most important one. His research has shown, he says, that too much sun causes previtamin D_3 to break down into a pair of biologically inert substances, preventing the overproduction of vitamin D.

Too much sun, of course, can also increase your risk of skin cancer and accelerate the aging of your skin. But Dr. Holick believes it may be time to "reevaluate the natural benefits of sunlight" for older people who may not get enough vitamin D in their diet. How much sun should you get? Well, 15 to 30 minutes of sun exposure twice a week in Boston in the summer should be "more than adequate" for lightly pigmented people over 60 years, Dr. Holick says.

Keeping your vitamin D stores in order really shouldn't be too difficult, even if you rarely venture into the sun. A recent study in Norway—at latitude 70 degrees north, where the sun hangs below the horizon a full two months of the year—is a case in point. Over a period of a year, serum 25-OHD levels were examined in 17 healthy adults living in Tromsö. Though the lowest concentration was found in March, blood levels overall remained "at a constant and fairly high level" throughout the year (*Scandinavian Journal of Clinical Laboratory Investigation*, vol. 40, 1980). The researchers attributed this sunny finding to good nutrition and the widespread consumption of dairy products fortified with vitamin D.

Actually, vitamin D isn't very common in the natural food supply. The foods that contain it in high amounts are all of animal origin, with the greatest amounts occurring in saltwater fish high in oil, such as salmon, sardines and herring. Fish liver oils are highly concentrated sources of vitamin D. Egg yolks and liver also contain substantial amounts.

Rickets on the Rise?

The fortification of milk and other milk products since World War II is one reason the childhood bone disease called rickets is today considered, in the words of one researcher, "a medical curiosity." In the days of the industrial revolution, when children were confined to sunless sweatshops in smoggy cities, it was a serious health problem and was still fairly common as late as the 1940s. But by 1969, a survey of over 6,000 children of low-income families showed only 0.1 percent had bowing of the legs (a symptom of rickets).

Yet, recently, some doctors have begun to worry that rickets "may still be a significant problem in some population groups." Over a period of a year, for example, four children from the Hartford, Connecticut, area were diagnosed as having rickets caused by poor diet. The youngsters exhibited classic symptoms of rickets, from bowing of the legs to general weakness, delayed motor development and low weight, but because their doctors were not familiar with the condition, a correct diagnosis wasn't made for months (*Pediatrics*, July, 1980).

After examining the youngsters' dietary histories, doctors concluded that "particular groups of children, namely vegetarians, children breastfed for an unusually long time, and black children, are at risk to develop the nutritional deficiencies of vitamin D and calcium metabolism that lead to clinical rickets." Vegetarians are at risk because they may not get enough milk and milk products, breastfed children because human breast milk may be inadequate in vitamin D—though this is still a controversial point—and black children because their dark skin blocks the ultraviolet light that triggers vitamin D_3 production.

One thing all four youngsters had in common: They turned up at the hospital at the end of winter. After months indoors, or outdoors only when they were buttoned up to the ears, they just hadn't been getting enough sunshine to keep their vitamin D batteries charged and humming. With that was coupled a diet deficient in vitamin D, and by winter's end they were in serious trouble.

Do You Live in the Colon Cancer Belt?

Another reason for keeping well supplied with vitamin D is the possibility that its lack could be linked to colon cancer.

Two scientists who conducted research at Johns Hopkins University in Baltimore have theorized that sunshine and a year-round supply of vitamin D might prevent this killer illness. No one has ever suggested that idea before.

"We have simply shown," says one of the reseachers, Cedric F. Garland, Ph.D., "that there is a predilection for colon cancer in areas that receive less sunlight. As far as we know, this is the first time that anyone has shown a correlation between vitamin D and colon cancer."

In late 1976, Dr. Garland and his brother Frank, a doctoral candidate in epidemiology, were comparing the rates of colon cancer and skin cancer in the United States. In the Sun Belt, skin cancer was common but colon cancer wasn't. In the colder regions, the reverse was true. Intrigued, they borrowed sunshine statistics from the U.S. Weather Service. The numbers pointed to an inverse relationship between sunshine and colon cancer. But Dr. Garland didn't know why.

"As epidemiologists," Dr. Garland told us, "we make a gross observation and hope to stimulate biochemists to find a mechanism. We discover associations long before we know the reasons behind them." He explains that epidemiologists, for instance, linked tobacco to lung cancer years before anyone knew the chemistry involved.

Colon cancer rates support the new hypothesis. A cattleman in sunny, sparsely populated New Mexico, for example, is much less likely to get colon cancer than a stockbroker in smoggy, crowded New York. Per 100,000 people, 17.3 New Yorkers will suffer from colon cancer, but only 6.7 New Mexicans will. (Nationally, there are about 120,000 new cases of colon cancer per year).

Inhabitants of cities are deprived of sunshine for several reasons. Ozone pollution deflects some of the urban sunlight. Tall buildings eclipse the sun even more. "Even in areas where sunlight is intense," Dr. Garland writes, "persons who live and work in cities may not receive much exposure to it. . . . Vitamin D deficiency occurs in large cities even in tropical and subtropical areas" (*International Journal of Epidemiology*, vol. 9, no. 3, 1980).

Dr. Garland's ideas may throw some new light on current wisdom about colon cancer. A high intake of beef and fats has been shown to increase the risk of colon cancer, and a high-fiber diet of fresh produce and whole grains has been shown to lower the risk. But Dr. Garland told us that, thanks largely to fast and processed foods, there aren't enough regional variations in the American diet to explain all the regional variations he found in colon cancer rates. To him, sunlight is a plausible additional factor.

How does Dr. Garland think vitamin D protects the colon? Working with the known fact that vitamin D enables the body to absorb calcium, he theorizes that calcium's presence somehow protects the lining of the colon from cancer-causing waste substances that pass through it.

As you can see, man (and woman) was not meant to live by fluorescent light alone. Sunshine and vitamin D are too important to give up. And you should do your best to get them year round. Vitamin D is not just for winter anymore.

VITAMIN E

CHAPTER

57

VITAMIN E— SCIENTISTS SAY IT WORKS

What must have been a very important moment in the history of vitamin E research took place in the auditorium of a fine hotel on Central Park South in New York City.

At the request of the New York Academy of Sciences, vitamin E experts from all over the world gathered together for three days to swap notes they'd been jotting down for ten years or more.

Armed with speeches, slides, graphs and charts, they all testified to the fact that vitamin E was no longer a "vitamin in search of a deficiency," as it had been called. Instead, it's a vitamin that can influence many illnesses and that provides a key to the healthy functioning of our muscles, eyes, blood, lungs and more.

What follows is a record of some of the research presented in New York by almost 70 physicians and biochemists from California to Boston, from Japan and China to Sweden, England, West Germany and Israel.

Severe pain in the lower legs while walking—caused by poor circulation below the knees—was the subject of a study reported by Knut Haeger, M.D., of Sweden, one of the pioneers in vitamin E research. When most of the medical community dismissed the vitamin as a fad, Dr. Haeger was already using it to promote circulation and relieve pain.

Since the mid 1960s, Dr. Haeger said, he has given 100 international units of vitamin E three times a day to a total of 122 people with "intermittent claudication," or calf pain that occurs only when the sufferer tries to walk. He also told the patients to take walks twice a day, to try gymnastic exercises at home and not to smoke cigarettes.

Of those who faithfully practiced this regimen, Dr. Haeger said, 82 percent reported they could walk at least 10 percent farther than before, and 50 percent said they could walk at least 30 percent farther. By comparison, only 11 percent of a non-supplemented control group was able to increase their walking distance by 30 percent.

"We were able to prove," Dr. Haeger reported, "that patients on alpha-tocopherol [vitamin E] had a significantly longer walking distance than patients given either vasodilator agents [drugs that widen the blood vessels] or anticoagulant therapy, or a regimen of multivitamins excluding vitamin E."

Dr. Haeger's system requires patience, however. He said it takes about 18 months of supplementation and regular exercise before circulation improves measurably. Of those patients who maintained his program, 73.4 percent improved, compared to only 19.2 percent of the control group.

For those who like walking, another of the conference lecturers reported that vitamin E is vital for physical endurance.

Lester Packer, Ph.D., of the University of California at Berkeley, said that E-deficient rats exercised to the point of exhaustion show a 40 percent decrease in endurance. Without vitamin E, he explained, there's increased damage to the mitochondria—the microscopic structures inside each cell where the body turns food into energy. "E-deficient animals just tire out earlier," Dr. Packer told us, adding that extreme vitamin E deficiency may cause a special form of muscular dystrophy.

Protecting the Eyes

The use of vitamin E for diseases of the eye was the subject of several papers at the conference. Representing the Mount Sinai School of Medicine in New York, Kailash C. Bhuyan, M.D., and colleagues were excited to talk about their finding that vitamin E could stop the growth of, and possibly reverse the damage caused by, cataracts in rabbits.

The researchers said they artificially induced the cataracts in the rabbits, then fed them vitamin E intravenously. The results were promising: "In rabbits having early cataract . . . there was an arrest and reversal of cataract in about 50 percent of the animals treated with vitamin E." Photographs showed that, when the rabbits were given vitamin E in the early stages of the disease, there was decreased clouding of the lenses.

Vitamin E may also keep the eyes young. Researchers from the University of California at Santa Cruz showed that, in rats deficient in vitamin E or deficient in selenium or chromium, fat droplets built up within the eye and the eye lost some of its ability to combat unwanted invaders. Most important, the light-sensitive nerve endings in the retina of the eye were destroyed or became abnormal when those deficiencies occurred. And that was a symptom of aging.

"Effects of deficiencies in vitamin E alone or in selenium alone suggest that each of those nutrients play an important role in the retina . . . and [a deficiency of either] appears to accelerate age changes in the retina," they concluded.

Healthier Blood

One of vitamin E's most important protective roles takes place in the blood, where there are two substances that must be carefully balanced—prostacyclins and thromboxanes. Prostacyclins inhibit clots from forming, and thromboxanes encourage clots to form. According to Rao V. Panganamala, Ph.D., of Ohio State University, diabetic rabbits suffer from abnormally high levels of thromboxanes, which makes them susceptible to cardiovascular disease.

But Dr. Panganamala found that, when he gave diabetic rabbits vitamin E supplements for two to three months, their thromboxanes dropped to a safer, normal level and their prostacyclins rose to normal levels or higher.

Two physicians who journeyed from Giessen, West Germany, reported that vitamin E helped them save the lives of certain intensive-care-unit patients. These people were in a state of shock after such things as auto accidents, poisoning or infection. Shock caused clots to form in the blood vessels of their lungs, threatening to cut off their breathing. The process is called *shock lung syndrome*. Vitamin E worked because it apparently prevented the clots from forming in the first place.

It was interesting how the physicians first came to use vitamin E. They discovered that the symptoms of shock lung syndrome were identical to symptoms of exposure to ozone and nitrogen dioxide. Knowing that vitamin E can protect the lungs from those atmospheric pollutants, they decided to give it to their shock lung patients—with success.

Several presentations at the conference dealt with cholesterol. In the blood, cholesterol attaches itself to low-density lipoproteins (LDLs) or high-density lipoproteins (HDLs). High levels of HDLs and low levels of LDLs have been associated with a lower risk of coronary heart disease and atherosclerosis.

A team of physicians from the Wood Veterans Administration Medical Center in Milwaukee tested the effect of vitamin E on the blood of 43 men and women. They gave each person 800 international units of the vitamin daily for four weeks. Results showed that the vitamin raised HDL levels, but only in those people who initially had low HDL levels.

William J. Hermann, M.D., a pathologist in Houston, came to similar conclusions. Dr. Hermann found that vitamin E was most effective in people who began with low HDL levels, who were under age 35, and who weighed no more than 10 percent more than their ideal weight.

A third group of physicians, from Sinai Hospital in Baltimore, used vitamin E to lower LDL levels in rats. They said the vitamin worked best when given early in an animal's life.

A Boost for Resistance

Researchers at the conference also showed that vitamin E may enhance our resistance to disease and pollution.

Ching K. Chow, Ph.D., of the University of Kentucky, exposed two groups of rats, one supplemented with vitamin E and the other not, to cigarette smoke. After three days of chain smoking, 5 of the 16 unsupplemented rats were dead, compared to only 1 of the 13 supplemented rats.

Dr. Chow said cigarette smoke contains more than 3,000 chemicals, many of which are highly reactive *free radicals* that may have altered certain essential enzymes in the rats. He concluded that it was the cigarette's visible smoke, rather than its invisible gases, that did the most harm.

Another speaker, Laurence M. Corwin, Ph.D., of the Boston University school of medicine, said that vitamin E boosts the body's *cell-mediated immunity*. This kind of immunity protects us from bacteria, viruses and, in some cases, cancer. His research showed that vitamin E stimulates the production of new defense cells and neutralizes substances that normally keep those cells in check.

Interestingly, Dr. Corwin commented that "as far as the immune response is concerned, normal dietary levels of vitamin E may not be sufficient to maintain an optimal host defense against disease."

Most of the researchers at the conference agreed that even fairly high doses of vitamin E—considerably higher than the current Recommended Dietary Allowance of 15 international units—are very safe. As a daily intake, the figures most often mentioned were between 300 and 800 international units daily. Bertram Lubin, M.D., of Oakland, California, who was cochairman of the conference, told us that he considers 200 to 400 international units to be a reasonable range for a daily supplement.

For Dr. Lubin, this conference signaled what he called "the turnaround in the acceptability of vitamin E that has taken place in the last ten years."

CHAPTER

58

VITAMIN E—
JACK OF ALL TRADES,
MASTER OF MOST

Vitamin E is a nutritional Swiss Army knife. The Swiss have a knack for making the greatest use of the smallest space, and with one of their military's pocketknives you can open cans, uncork bottles, clip your nails, balance your checkbook, practically everything short of squaring the circle.

The thing's amazing, but it's nothing next to vitamin E. The vitamin modifies blood fats so that they protect against heart disease. Vitamin E may also promote a healthy circulatory system by preventing the formation of dangerous blood clots and by protecting red blood cells from damage by oxidation.

If vitamin E worked just to prevent heart disease, it would be impressive enough. But on top of that, scientists are finding that vitamin E protects health in a lot of other ways, as well. It's the sheer variety of E's protective action that is most astonishing.

At a conference of the American Chemical Society, Robert P. Tengerdy, Ph.D., reviewed work he and researchers at Colorado State University did, plus research by scientists at other institutions, on the effects of vitamin E on the immune system.

The most intriguing aspect of that research is that it involves levels of vitamin E higher than the Recommended Dietary Allowances.

Dr. Tengerdy and Cheryl Nockels, Ph.D., professor of animal science at Colorado State University, used what he calls high doses of vitamin E to discover how much is needed for the optimal performance of the body.

"When animals are fed vitamin E at a level three to six times exceeding what is available in normal diets, the most noticeable improvement in their defense against infectious diseases is a significantly enhanced immune response," he says. "In this case, it is manifested by an increased production of antibodies, the protein molecules that help eliminate invading microorganisms."

Increased production of antibodies with high vitamin E diets has been observed in mice, chickens, turkeys, guinea pigs, rabbits, pigs and sheep.

Can a "Good" Diet Still Benefit from Supplements?

While many nutritional studies compare the effect of a deficient diet to that of one with an "adequate" supply of the vitamin involved, these researchers organized things a bit differently. They gave some animals their normal laboratory diet— which supplied the Recommended Dietary Allowance of everything, including vitamin E. To others they gave the same diet plus a supplementary amount of vitamin E. It's like comparing a group of people who eat "a good diet" with another group who eat a good diet with vitamin E supplements.

"I tried to determine whether supplements of vitamin E, given in excess of what is required for normal growth and reproduction, increase immunity to infection," Dr. Nockels told us.

In one experiment, she said, researchers gave one group of mice their normal diet and another a diet supplemented with 60 international units of vitamin E per kilogram of food (1 kilogram is about the amount of food you probably eat in a day). They injected both groups with sheep red blood cells. Four days later, the mice were examined.

When mice are injected with sheep red blood cells, their bodies react to them the way they'd react to bacteria—by producing the chemicals, called antibodies, that take invaders out of action. That vital defensive process was significantly stronger in the mice who received the vitamin E supplements. For one thing, the weight of their spleens was greater (a sign of increased antibody production). And when the researchers measured the amounts of antibodies in the blood of both groups, the supplemented mice tested considerably higher.

Dr. Nockels and her co-workers then tested the effect of vitamin E on immunity in guinea pigs. She gave one group of the small rodents injections of vitamin E in amounts well above the standard dietary level, another group got no injections. Then she vaccinated them with the virus that causes a serious strain of encephalitis.

Here, too, the animals who received supplemental vitamin E protected themselves with significantly higher levels of antibodies than those who did not.

Active immunity, the body's ability to manufacture antibodies against invading organisms, provides important protection at any age. But newborn animals (and this includes human infants) don't have this ability. Until they can establish it on their own, they are dependent on the antibodies transferred to them as they grow in embryo and, after birth, in their mothers' milk.

According to another of the Colorado State experiments, vitamin E can effectively boost the process of *passive transfer* that keeps defenses up at this particularly vital time for newborns. The researchers gave one group of hens a diet supplemented with 150 international units of vitamin E per kilogram of food, the other just the normal feed. After four weeks, they incubated the hens' eggs.

Researchers took blood samples when the chicks were two days and seven days old and measured the antibody levels. The offspring of hens given vitamin E supplements, it was found, had higher levels of antibodies than the controls. The vitamin E their mothers received, it seems, gave them a better start in life.

Putting Vitamin E to the Real Test

While laboratory measurements of immune reactions are important, they must be judged with care. Resistance to disease is a complex thing, and a higher level of antibodies does not automatically mean better defense against infection. A small but significant number of antibodies, for instance, might not make any practical difference when real bacteria and viruses are involved. To determine whether vitamin E supplements effectively help to prevent infection, the Colorado researchers performed a series of experiments with chicks, turkeys and sheep. Using a number of different species, they explained, "makes generalizations sounder. It strengthens the likelihood that findings will also apply to humans."

Groups of chicks and turkeys were fed either the normal chick or turkey feed or that plus vitamin E supplements ranging from 100 to 300 international units per kilogram of food. They were then injected with disease-causing bacteria. Among both the chicks and the turkeys, vitamin E supplements meant a lower mortality rate: Fewer animals succumbed to the disease.

What was more, there was a significant connection between the size of the supplement and the degree of protection. Twenty-five percent of the chicks who received no supplements died of the infection, for example; 10 percent of those who received 150 international units of vitamin died, and only 5 percent of those who received 300 international units died.

In another experiment, the researchers fed a group of lambs large doses of vitamin E, then inoculated them and an unsupplemented group with *Chlamydia*, a germ which induces pneumonia in sheep.

Later examination of the animals showed less damage to the lungs of those who had received vitamin E supplements than to those of the controls. Also, the supplemented animals showed no traces of the bacteria in their bodies, while the pathological organisms could be found in 40 percent of the controls.

In all three species, Dr. Nockels concluded, vitamin E significantly improved resistance to disease.

This particular aspect of vitamin E may be worthy of greater attention, Dr. Nockels says. "I think that further research may show that vitamin E provides positive improvement of immune capability in humans, too."

Such research may show, among other things, that the RDA— what is normally considered "enough" vitamin E—is far too low.

"The RDA does not appear to maintain immunity at full strength," says Dr. Nockels. "In every case, I found that an amount of vitamin E greater than the RDA for the animal was required to stimulate improved immune response. And with elderly animals, the allowances might have to be even higher."

Vitamin E has also been shown to be involved in the prevention of a number of specific problems unrelated to bacterial infection. Patients with vitamin E deficiency have developed serious nerve degeneration. Recent research indicates that vitamin E may also prevent cortical cataracts, the most common type of cataract among older people.

Cortical cataracts are a clouding of the outer part of the lens of the eye. The condition often afflicts older diabetics and can result in partial or total blindness. John R. Trevithick, Ph.D., a biochemist at the University of Western Ontario, has shown that large doses of vitamin E can prevent the formation of cortical cataracts in animals.

Vitamin E's protective action may cover cancer, as well. E has been shown to inhibit the breast-cancer-causing action of the chemical daunorubicin in rats and the colon-cancer-causing effects of dimethylhydrazine in mice.

That result clearly supports the idea that vitamin E blocks the formation of nitrosamines and nitrosamides, a family of chemicals that are strongly suspected to cause colon cancer in humans, and researchers at the Ontario Cancer Institute in Canada are now testing vitamin E to determine if it can block the recurrence of threatening growths (called polyps) in patients with cancer of the colon and rectum.

Those researchers have already shown that the wastes of people eating a normal diet contain chemicals that cause mutations in a special strain of test bacteria. Scientists know that chemicals which cause the mutations very often also cause cancer, and results of various tests led the Canadian researchers to believe that the chemicals they found in the feces were probably nitrosamines and nitrosamides (*Environmental Aspects of N-Nitroso Compounds*, International Agency for Research on Cancer, 1978).

The most interesting developments came when the researchers tested the effects of vitamin E on the levels of the suspected cancer-causing chemicals. Supplementation of people's diets with 120, 400 and 1,200 international units of E a day led to significant reductions in the amounts of the chemicals in feces (*American Association for Cancer Research Abstracts*, March, 1980).

Cramp Relief with E

Another problem that succumbs to vitamin E is the pain of cramps.

When a team of Los Angeles doctors gave vitamin E to 125 patients with nighttime leg and foot cramps, 103 had complete or nearly complete relief *(Southern Medical Journal)*.

"More than half of the patients had suffered from leg cramps longer than 5 years and many of these had had cramps for 20 to 30 years or longer," Samuel Ayres, Jr., M.D., and Richard Mihan, M.D., reported. "Approximately one-fourth of the patients had cramps every night or several times a night, and in about 65 percent of the cases the cramps were severe."

About half of the patients found relief by taking 300 international units or less of vitamin E a day. The other half needed

400 international units or more to control their cramps. And, the doctors note, many patients had to continue taking vitamin E to stay free of cramps: "In a number of instances it was learned that cramps recurred when treatment was stopped or greatly reduced, but promptly responded again when treatment was resumed."

After treating so many patients with vitamin E, the doctors believe the nutrient is practically a cramp medicine: "The response of nocturnal [nighttime] leg and foot cramps to adequate doses of vitamin E is prompt, usually becoming manifest within a week, and occurs in such an overwhelming number of cases that it appears almost specific for this ailment."

But doctors have treated more than nighttime foot and leg cramps with vitamin E.

They have also treated nighttime rectal cramps, cramping of abdominal muscles and cramps from heavy exercise.

One particular type of cramp that may occur after exercise—heavy or mild—is intermittent claudication, a cramp of the calf. Scientific evidence shows that this cramp, too, may yield to vitamin E.

A doctor studied 47 men with severe intermittent claudication, giving 32 of them vitamin E and the rest drugs to improve their circulation. After about three months, he tested the men to see how far they could walk. In the vitamin E group, 54 percent of the men could walk the test's maximum distance, a little more than half a mile. But only 23 percent of the drug group completed the test (*American Journal of Clinical Nutrition*).

Vitamin E may have treated intermittent claudication by doing what the drugs failed to do—improve circulation. After about 18 months of taking vitamin E, 29 of the 32 men showed an increase in the flow of blood to their calves. During those same months, most of the men in the drug group had a decrease in their flow. But exactly how vitamin E works continues to puzzle doctors.

An Australian physician, who tried vitamin E "with remarkable success" on approximately 50 patients, wrote to a medical journal saying he was "unable to explain the physiological reason why vitamin E should control muscle cramp'' and asked his colleagues to "give me an explanation" *(Medical Journal of Australia)*.

Well, it doesn't really matter why. What matters is that vitamin E does work in many cases to relieve cramps. If you should ever have a cramp, that's all you need to know.

And given the extra threats to health we all encounter in today's environment, it's a good idea to make sure your diet contains the vitamin E you need. Most grains, nuts and seeds are high in vitamin E. Sunflower seeds and wheat germ are two particularly good sources of the vitamin, and supplements can help you attain the optimal levels necessary for good health. When just one nutrient boosts the body's well-being in so many different ways, you should take full advantage of it.

59

VITAMIN E LUBRICATES THE CIRCULATION

Some people don't need convincing.

People like Drs. Evan and Wilfrid Shute—pioneers in the vitamin E field—who for more than 30 years have been advising patients to take vitamin E to dissolve painful blood clots and prevent heart attack and stroke.

Or Alton Ochsner, M.D.—a leading surgeon and teacher for many years at the Tulane University school of medicine in New Orleans—who was giving his patients the edge against post-surgical blood clots back in 1950 by prescribing vitamin E.

But for those who haven't tried it and who still have to be convinced of the anticlotting benefits of vitamin E, your time has come. We've now got scientific evidence that vitamin E can reduce clotting at its earliest stages. And why.

But first, you may be wondering how this research may affect you. After all, aren't blood clots basically good guys that could save your life in a pinch?

Yes, that's true. When you nick yourself with a razor or slit your finger on the razor-sharp edge of a piece of paper, tiny saucer-shaped blood cells (appropriately named platelets) are immediately called to the rescue.

Normally, platelets are pretty independent characters that

slip and slide through the bloodstream with no real desire to latch on to other blood cells. But when the word is out that there's been damage to a vessel wall, they stick together—literally.

Within seconds, they're clinging to the crack in the vessel and sticking to each other to build up a thickened, gooey mass— just perfect for plugging the gap in the vessel wall and preventing further blood loss.

It is this clumping of platelets—the first most crucial step of blood clot formation—that scientists refer to as *platelet aggregation.* Usually, it takes only a few minutes after injury for other substances to get caught up in this sticky mass and form a clot.

But sometimes something goes amiss. Instead of clumping on cue, the platelets begin to congregate on a healthy artery wall. If they grow into an unruly mob and are joined by other chemical agitators, a blood clot could form within the blood vessel and cause real trouble.

Deep vein thrombosis (a medical term for a blood clot in the leg) and phlebitis (another condition of the legs, characterized by inflamed blood vessels and clot formation) are caused by spontaneous clotting. Both conditions can be painful. But the real problem arises when the clot journeys up the leg and gets caught in a major blood vessel of the heart, lungs or brain.

If a blood clot gets stuck in a coronary artery that is obstructed by cholesterol deposits and blocks blood flow, a heart attack could result. Similarly, a clot may lodge in the lungs (pulmonary embolism) or brain (stroke) and again pose fatal possibilities.

There is also a growing number of studies which link increased platelet aggregation with migraine headaches. Writing in the *Journal of the American Medical Association,* Donald J. Dalessio, M.D., of the Scripps Clinic and Research Foundation in La Jolla, California, notes, "There is a substantial increase in platelet aggregation during the pre-headache phase of migraine." He also suggests that this apparent tendency toward clotting may explain the slight increase in incidence of stroke among patients with migraine.

It stands to reason, as Dr. Dalessio points out, that any

substance which might interfere with platelet aggregation could act as a protective measure against recurrent migraines as well as strokes.

And that substance is vitamin E.

One of the links between vitamin E and platelet aggregation was published in the *Proceedings of the Society for Experimental Biology and Medicine*. Lawrence J. Machlin, Ph.D., and a group of researchers at Hoffmann–La Roche, Nutley, New Jersey, compared blood samples taken from vitamin E–deficient rats to those taken from animals receiving extra doses of the vitamin.

Not surprisingly, the supplemented animals had the edge against clotting. For one thing, platelet aggregation was significantly reduced in all the rats of the vitamin E group. In addition, after 15 to 16 weeks, the rats on a deficient diet began producing more and more platelets. And this, researchers speculate, may also contribute to the increased clotting: The more platelets you've got bumping into each other in the bloodstream, the greater the chance of them sticking together and setting off the series of reactions leading to a blood clot.

Pediatricians at the State University of New York's Upstate Medical Center have reported a similar correlation in two children seen at the center. Blood samples taken from both girls were found to be extremely low in vitamin E and abnormally high in platelets.

To test the clotting capacity of the blood samples, the physicians added certain chemicals, which cause platelet aggregation, to test tubes of the blood and compared them to similarly treated samples taken from healthy children.

As expected, the platelets from the deficient girls clumped more readily than those from the control group.

However, both the platelet count and the high clotting tendency were reduced to normal following vitamin E supplementation *(Journal of Pediatrics)*.

This finding falls in line with the results of studies conducted by Manfred Steiner, M.D., Ph.D., a blood research specialist and associate professor of medicine at Brown University in Providence, Rhode Island.

In one of Dr. Steiner's earlier works, blood samples taken from several healthy volunteers were similarly exposed in test tubes to chemical agents, to stimulate the type of platelet clumping that might occur spontaneously in a blood vessel. When vitamin E was added to the test tubes, however, this clumping was kept to a minimum.

In another similar study, Dr. Steiner first put the volunteers on a vitamin E regimen (1,200 to 2,400 international units daily) for a few weeks and then took the samples, which he exposed to the same chemical agents used above. Again, he reported, vitamin E minimized platelet sticking *(Journal of Clinical Investigation)*.

Dr. Steiner was convinced, but not satisfied that his work was completed. "There's no question that vitamin E does have a profound effect on platelet aggregation," the Rhode Island researcher says. "But that's only the beginning. We wanted to know whether we could explain the molecular basis of that effect." And, he indicated, he had a hunch that the answer might be found in the outer coating, or cell membrane, of the platelets.

Vitamin E Protects Cell Membranes

And why not? Other researchers have found that vitamin E protects cell membranes, especially, from the destructive effects of oxygen.

For example, a biochemist from the University of Puget Sound in Washington, Jeffrey Bland, Ph.D., found that the membranes of red blood cells (not platelets) became weakened when exposed to the circulating oxygen in the blood. But vitamin E protects against this weakening and increases the life expectancy of the cell.

"When cells are subjected to oxidative damage, it is as if they have been hit with a tiny hand grenade," Dr. Bland told us. "There is little question that damage is being done.

"But vitamin E has a great affinity for cell membranes because these membranes contain large amounts of unsaturated fatty acids and other fats, and vitamin E is a fat-soluble vitamin."

In Dr. Bland's research, 24 volunteers were instructed to take 600 international units of vitamin E a day for 10 days. Then blood samples were taken and these samples exposed to oxygen and sunlight for 16 hours to hasten oxidation. Normally, a great many of the cell membranes would have shown signs of damage. But with the vitamin E, Dr. Bland reports, "only a very small number" of cells were harmed.

Is it possible to relate this finding on red blood cells to blood platelets? "I think there is enough consistency in cell membranes to say that this is going to hold true," Dr. Bland told us. "We have done a little bit of research on platelets and, so far, we've found that, the higher the concentration of vitamin E, the greater the stability of the platelet membranes. There is less chance of developing binding sites on the platelet membranes."

Dr. Steiner agrees. "Many nutrition biochemists say that vitamin E does have a stabilizing effect on the cell membranes. I have tried to investigate this possibility by measuring the membrane fluidity, that is, measuring the motion of molecules in the platelet membrane.

"Let me explain it this way: The cell membrane consists of lipids [fats] and proteins. The lipids act like an oily sea in which the proteins are inserted. Think of it as cooking oil: As you heat it or cool it, the consistency changes. The lipid sea reacts the same to temperature change. And it's possible to monitor these changes by measuring the movement of the protein molecules; the thicker the sea, the slower the movement of the molecules. And, of course, the thinner the sea, the faster they will move.

"Vitamin E affects the fluidity of the membrane much in the same way that temperature does. I've found that, under any temperature conditions—even at body temperature—vitamin E permits the proteins to move about more freely. And in blood platelets, it is this increased fluidity that reduces the stickiness of the platelets."

How much? Well, in volunteers taking 1,200 to 1,600 international units of vitamin E a day for four weeks, Dr. Steiner reports a 30 to 45 percent reduction in the stickiness of the platelets. And in those who kept up with the E regimen for more than a year, platelet adhesiveness was cut 50 percent.

But there's a second wave in platelet aggregation that we haven't discussed yet but which plays a very important part in the development of dangerous blood clots.

Apparently, when platelets first stick together, they look very much like a cluster of grapes. And they're just as fragile. At any time, they can break apart and slip back into the blood-stream unnoticed. Under these circumstances, a blood clot doesn't have a chance to develop.

However, if the platelets hold on long enough, they eventually release a chemical substance which draws them closer—and tighter—together. The cluster of grapes we had before becomes one solid piece of fruit. And now there's no turning back.

According to Dr. Steiner, a blood clot is inevitable at this point—unless you're fortified with vitamin E.

"During platelet aggregation, subtle changes occur in the platelet membrane which activate certain enzymes in the membrane to link up with those fatty acid molecules we talked about earlier," Dr. Steiner explains. "Somewhere in the process of this union, a powerful chemical substance is released into the surrounding platelets which significantly increases the stickiness of the membranes. The clump then becomes permanent."

But here, again, vitamin E can block a potential tragedy. "The molecular structure of vitamin E is just perfect for linking up with the polyunsaturated fatty acid molecule," Dr. Steiner explains. "And if vitamin E links up with it first—which it will if you keep yourself supplemented with E—then the fatty acid molecule is unavailable to the enzyme. No chemical agent is released. The platelet clump is able to dissolve. And no clot forms.

"Based on these findings, I feel that vitamin E should be considered a worthwhile preventive measure against such clot-related disorders as heart attack and stroke," Dr. Steiner says. "I take 1,200 international units of vitamin E every day."

A Sticky Problem

Dr. Bland is convinced of the importance of this vitamin E research. "Preventing platelet adhesion is a very big concern of medical researchers these days."

One of those researchers is R. V. Panganamala, Ph.D. He's seeing firsthand how vitamin E works. Dr. Panganamala, of the department of physiological chemistry at the Ohio State University school of medicine in Columbus, has conducted experiments with rabbits and rats to show how and why vitamin E is so crucial to the health of blood vessels.

"Any time platelets stick together inside an intact blood vessel, it's a problem," explains Dr. Panganamala. "But that can happen when the platelets produce too much thromboxane, a substance that enhances their stickiness. It can also happen if the vessel wall doesn't produce enough prostacyclin. This chemical has the opposite effect on platelets—that is, it keeps them free-flowing and slippery.

"In our experiment," Dr. Panganamala told us, "we wanted to see what effect vitamin E had on those two chemicals. We used animals that were normal and healthy to begin with and divided them into two groups. One group received a diet high in vitamin E while the other's diet had no vitamin E at all. After 10 to 12 weeks, we tested the levels of thromboxane and prostacyclin in the animals. We found that those deficient in vitamin E had significantly higher amounts of thromboxane while, at the same time, their vessels lost the capacity to produce prostacyclin.

"It's our current understanding that the proper ratio of thromboxane to prostacyclin is imperative if platelets are to move through the blood without aggregating at the wrong time. If the ratio's out of balance, there is a far greater chance of thrombosis [blood clots] to occur. Vitamin E helps keep these substances in precise, proper balance."

Because of the success of that experiment, Dr. Panganamala wanted to try a similar experiment using diabetic animals.

"We know that people with diabetes are particularly vulnerable to circulatory problems," he told us. "So we decided to see if the thromboxane and prostacyclin balance was adversely affected in animals with that condition.

"First, we created diabetes in a group of experimental rats. After the diabetes was established, we tested their levels of thromboxane and prostacyclin and found that they were out of balance—too much of the first and too little of the second.

"Next, we supplemented the rats' diet with vitamin E. Within eight to ten weeks, the two chemicals were back to their normal levels."

Diabetics may gain an extra benefit from vitamin E. Research has shown that excessively sticky platelets and diabetic retinopathy (disease of the retina) go hand in hand.

A study done in Israel has shown that vitamin E may counteract the damaging effects of diabetic retinopathy (possible blindness) by inhibiting platelet aggregation and, consequently, improving circulation to that area (*Acta Haematologica,* vol. 62, no. 2, 1979).

IV Patients May Need Extra E

When hospital patients are fed intravenously, they are particularly susceptible to vitamin E deficiency and excessively sticky platelets, according to Peter M. Thurlow, M.D., and John P. Grant, M.D., of the department of surgery at the Duke University medical center in Durham, North Carolina. They studied 13 patients who were on total parenteral (intravenous) nutrition (TPN) for two or more weeks, and they found that, even with standard vitamin supplementation, TPN is associated with a gradual decrease in serum vitamin E concentrations.

And as serum vitamin E levels decrease, platelet aggregation becomes abnormal. One patient, whose vitamin E concentration and platelet aggregation were normal initially, developed a deficiency and platelet hyperaggregation (overly sticky platelets) after 15 days of TPN. In fact, every patient with low vitamin E levels also had abnormal platelet aggregation. Extra supplementation raised the plasma vitamin E levels and returned platelet aggregation to normal in most of those patients.

Because platelet hyperaggregation has been implicated in the development of both thrombosis and atherosclerosis, the doctors recommend supplemental vitamin E during TPN to maintain normal vitamin E levels and platelet function (*Surgical Forum*, vol. 31, 1980).

Actually, that's good advice for just about everyone, not just those fighting off illness. Smooth-flowing blood vessels mean a healthier circulation, no matter what your present state of health. Let vitamin E be the plumber that helps clean up your internal pipes.

CHAPTER
60

HELP YOUR HEART
WITH VITAMIN E

Medical discoveries are often the results of fortunate accidents. When, by coincidence, a 33-year-old Houston pathologist tested his own blood cholesterol while taking daily doses of vitamin E, he stumbled on what he thinks might be an important new method for preventing atherosclerosis, or hardening of the arteries.

In the summer of 1978, William J. Hermann, M.D., a pathologist at Memorial City General Hospital in Houston, was setting up new tests to study the distribution of cholesterol in the blood of the hospital's patients.

The tests showed more than just how high a person's cholesterol level was. In the blood, cholesterol is transported by complexes of fats and proteins called lipoproteins. Low-density lipoproteins (LDLs) carry cholesterol to the cells, and high-density lipoproteins (HDLs) carry cholesterol away from the cells. A high proportion of LDLs has come to be associated with a high risk of atherosclerosis, and a high proportion of HDLs is associated with a low risk. On sampling his own blood—which happened to be handy—Dr. Hermann found only 9 percent HDLs, a sign of a higher than average risk.

At about the same time, with no idea that it would eventually affect his laboratory work, Dr. Hermann urged his father to start taking vitamin E. The elder Hermann, a man of 60 at the time, was in good health. But there was a family history of cardiovascular problems, and Dr. Hermann had seen evidence that vitamin E can prevent unsaturated fats in the body from turning into bulkier, "stickier," potentially more harmful saturated fats. His father agreed, but he also persuaded his son to start vitamin E therapy. Dr. Hermann began taking 600 international units of vitamin E per day.

The dog days of August passed by. Dr. Hermann went on vacation, where he drank almost no alcohol (alcohol might have increased his HDL fraction) and even gained a little weight (which can decrease HDL). When he got back to his lab, he tested his blood again. He found "with astonishment" that, after taking vitamin E for 30 days, 40 percent of his blood cholesterol was now attached to HDL.

Vitamin E Lowered Cholesterol

"I came back from vacation and the results had changed so dramatically that for two days I thought the experiment had failed," Dr. Hermann told us. Then he realized that the vitamin E had apparently shifted the cholesterol, taking him from what is considered a higher than average risk to a lower than average risk of atherosclerosis.

Although he is frequently skeptical of vitamin therapy claims in general, Dr. Hermann was excited by his discovery. He decided to put the accidental discovery to a test. In the fall of 1978, he picked five people with average amounts of HDL cholesterol and five with high risks of atherosclerosis (low HDL cholesterol) and placed them all on 600 international units of vitamin E per day. The results: All five people with cholesterol problems improved radically within a few weeks. And though the experiment was small, Dr. Hermann was impressed because vitamin E even had a positive effect on four of the five healthy volunteers.

In publishing his findings, Dr. Hermann wrote, "The results were so obviously significant and of potential value to the medical community that we wish to report them in their somewhat tentative form" (*American Journal of Clinical Pathology,* November, 1979).

What does Dr. Hermann's experiment mean to someone who's concerned about preventing or delaying the onset of atherosclerosis? It means that he or she may be able to use vitamin E as another defense against cholesterol buildup in the arteries. Exercise, such as long-distance running, has been shown to decrease the risk of atherosclerosis (*New England Journal of Medicine,* February 14, 1980). Both exercise and vitamin E seem to raise the amount of cholesterol in the HDL complexes. That indicates that excess cholesterol is leaving the cells and getting dumped out of the body in a healthy way.

In Dr. Hermann's experiment, the three men and two women who started out with very low levels of HDL cholesterol all raised their levels by between 220 and 483 percent. The effect of vitamin E was consistent, even though the volunteers ranged in age from 28 to 55 and had widely varied exercise and eating habits. One woman of 55, who was overweight, took longer to respond and needed 800 international units per day, but her results were ultimately the same.

All five of these high-risk subjects moved within seven weeks or less to an average or even above average level of HDL cholesterol—a good sign that they were reducing their chances of developing atherosclerosis. They also lowered the levels of very-low-density lipoproteins (VLDL) and triglycerides (another fatty acid complex) in their blood by about one-quarter and one-fifth, respectively, thereby mitigating two more warning signs of impending atherosclerosis.

Of the five volunteers with average initial cholesterol distribution, four saw their HDL fraction rise to between 127 and 237 percent of its original value. The only person who did not seem to benefit from the vitamin E therapy was a 33-year-old man with an average HDL cholesterol level. His HDL fraction stayed the same after 30 days.

The total amount of cholesterol in the blood hardly changed at all for any of the subjects. But that didn't matter, Dr. Hermann stressed. "What matters," he said, "is whether the cholesterol is on the way in (bound to LDL) or on the way out (bound to HDL)."

When the body is functioning properly, Dr. Hermann explained, cholesterol is manufactured in the liver and sent through the bloodstream to the cells. It is essential for the synthesis of hormones, for the formation of cell membranes and even for protection against cancer. The cells can make their own supply of cholesterol, or they can pick it up from the blood. What they don't need, they send back into the blood, on to the liver and out of the body.

VLDL, LDL and HDL, as mentioned before, are the complexes of fats and proteins that carry cholesterol through its cycle. The VLDL carries it out of the liver, where it is made. Then the VLDL, with cholesterol still on board, degrades into an LDL. The LDL delivers the cholesterol to the cells along the artery walls. After an intricate digestive process, the cells spit out any excess cholesterol. This is where the all-important HDL plays its role. Acting as, in Dr. Hermann's words, "a garbage collection mechanism," the HDL picks up the discarded cholesterol and packs it off to the liver.

The delicate balance of the cycle, however, can get derailed. A family tendency toward circulatory problems, a high-fat diet, smoking or a sedentary life style can increase the level of LDL and decrease the level of HDL. When that happens, too much cholesterol is being fed to the cells, and not enough is being eliminated. Clogged with cholesterol, the cells die, eventually forming fatty streaks, or plaque, along the artery walls. And plaque is what promotes clotting and narrowing, eventually blocking the artery and causing heart attack and stroke.

Vitamin E, according to Dr. Hermann, may help maintain a healthy LDL-HDL balance. At some point in the biochemical process, the vitamin seems to enhance the metabolism of cholesterol. But Dr. Hermann wasn't sure where. His best guess was that vitamin E enables cell membranes to let cholesterol pass out of them more easily, making it available for HDL pickup.

Dr. Hermann believes that this was the first experiment to show a direct relationship between the use of vitamin E and a higher level of HDL cholesterol in the blood.

Dr. Hermann's preliminary findings about vitamin E can be summed up as follows. First, the vitamin seems to improve cholesterol metabolism. Second, it seems to have this effect regardless of age, sex or diet. Third, it seems to begin working within 20 days (or longer for those who are overweight).

These effects do require a maintenance dose. Dr. Hermann found that, when he stopped taking vitamin E for one month, his HDL cholesterol level dropped from its high of 40 percent down to 16 percent—close to where it started. But when he renewed the therapy, this time at 400 international units per day, his HDL fraction rose within a month to 27 percent.

Dr. Hermann won't go so far as to prescribe an exact dosage of vitamin E. But he does say that the 15 to 50 international units of vitamin E often found in multivitamin preparations probably aren't enough to have an effect on cholesterol metabolism. He suggests 400 international units as a good maintenance dose for the average person. He recommends higher doses—600 or 800 international units—at first for people with cholesterol imbalances.

Dr. Hermann is hoping that his discovery will inspire more research on vitamin E. "I'd like to see people get excited about this effect, study the mechanism of it and verify these preliminary findings," he said.

If new studies confirm what Dr. Hermann has found, he will have added significantly to the growing body of clinical evidence of vitamin E's healthy effect on the human circulatory system.

CHAPTER
61

VITAMIN E—
STRONG MEDICINE
FOR RARE DISEASES

Here's a health quiz that few people outside of the medical profession could be expected to pass. But you might want to try it, anyway.

What is discoid lupus erythematosus? Sickle cell anemia? Thalassemia? Bronchopulmonary dysplasia? Retrolental fibroplasia?

Give up? Unless they've touched you personally, or a friend or someone in your family, it's not likely that you would recognize many (or any) of the above health problems. But to the tens of thousands of individuals afflicted, the consequences of those obscure disorders are all too real.

Here's something you *have* heard of, though: vitamin E. And the important thing to know about this last item is that it's helping doctors to come to grips with all of those problems we've just mentioned.

Consider discoid lupus erythematosus (DLE), for example. It's a chronic disease of the skin which torments its victims with red, circular blotches, or plaques. Pore openings widen and become plugged with scale. Although not as serious and deep-seated as the related malady systemic lupus erythematosus (which attacks and breaks down connective tissue throughout the body), DLE can be quite an ordeal.

That's why a report by two Los Angeles dermatologists, Samuel Ayres, Jr., M.D., and Richard Mihan, M.D., is so noteworthy. Dr. Ayres, who is emeritus clinical professor of medicine at the University of California at Los Angeles (UCLA), and Dr. Mihan, a clinical professor at the University of Southern California school of medicine, have had excellent results treating patients with vitamin E (*Cutis*, January, 1979).

Current therapy of lupus, they point out, "depends almost entirely on three categories of drugs: antimalarials, corticosteroids and immunosuppressives, all three of which may be helpful, but which also carry serious risks of undesirable side effects, including infections and malignancy.

"Vitamin E, on the other hand, when properly used, is essentially free of such side effects. However, it must be employed in potent form, in adequate amounts, and over an extended period of time, sometimes indefinitely, to achieve maximum therapeutic benefits."

Blotches Disappeared

Drs. Ayres and Mihan described seven patients treated with vitamin E. One, a 63-year-old woman, had been troubled by discoid lupus for about eight months. Reddish, scaly and crusty blotches the size of nickels and quarters marred her skin. She was started on a supplement of 800 international units of vitamin E daily, later increased to 1,200 international units, and a special cream containing vitamin E was applied directly to the skin twice a day. "Five and a half months later, the patient's skin was completely cleared," the doctors report. "Her response was excellent."

Another woman, 37 years old, had suffered with lupus symptoms on and off for 23 years. Pea-size and larger scaly plaques were scattered over her upper back, chest, arms and face. She began taking 800 international units of vitamin E daily, with the dosage later stepped up to 1,600 international units. Vitamin E was also applied directly to the skin. "After nine months, all lesions were clear," according to Drs. Ayres and Mihan, "except for six tiny inconspicuous remnants on the face and left neck."

Still another patient, a 33-year-old woman, had on-and-off symptoms for 20 years. There were plaques on her cheeks, chin and neck, along with some withered areas on the scalp with associated hair loss. After taking vitamin E and 50 micrograms of selenium daily—the doctors observed that this trace mineral enhanced vitamin E's effect—the woman showed almost no remaining signs of redness after seven months, and there was "considerable new hair growth in previously bald areas on the scalp."

Not all responses were so dramatic. A 54-year-old woman with rough plaques on her face, nose, neck and chest also tried vitamin E. "There was definite improvement six months later, compared to photographs taken at her first visit. All lesions were flatter, paler, and some showed areas of normal skin." Her response was "good."

Others in the group who took the lowest amounts of vitamin E—only 300 international units daily—showed the poorest response, leading Drs. Ayres and Mihan to conclude that the preferred dosage is between 1,200 and 1,600 international units daily.

Protecting Cell Walls

How does vitamin E accomplish its results? The doctors aren't entirely sure, but they suspect vitamin E acts at the cellular level. "Theoretically, vitamin E functions as a first line of defense by protecting cell membranes from destructive lipid peroxidation. . . ." In other words, fatty components in the cell wall may be shielded from harmful oxidation or breakdown when sufficient vitamin E is present.

Unfortunately, the cards are normally stacked against vitamin E being present in any abundant quantity. According to Drs. Ayres and Mihan, "deficiencies of vitamin E may be actual, due to an inadequate intake, but are probably more often due to inadequate absorption, defects in utilization or increased requirements. Unsaturated fats, laxatives and mineral oil, inorganic iron, white bread and cereals 'enriched' with iron, and estrogen exert an antagonistic effect on the utilization of vitamin E.''

Overcoming such obstacles require larger amounts of the nutrient than diet alone could ever supply. "We would like to emphasize," they point out, "that we have prescribed vitamin E for patients with lupus and other diseases not as a simple nutritional supplement but as a potent therapeutic agent."

What does the future hold? In light of their good results, Drs. Ayres and Mihan would like to see larger clinical studies begun in which vitamin E would be pitted against not only the discoid, but also the much more serious systemic form of lupus erythematosus.

They are hopeful that such investigations will establish the value of this simple innocuous form of therapy for managing an otherwise recalcitrant, disfiguring and sometimes fatal disease.

Another little-known but serious disease which may someday yield to vitamin E is sickle cell anemia. People with this inherited disease suffer from an abnormality of hemoglobin which affects their circulating red blood cells, with sometimes disastrous results.

Hemoglobin is the iron-rich reddish pigment inside the cells which carries vital oxygen to all the tissues of the body.

Unfortunately, sickle cell victims have an unusual molecular form of hemoglobin which can actually cause the red blood cells to bend into a distorted crescent or sickle shape.

The sickle shape makes it possible for the red cells to slip through the tiniest of blood vessels (called capillaries). Those vessels are so small in diameter that even normal blood cells have to march through in single file. Sickled cells get caught and hopelessly jammed.

Sickle cell victims suffer from recurring attacks of fever and pain in the arms, legs and abdomen as sickled cells back up in blood vessels, causing painful sickling crises.

"Sickle cell anemia afflicts 1 black person out of every 500, or 50,000 American blacks," according to Danny Chiu, Ph.D., a researcher at the Children's Hospital medical center in Oakland, California.

Dr. Chiu and a colleague, Bertram Lubin, M.D., have now discovered that patients with sickle cell anemia also have a vitamin E deficiency. As Dr. Chiu suggested at the Federation of American Societies for Experimental Biology's annual meeting in Dallas in April of 1979, inadequate levels of vitamin E in sickle cell patients' blood plasma and red blood cells may contribute to the sickling process.

For one thing, the scientists found that the extreme susceptibility of red blood cells from sickle cell patients to lipid peroxidation can be prevented—at least in the test tube—by vitamin E. Dr. Chiu speculates that vitamin E's action as an antioxidant may alter the red blood cell membrane's stability, making it less vulnerable to bending and distortion.

Next, Dr. Chiu plans a clinical trial—in which sickle cell patients will receive 400 international units of vitamin E daily for a year and a half—to see if the nutrient can relieve sickling symptoms, as well.

"Normally, most cells of sickle cell patients only sickle under certain circumstances," he explains. "Otherwise, the molecular defect isn't expressed clinically. But some cells, which we call ISC, or irreversibly sickled cells, always sickle. The amount of these cells varies from one patient to another, from 5 to 30 percent."

Already, another study has discovered that supplemental vitamin E can reduce the percentage of ISC by more than half. Researchers from Hoffmann–La Roche and Columbia University told the same Dallas conference that, when 13 sickle cell patients took 450 international units of vitamin E a day, the proportion of irreversibly sickled cells dropped from 25 to 11 percent.

While individuals of African origin are at risk for sickle cell anemia, those from Mediterranean countries like Greece and

Italy sometimes inherit a blood disorder known as thalassemia. Here, too, vitamin E seems to be involved.

People who are born with thalassemia are not able to produce normal hemoglobin. Their red blood cells are misshapen, defective and rapidly destroyed. In its severe form, the disease requires blood transfusions to sustain life.

When a group of patients with thalassemia took supplemental vitamin E (750 international units for three to six months), "encouraging" changes occurred in their red blood cell membranes. This may indicate that vitamin E helps the membranes to better withstand oxidative stress, according to the researchers from Hebrew University–Hadassah Medical School and the Hadassah University hospital, Jerusalem (*Israel Journal of Medical Sciences*).

Protecting Premature Infants

It's too soon to tell if vitamin E will someday be routinely prescribed for treating thalassemia. But the vitamin is already being used in some hospitals to prevent another killer with an unfamiliar name—bronchopulmonary dysplasia, or BPD, for short.

BPD's victims are much too young and helpless to defend themselves. They are premature infants, placed on mechanical respirators because of acute difficulty in breathing. Researchers now believe that this prolonged exposure to high oxygen concentrations under pressure can cause the serious and often fatal structural changes in the lungs called BPD.

However, in a trial at Yale–New Haven Hospital in Connecticut, Joseph B. Warshaw, M.D., and several associates demonstrated that, when such infants were injected with vitamin E, they were far less likely to succumb to BPD. Six of 13 babies who did not get the injections experienced lung changes indicative of BPD, and 4 died. But none of the 9 infants who received supplemental vitamin E showed any signs of BPD, and all survived (*New England Journal of Medicine*).

Finally, vitamin E is believed to protect against another threat to the newborn—retrolental fibroplasia. Again, as with BPD, the premature baby is the target, and life-saving oxygen delivered under pressure is the culprit. The artificially high concentrations of oxygen cause spasm and rupture in tiny blood vessels inside the eye, which can lead to detachment of the retina and a halt to eye growth. For this reason, retrolental fibroplasia is the chief cause of blindness in the newborn.

Researchers at the University of Pennsylvania have found that, when supplemental vitamin E is given, fewer premature babies develop retrolental fibroplasia, and those who do are affected less severely than would otherwise be expected *(Pediatric Research)*.

It's just one more example of the many ways this special nutrient is helping those with special health problems.

62

NUTRITION THAT STARTS AT SKIN LEVEL

Versatile might be a good label for them. They're the nutrients that not only help to keep you healthy on the inside, but go to bat for you when you're hurting on the outside, too. And they go to work directly, right where the hurt is—whether it's a burn, cut or abrasion—because they're applied topically, just like any other salve or ointment. Take a look at vitamin E, for example.

"We've been using vitamin E here for years," says John Flanigan, M.D., a surgeon and director of the enterostomal therapy unit at the Pottsville Hospital and Warne Clinic in Pennsylvania. Dr. Flanigan uses vitamin E ointment or oil in conjunction with oral supplements of E and zinc to promote the secondary closure of wounds.

A primary closure is when a cut is sewn up and it heals, explains Dr. Flanigan. A secondary closure means there is a gaping wound in which some skin has been lost and the tissue underneath is exposed. "Then I give patients the supplements and use vitamin E ointment or oil." Applying vitamin E helps the tiny red particles of new capillaries form on the surface of the wound to patch it together and heal. Doctors call this process granulation. Dr. Flanigan told us, "The tissue is fresher and the wound heals better when vitamin E is applied to it. But you have to have a good range of vitamin E systemically (inside the body) as well as locally." Healing time may be cut in half when vitamin E ointment or oil is used, he said.

The results obtained by using vitamin E can be "very impressive," Dr. Flanigan says, relating the case of a patient whose leg was gangrenous and required amputation. Doctors had decided to amputate above the knee because the leg would heal better. But instead of healing, the leg became gangrenous again and required reamputation higher up on the thigh.

After the second operation, the patient was given vitamin E and zinc supplements, while vitamin E was applied locally on the granulating surface of the wound. The wound began to heal nicely, but the patient broke out in hives. The doctors believed the reaction was an allergic response to the vitamin therapy, so they discontinued it. Within two or three days, the surgical wound began to get worse.

"We decided it wasn't the E and zinc causing the allergy and put the patient back on the program. The wound healed beautifully," says Dr. Flanigan.

Dr. Flanigan says vitamin E ointment and oil are effective on bedsores, too, and can be used in the home for minor first-aid problems. They may be used "indiscriminately" for minor cuts, abrasions and burns, he says, since "vitamin E is never going to hurt anybody." If you should fall and scrape yourself, for instance, thoroughly clean the wound, apply an antiseptic and then reach for the vitamin E, says Dr. Flanigan. The wound should be recleaned and the vitamin E should be reapplied daily for the problem to heal quickly and safely, he says.

Dr. Flanigan credits the late Evan V. Shute, M.D., as one of the people who first convinced him to try vitamin E. Dr. Shute, with his brother, Wilfrid E. Shute, M.D., pioneered research in vitamin E more than 50 years ago. Together they founded the Shute Institute in Canada, which has treated more than 40,000 patients for a variety of diseases with vitamin E.

Vitamin E Should Be in Every Kitchen

In 1975, Dr. Evan Shute, writing in his annual publication for doctors, proclaimed, "Vitamin E should be in every kitchen for convenient use. . . . Burns, abrasions, lacerations respond well to alpha tocopherol [vitamin E]. It should be given promptly, both orally and locally. This minimizes the scarring and deformity seen so often when burns and other wounds heal" *(Summary)*.

In one of several cases documented, Dr. Shute writes of a man who had suffered a second-degree burn of his right forearm. He had come to Dr. Shute 7 days after the accident, his burns severely blistered. He was given 300 international units of vitamin E to take daily by mouth. Vitamin E ointment was applied locally, as well. Within 5 days, the patient's wounds were 90 percent healed. He was completely healed in 11 days without the slightest impairment of his arm's bending ability, notes Dr. Shute.

"The most puzzling yet helpful feature of patients treated for burns with alpha tocopherol is the quick relief of pain," he writes. "When skin grafts fail, they are merely repeated, for that is the end of the line. We rarely send a patient for grafting and never repeat it. Since vitamin E is slightly anti-infective, wounds are usually very clean, an important factor in the 'take' of grafts."

Relief from Cold Sores

Vitamin E also has been reported successful in the treatment of another skin problem, cold sores (herpes simplex). At the health facilities of two industrial firms in Liverpool, England, an "unusually large number of patients" were seen suffering from cold sores, many of which were failing to respond well to standard treatment. Vitamin E capsules were handed out to the patients with instructions to apply the liquid contents to the lesions every four hours.

"The most striking results were: (a) quick and sustained relief of pain, and (b) early disappearance of the lesion," say the report's authors, who have treated at least 50 patients successfully with the method. "Now, as a matter of routine," patients with cold sores are given a capsule (and a pin!) and told how to apply the oil," they write (*British Dental Journal*, vol. 148, no. 11-1, 1980).

CHAPTER

63

VITAMIN E, WHEN IT'S SINK OR SWIM

We're all swimming in a sea of stress—physical, emotional, chemical. And some of us are in over our heads. How about you?

Air pollution is dragging your lungs down for the third time. Some scientists say that radiation—microwaves, X rays, nuclear power—is a hidden riptide that can wash your health out to sea. And the doughnuts tossed at you by the neon lights of your local fast-food strip aren't exactly life preservers.

Have a sinking feeling about all that stress? Then swim—with vitamin E.

When researchers want to find out about stress, they don't kid around. One of their favorite tests is to throw rats into a tub of cold water and see how long they can swim before sinking. The test packs a lifetime of stress into an hour (the rats even develop ulcers).

A researcher from the California State University in Hayward recently conducted such a test. But first, he divided the rats into a few groups and, for 18 days, supplemented the diets of some groups with vitamin E. He found that the vitamin E rats swam longer and had milder ulcers than the animals who weren't fed vitamin E (*Clinical Research*, vol. 27, no. 1, 1979).

But does this test hold water for you? After all, you're probably not a member of the local Polar Bear Club or an English Channel swimmer who likes to make January crossings. But you are someone who breathes, and that means coping with a source of stress that can give cold feet to anyone who's striving for better health—air pollution. Vitamin E can guard against that, too.

Daniel Menzel, Ph.D., a researcher at the Duke University medical center in Durham, North Carolina, continuously exposed three groups of mice to ozone, one of the deadliest air pollutants. One group, however, received a large amount of vitamin E with its diet, another group got a smaller amount and the third group got no vitamin E. The group receiving the large amount of vitamin E survived an average of two weeks longer than the other groups (*Toxicology and Applied Pharmacology*).

In another experiment, Dr. Menzel exposed two groups of mice to nitrogen dioxide, a pollutant just as deadly as ozone. He gave one group a daily amount of vitamin E equivalent to what a person would get if he took 100 international units. The other group received the equivalent of 10 international units of vitamin E, the amount found in the average American's diet. After three months of exposure to nitrogen dioxide, both groups of mice had lung damage "very similar to what occurs in the early stages of human emphysema," said Dr. Menzel. But the 100 international unit mice had significantly less lung damage (*Medical Tribune*).

In yet another study, Ching K. Chow, Ph.D., of the University of Kentucky, exposed two groups of rats, one supplemented with vitamin E and the other not, to cigarette smoke. After three days of chain smoking, 5 of the 16 unsupplemented rats were dead, compared to only 1 of the 13 supplemented rats.

Dr. Chow said cigarette smoke contains more than 3,000 chemicals, many of which are highly reactive and may have altered certain essential enzymes in the rats. He concluded that it was the cigarette's visible smoke, rather than its invisible gases, that did the most harm.

Well, you're not a rat or a mouse. But you are a guinea pig in an experiment called the 20th century—continuous exposure to ozone, nitrogen dioxide and a menacing mix of other air pollutants. And you don't want to be in the 10 international units' group—even if you live where the air seems clean.

Pollution Is Inescapable

"Air pollution is not confined to metropolitan areas," Dr. Menzel told us. "Rain made highly acidic by air pollution is a uniform phenomenon east of the Rocky Mountains. The amount of ozone in certain rural areas of New Jersey is greater than in downtown Manhattan."

To protect his own health, Dr. Menzel takes 200 international units of vitamin E every day. "A study I'm now completing may show if a higher amount is needed," he says. "But 200 international units should help protect the body from the stress of air pollution."

Why can't your body go it alone? Oxidation is why.

Oxidation is happening all around you—a rusted-out car, a rotten banana, yellowed newspapers in the attic. All have been oxidized, slowly sizzled by oxygen. Ozone and nitrogen dioxide can turn the scorch of oxidation into a four-alarm blaze—and turn your lungs into a burned-out ruin. Vitamin E douses the fire.

But that's not the whole story. Free radicals are chemical maniacs, out-of-control molecules that roam around looking for something to destroy. Oxidation creates the free radicals and they do the dirty work—but not if they meet their match in vitamin E. Oxidation isn't the only process that creates free radicals, however. So does radiation.

Radiation—the energy that beams out of X-ray machines and pulses at the core of nuclear reactors. Like an atom-size bullet racing at nearly the speed of light, radiation can rip into the very center of a cell. The wound is called cancer. Some scientists believe that free radicals are responsible for radiation-caused cancer. And with various kinds of radiation in the living room (color TV), the bedroom (luminous clock dial) and the kitchen (microwave oven), vitamin E may help keep your home a sweet home.

Researchers from the Netherlands grew cell cultures in their laboratory, adding vitamin E to some of the cultures. After several weeks, they bombarded all the cells with X rays—and more of the vitamin E cells survived *(British Journal of Radiology)*.

Radiation is a typically modern—and typically dangerous—stress. Mercury is another.

Mercury made the headlines in the late 60s and early 70s when a Japanese industrial firm dumped it into a bay and severely poisoned many of the people living near there. Their symptoms—lack of coordination, blindness, deafness, slurred speech—marked mercury as one of the most toxic substances around. And even though you don't hear much about mercury these days, each year in America 310 tons are spewed into the air and 80 tons dumped into the water. But E can help.

Scientists from the National Medical Center for Toxicological Research in Jefferson, Arkansas, gave laboratory animals either mercury alone or mercury with vitamin E. The animals who got mercury alone suffered severe damage to their brains and central nervous systems. But vitamin E, said the researchers, "showed a remarkable protective effect"—the animals who received it remained in almost perfect health *(Environmental Research)*.

Mercury, radiation, ozone—vitamin E takes them all on. And it even tussles with the toughest customer there is—aging.

Extending the Life Span

Scientists are just beginning to understand what makes people age. One widely accepted theory lays the blame on free radicals. Denham Harman, M.D., Ph.D., a professor at the University of Nebraska college of medicine and the chief proponent of this theory, believes that cancer, heart disease, high blood pressure and senility are all caused, in part, by free radicals. He told us that a diet which includes ample amounts of vitamin E could "lessen the possibility of those health problems occurring." Such a diet, he says, "may reasonably be expected to add five to ten or more years of healthy, productive life to the life span of the average person.''

Another scientist who studies aging, Johan Bjorksten, Ph.D., says the RDA for vitamin E is the amount "necessary to avert obvious deficiency symptoms, but by no means the optimal range for longevity." He thinks that a daily supplement of 200 to 300 international units could conceivably extend a person's life span by 5 to 15 years *(Rejuvenation)*.

And Dr. Menzel told us that the amount of vitamin E in the typical American diet—9 international units—is probably too low to maintain good health, let alone shield a person from stress.

Diet Alone Can't Do It

The daily amounts of vitamin E recommended by these scientists—anywhere from 100 to 600 international units—are much higher than found in even the most natural and wholesome diet. But one study shows that there are no harmful effects from taking 800 international units a day for many years, so if you want to use that much vitamin E, you can do so with confidence *(American Journal of Clinical Nutrition)*.

Of course, even if you take a vitamin E supplement, you still want to get as much vitamin E from your food as you're entitled to. And it's simple to do: Avoid processed and refined foods.

Canned and frozen foods lose up to 65 percent of their vitamin E. Grains are a good source of the vitamin, at least until they're milled. Corn flakes, for instance, have lost 98 percent of their vitamin E. Whole wheat bread has seven times more vitamin E than white bread, and brown rice has six times more than white rice. Nuts, another good source, lose up to 80 percent of their vitamin E when roasted. Oils, too, provide plenty of vitamin E—unless they're hydrogenated. For the most vitamin E, eat whole foods.

You have to swim against the stream of stress, but you don't have to drown in it. Buoy yourself up—with vitamin E.

CHAPTER

64

VITAMIN E HELPS PROTECT THE BREASTS

"Given the results of this study, we can conclude that vitamin E may help prevent cancer of the breast."

So says Robert London, M.D., director of obstetrical and gynecological research at Sinai Hospital in Baltimore, Maryland. The study he's talking about is one he conducted in which vitamin E was used to treat not cancer, but fibrocystic disease of the breast. That's a disease in which cysts, tiny sacs filled with liquid, poke out through the skin of the breast, tearing tissue and forming hard lumps and sores.

In an interview with us, Dr. London emphasized that these lumps are not cancerous. However, he did point out that "50 percent of all women have this disease sometime in their lives, and there is a much higher incidence of cancer of the breast—about two to eight times greater—among women who have had fibrocystic disease."

With this in mind, Dr. London reasons that anything that would effectively treat fibrocystic disease might prevent breast cancer in thousands of women.

And according to his study, vitamin E does just that.

Dr. London first reported the results of his study to a meeting of the American College of Obstetricians and Gynecologists held in Washington, D.C. *(Ob. Gyn. News)*.

Dr. London told the physicians that, for his study, he selected 12 of his patients, menstruating women with fibrocystic breast disease. These women ranged in age from 16 to 42 years old. Every day for three months, he gave these women a placebo—a pill with no real potency. Then, for two months, they received a daily dosage of 600 international units of vitamin E. Eight healthy women, chosen as controls, also were given placebos and vitamin E.

Of these 12 patients, 10 improved. Seven had what Dr. London called a "good" clinical response. Three had a "fair" response. But when these 10 women were taken off the vitamin E treatment, their disease returned full force—within just six weeks, the women's breasts "had the appearance they did before the treatment," Dr. London told the conference.

This finding alone is dramatic evidence that vitamin E treats fibrocystic breast disease—and so could prevent breast cancer.

But Dr. London also discovered the biological mechanics behind vitamin E's rapid healing of cysts and sores, and this discovery gave him a hint as to how vitamin E might stop breast cancer before it starts.

Dr. London found increased amounts of a hormone secreted by the adrenal gland in the women with fibrocystic disease after they started taking vitamin E. But why is this so important?

Boosting hormonal levels is a classic treatment for women who already have breast cancer. An article in the *Journal of the American Medical Association* states that "alteration of the hormonal milieu is still one of the major and most successful methods for treating advanced breast cancer." And another article in *Science* points out that, in some cases of breast cancer, "tumor growth is regulated by the hormonal environment and that a change in this environment will cause tumor regression."

Dr. London told the conference that vitamin E, by altering the level of a certain hormone in women with fibrocystic disease before they get breast cancer, "might alter the subsequent development of breast carcinoma. . . ."

But in spite of all this fanfare, do we really need to enlist vitamin E in the fight against breast cancer? After all, isn't the American medical establishment slowly but surely conquering this disease? What about those highly touted early detection programs that supposedly save the lives of thousands of women? What about those new drug treatments hailed in a prestigious medical journal as "nothing short of spectacular?"

Conventional Therapy Inadequate

Norman Simon, M.D., and Sidney Silverstone, M.D., professors at the Mount Sinai School of Medicine, provide one thoughtful answer to these questions: "Despite recent great advances in medical care, the mortality rate for cancer of the breast in the United States is essentially unchanged. Even if there has been some improvement in the survival of patients with cancer of the breast through modern, presumably more effective management, this improvement is hardly commensurate with the announced advances in therapy and early detection" *(Bulletin of the New York Academy of Medicine)*.

Breast cancer is still the most feared cancer among women. And for good reason. The major killer of American women between the ages of 33 and 55, breast cancer will strike at least 88,000 American women this year. Thirty-three thousand will die. But these facts and figures don't tell the whole story.

Cancer specialist Henry M. Lemon, M.D., professor of medicine at the University of Nebraska medical school, speaking to an American Cancer Society seminar for science writers, warned that eight million American women will develop breast cancer sometime in their lives, and "the majority of these women will ultimately die of their disease with current diagnostic and treatment methods."

"Although there is no current therapeutic regimen for fibrocystic disease of the breast," Dr. London suggests, "vitamin

E under controlled circumstances may be a valuable adjunct to therapy.'' And he says that he has seen no harmful side effects from taking the vitamin, either in his own practice or reported in medical journals.

"It may be doing women with fibrocystic disease some good,'' Dr. London told us, ''and certainly is relieving their symptoms of lumps, sores and tenderness.''

At least for 50 percent of the women reading this book, that's good to hear.

CHAPTER

65

CF KIDS REQUIRE EXTRA VITAMIN E

Coping with cystic fibrosis (CF) generally means pulling out all nutritional stops. But now there's evidence that vitamin E may be the most critical consideration.

The idea that CF kids may be deficient in vitamin E isn't new. It's been suspected for some time, since the body's uptake of vitamin E depends largely on its ability to digest and absorb fats. And many—if not most—CF patients have trouble absorbing fats due to a complication involving the pancreas.

Yet, until now, researchers had a hard time making that theory stick. For one thing, traditional blood tests which measure the total vitamin E levels never show much difference between CF patients and healthy controls. And even if they did, the doctors would tell us that vitamin E deficiency wasn't much to worry about.

Researchers at the National Institutes of Health in Bethesda, Maryland, suggest otherwise. Singling out alpha tocopherol (the most important component of vitamin E) in blood samples taken from CF patients, they found that all of 52 patients suffering from intestinal dysfunction were deficient in the vitamin. And—more important—they discovered that this deficiency had a decided effect on the red blood cells.

Red blood cells taken from vitamin E–deficient CF patients had a much shorter life span than those taken from healthy persons with adequate vitamin E levels. This reduced survival rate was boosted back up to normal with vitamin E supplementation in doses ranging from 50 to 400 international units per day, the researchers noted (*Journal of Clinical Investigation*).

What does this mean to the CF patient? We asked Philip M. Farrell, M.D., Ph.D., head of these investigations.

"Taking vitamin E isn't going to cure CF," he explained. "But I'd say it's likely to be of some benefit.

"It's conceivable, for example, that the severe lung disease associated with CF puts stress on the red blood cells, which—as you know—are involved in transporting oxygen. Since vitamin E provides protection of these blood cells, it's likely that a vitamin E–supplemented child will have the edge in fighting CF.

"And there's another thing that we didn't mention in the report but which I think you should know," Dr. Farrell confides. "The vitamin E content in lung tissues is normally high. In view of the pulmonary problems in CF patients, I think that says something!"

Of course, Dr. Farrell is just speculating on the implications of a vitamin E deficiency, at this point. But he is sure of one thing—"patients with CF should be given daily doses of a water-soluble form of vitamin E."

How much?

"We gave our patients five to ten times the Recommended Dietary Allowance," he replied. "The RDA for children is 5 to 10 international units per day."

VITAMIN K

CHAPTER

66

YOUR FOUNDATION NEEDS VITAMIN K

What vitamin is found in such large quantities in nature, and required in such small amounts by the body, that deficiencies were always thought to be rare? Most people haven't even heard of it. It's not commonly available in supplemental form because we apparently need no more of it than is available in a good, sensible diet. And part of our supply of the vitamin is produced in the body itself, by bacteria in the intestinal tract.

Although most people don't even know it exists, there is such a thing as vitamin K, and we'd all be in deep trouble without it.

Vitamin K is required for the production of a number of coagulation factors, substances in the blood which are essential for normal blood clotting. Nosebleeds, bleeding in the intestines and stomach, and blood in the urine are all common in vitamin K deficiency. Bleeding may occur within the brain, and the deficiency can result in death.

But if vitamin K deficiency is so rare, what's the problem? Scientists used to believe there was no problem at all, but now they're not so sure. Until a few years ago, the only role vitamin K was known to play in maintaining good health was its assurance of proper blood clotting. And people were certainly not bleeding to death because of vitamin K deficiencies. Indeed, it was hard to find even minor problems caused by a lack of vitamin K.

Now, however, a body of evidence is building which indicates that vitamin K may do more than promote coagulation. Research at Harvard University, the University of California at San Diego, and other scientific centers suggests that vitamin K is necessary for the maintenance of healthy bones, as well. There is evidence, a spokesman for the Harvard research team told us, that slight vitamin K deficiencies in older people may be contributing to the degeneration of bone that is so common at that time of life.

"The work so far," the spokesman told us, "is only a suggestion that vitamin K is important. Vitamin D has long been known to be involved in calcium uptake and turnover in bone. Now, evidence suggests that another vitamin may also play a role, but by a totally different mechanism."

Research has already demonstrated a possible connection between vitamin K and strong bones in animals. Scientists at the University of North Carolina at Chapel Hill found that chicks fed a vitamin K–deficient diet suffered a 10 percent reduction in the mineral content of their bones after only five days on the diet *(Journal of Dental Research)*.

That study was prompted by, and supported, work the Harvard team did in 1975. "What we did first," one of the Harvard researchers told us, "was to isolate from chick bone a protein which binds calcium and does so only through the action of vitamin K. The protein is called osteocalcin, and it's also abundant in human bone."

The binding of calcium around a protein framework is a crucial step in the building of healthy bones. "The bone is a complex mixture of minerals," the spokesperson told us, "primarily calcium phosphate, precipitated in and around a protein matrix. The protein matrix is about 90 percent collagen and 10 percent other proteins. Possibly the most important of those other proteins is osteocalcin, which makes up 1 percent of the total protein in the bone.

"Osteocalcin doesn't bind all the calcium in the bone, only a small fraction of it, in fact. But osteocalcin plays an important role when the bone is first taking shape. Just as bone starts to mineralize, this protein appears on the scene. Vitamin K is required for the synthesis of osteocalcin, or rather, for an important modification of osteocalcin once it has been synthesized. After the protein has been modified by vitamin K, it can bind calcium, even if vitamin K is no longer present."

Vitamin K gives osteocalcin its special chemical gift, and that might be the spark which sets the whole process of bone mineralization in motion. The scientists in North Carolina found that the initial binding of calcium by the protein matrix was either severely reduced or totally absent in the bones of chicks deficient in vitamin K.

Bone mineralization is an ongoing process, though, and it may be that vitamin K is continually needed for the process to go on. The skeleton is a living, constantly changing organ, the Harvard spokesman stressed. "The structure of bones is like reinforced concrete, in that the protein matrix supports the mineral structure around it. But I hesitate to use that analogy because bone is a very dynamic organ. Unlike concrete, it's constantly being replaced. The whole structure turns over in the course of time. In some parts of the skeleton, the turnover is as little as 1 percent in a year, but in babies the entire skeleton is replaced in that time."

As we grow older, and particularly as women undergo menopause, something happens to disrupt the healthy turnover of bone. A condition called osteoporosis may set in, causing loss of bone mass and increasing fragility of the bones. The condition affects three out of every four women after menopause, resulting in a frightening increase in broken bones. By the age of 90, one woman out of every five fractures a hip, and one of every six of those women dies within three months of the injury. Studies have already shown that extra calcium in the diet can help prevent osteoporosis.

But scientists in Japan have also used vitamin K to reduce the loss of calcium from bones that occurs in osteoporosis, the Harvard researcher told us. "The Japanese study was published in 1971, well before our knowledge of the connection between osteocalcin and vitamin K. We dug it out of the literature only after we isolated osteocalcin in bone in 1975. Once we had done that, we wanted to see if vitamin K had ever been associated with bone mineralization before.

"The Japanese scientists looked at three osteoporosis patients. In three women, vitamin K reduced calcium loss in the bone, by 18 percent in one patient, 50 percent in another and 21 percent in the third.

"But such evidence is very preliminary in nature. The studies of vitamin K and bone formation have mostly been done with animals and are just now expanding to clinical research, to relate the ideas developed with animals to human problems."

Work with humans has established one other bit of evidence indicating a link between vitamin K and bone formation. Anticoagulant drugs, which prevent blood clotting, are antagonists of vitamin K. They block its coagulant effects. They may also block its possible effects on bone formation.

"When pregnant women are given anticoagulant drugs in the first three months of pregnancy," the Harvard spokesman said, "many have given birth to babies with bone defects. Conceivably, this syndrome involves an abnormal synthesis of osteocalcin.

"Of course, it will be years before the facts are established in humans. But having the power to speculate, when you reach certain conclusions in animal studies, you begin to look at the possibilities for humans. After all, that's the reason we study animals, to get clues for applications in clinical situations with human patients."

One of the most tantalizing possibilities would be the use of vitamin K to fight osteoporosis. The Harvard spokesman told us there are plenty of hints that such therapy might help.

"Osteoporosis occurs mainly in older people. Those people often eat soft, bland foods and fail to eat enough green vegetables, which are rich in vitamin K. Studies in England have shown that older people are commonly slightly vitamin K–deficient, in that their blood coagulation activity is slightly reduced.

"Older people also often take mineral oil as a laxative, which interferes with the way vitamin K is absorbed into the body.'' Other drugs which older people are more likely to use—including anticoagulants, antibiotics and cholestyramine, a drug used to lower cholesterol levels in the blood—may all contribute to vitamin K deficiency.

Beyond the problem of calcium loss in bones, there are larger possibilities for vitamin K suggested by current research. Calcium is involved in a host of biological processes other than bone formation, such as muscle contraction, the transmission of nerve impulses and the release of hormones. All those processes involve a chemical reaction called calcium binding.

Just as vitamin K is involved in the formation of the calcium-binding protein osteocalcin in bones, scientists have found, it triggers another calcium-binding protein in the blood. That reaction has been shown to be the key to vitamin K's promotion of blood clotting. And the researchers at Harvard have found similar proteins, dependent on vitamin K, in the kidneys and human placenta (*Biochemical and Biophysical Research Communications; Biochemica et Biophysica Acta*, vol. 583, 1979).

In the placenta, a vitamin K deficiency may produce the bone defects seen in the babies of mothers taking anticoagulant drugs. ''The placenta provides all the calcium to the fetus from the mother's circulation,'' the Harvard spokesman explained. ''It's the exchange mechanism through which the fetal skeleton gets all its calcium.'' If, according to the theory, a vitamin deficiency produced by anticoagulant drugs upsets this vital link, the fetus fails to get the calcium it needs.

A vitamin K deficiency acting on the kidneys could cause problems for adults. ''The kidneys are involved in determining how much calcium is excreted from the body,'' the spokesperson told us. ''The vitamin K–dependent protein we found in the kidney may have an important role in the retention of calcium in the body.'' A failure of that protein, caused by a lack of vitamin K, might disrupt the supply of calcium to the entire body. That, of course, would throw a variety of essential biological systems on the blink.

''A daily requirement for vitamin K has not yet been established,'' the Harvard spokesperson said, ''but diets containing plenty of fresh green vegetables will provide adequate vitamin K.'' Broccoli, cabbage, lettuce, turnip greens and spinach are all good sources of the nutrient.

People taking anticoagulant drugs should keep their physicians posted on any changes in their diets, particularly any increase in foods rich in vitamin K. The amounts of those drugs required to produce a desired effect vary with intake of the vitamin, since K promotes the blood clotting the drugs are meant to stifle. A radical change in diet could produce health hazards for people using those drugs.

Though no one knows for sure exactly how much vitamin K the average adult needs, there have been some estimates. The National Research Council, which draws up the Recommended Dietary Allowances for nutrients used by the government, does not have an official RDA for vitamin K, but they do make a ball-park guess.

They say the average adult needs between 70 and 140 micrograms of K each day. That's not too difficult. For example, to get 140 micrograms of vitamin K, you would have to eat about 2½ ounces of broccoli. (You'd probably be better off with a bit more vitamin K, especially if you're over 60 or so.) Sounds like a very sensible approach, indeed, to avoiding what could be some very complex health problems.

BOOK III

Vitamin Therapy for Disease

INTRODUCTION

One doctor we talked to called it "medical schizophrenia."

On the one hand, scientific study after study shows that vitamins have *therapeutic* power—that they can prevent or cure disease. And these studies are published in medical journals that doctors read as regularly as you read the morning paper.

On the other hand, when someone walks into a doctor's office and says he has kidney stones, he gets a drug—not magnesium and vitamin B_6. A person with intermittent claudication (leg cramps during walking) gets a drug—not vitamin E. And a woman on the Pill who has depression gets a drug—not vitamin B_6. Yet all these vitamins are *proven* treatments that many doctors know about. Not only that, they're often safer and more often effective than drugs. So why don't doctors use them? Why this medical schizophrenia?

No one really knows for sure. But what we do know is that you shouldn't be cheated out of using vitamins when they could help your disease or condition. That's what book 3—Vitamin Therapy for Disease—is all about. It will describe scores of scientific reports that show vitamins can help everyday problems like colds or fatigue and health disasters like cancer or heart disease. In many cases, the vitamin will be preventive, a way of stopping those illnesses before they start. But you'll also read about vitamin therapy for people who are already sick. Not that you should stop seeing your doctor and switch to vitamins. These therapies are meant to be used in conjunction with medical treatment and with your doctor's approval. That's why throughout the book we've included the names of the medical journals in which these studies appeared and the scientists who conducted them—if you tell your doctor that information, he can read those studies for himself in a source he's sure to respect. And maybe *you* can cure *him*—of medical schizophrenia.

ACNE

CHAPTER

67

VITAMIN A FOR ACNE

Most people suffer from acne during adolescence. The passage of time heals them. But for a few unlucky people, acne persists, covering their faces, necks and shoulders with weltlike sores and inflamed sacs that can leave permanent scars. Dermatologists have tried helping them with X rays, antibiotics, female hormones, anti-inflammatory corticosteroids and even steel brushes for scouring off the scars. Unfortunately, serious side effects often accompany the long-term use of those treatments.

There are promising new alternatives, however. In experimental trials, a man-made cousin of vitamin A, called 13-cis retinoic acid, has cured even the most stubborn acne in many cases.

One study of 13-cis retinoic acid (*13-cis* identifies its molecular structure) comes from Leeds, England, where doctors used it to treat eight patients between the ages of 18 and 32. The patients suffered from severe acne—ranging from small pimples to deeply inflamed cysts—that therapy with antibiotics hadn't helped.

The patients took oral 13-cis retinoic acid daily for four months. After one month, the amount of sebum (the skin oil that causes pimples when it's trapped under the skin by clogged ducts) produced by their sebaceous glands declined by 75 percent. After four months, the patients' acne conditions improved by 80 percent (*Lancet,* November 15, 1980).

The researchers described the improvement as "dramatic." "By 16 weeks there was an 80 percent improvement in the overall grade and 80 percent reduction in non-inflamed lesions, 90 percent reduction in small inflamed lesions, and 90 percent reduction in deep inflamed lesions."

According to the researchers, this synthetic form of vitamin A does what vitamin A does—normalizes all the epithelial tissues, including the skin—but does it much more efficiently.

Side effects from the therapy included dryness of the eyes and inflamed lips, but they weren't severe enough to make any of the patients drop out of the program. In fact, the researchers were able to minimize the side effects by cutting the dosage down without sacrificing the therapeutic effect.

Most important, 13-cis retinoic acid seems to keep on working after the patients stop taking it. In experiments at the National Cancer Institute, 13 of 14 previously untreatable acne patients were totally cleared of acne, and the other one improved by 75 percent. After the treatment ended, the patients remained acne free for between 12 and 20 months (*New England Journal of Medicine,* February 15, 1979).

Thirteen-cis retinoic acid is not to be confused with vitamin A or vitamin A acid. Natural vitamin A is necessary for healthy skin, and some dermatologists prescribe it for their acne patients. But many physicians feel that in the doses required for long-term acne therapy—as much as 300,000 international units a day—vitamin A isn't safe.

Vitamin A acid, also called retinoic acid, is commonly applied as an ointment for acne. It dissolves the comedo—better known as a plug or blackhead—so that the acne sores can drain. Some doctors avoid retinoic acid because it can irritate the skin, making it more vulnerable to sunburn and to sunlight-induced skin cancer.

Vitamin A levels in the body are dependent on a good supply of zinc, and some researchers have studied the combined effects of zinc and vitamin A on acne.

Gerd Michaelsson, M.D., of Uppsala, Sweden, has found that "boys with severe, but not mild, acne have significantly lower serum zinc levels than healthy controls" and that "both boys and girls with severe acne have significantly lower levels of retinol-binding protein [an indicator of the amount of vitamin A in the blood] than healthy controls.

"A low-zinc diet may worsen or activate acne, especially the pustular reactions," Dr. Michaelsson says. "This is seen after 10 to 14 days in acne-prone patients" (*Nutrition Reviews*, February, 1981).

Dr. Michaelsson first linked zinc to acne while treating a patient who suffered from a disease called acrodermatitis enteropathica and also from acne. He prescribed zinc for the acrodermatitis and, unexpectedly, his patient's acne cleared up. Dr. Michaelsson later began experimenting with zinc and acne.

None of the researchers know exactly how zinc works. Dr. Michaelsson found that acne recurred when the zinc treatment was discontinued. He theorizes that zinc may induce the release of vitamin A in the body, that it may have an anti-inflammatory effect, that a deficiency of zinc causes enlargement of the sebaceous glands. He also thinks that a widespread zinc deficiency may contribute to acne.

Two dermatologists who use vitamin A as well as zinc in their practice are Milton Saunders, Jr., M.D., and Irwin I. Lubowe, M.D. Dr. Saunders is the president of the Optimum Health Foundation in Virginia Beach, Virginia. Dr. Saunders advises against an excess of whole milk and fried foods. He also discourages the use of coffee, tea or very hot and spicy foods because they may dilate blood vessels of the face and aggravate acne.

Stress Can Be a Factor

About 20 percent of his patients are adults, Dr. Saunders says, and their therapy differs from adolescents'. "In many teenagers, diet is the key to acne, but among adults, stress is the key factor."

Women schoolteachers, Dr. Saunders has found, often come to him with stress-related acne. He finds that when they spend time away from the classroom their acne begins to clear. Salesmen are another high-risk group. Their regimen of travel, restaurant food and social drinking tends to give them pimples. Athletic stress, if it triggers the release of male hormones (in men or women), is also suspected of making acne worse.

Dr. Saunders uses antibiotics, vitamin A acid ointment, zinc supplements and water-soluble vitamin A (since fat-soluble vitamin A may be harmful in large doses) in an effort to heal the skin as soon as possible. "There's no point in fooling around," he told us. "These people want results yesterday."

Dr. Lubowe, who practices in New York City, also prescribes water-soluble vitamin A. In addition, he advises his patients to take 400 international units of vitamin E and 50 milligrams of zinc daily. And in his book, *A Teenage Guide to Healthy Skin and Hair* (E. P. Dutton, 1979), he expresses his own opinions on diet and acne:

"Too many fats in your diet are a common cause of acne. Since the sebaceous glands need food to function, they draw upon the daily intake of food that is transported to the skin by the blood. The worst villains are fatty meats, carbohydrates, chocolate, cocoa, spices, iodized salt and shellfish."

The outlook for acne treatment has never been better. In the past, acne sufferers faced difficult and confusing choices between treatments of questionable value. But now there are promising alternatives, including options as simple as switching from saturated to unsaturated fats and eating foods rich in vitamin A and zinc.

CHAPTER

68

ANTIOXIDANT VITAMINS VS. PREMATURE AGING

Oxygen. You can't live without it. But each breath you take, drenching every cell in your body with life-sustaining oxygen, carries you one step closer to old age and possible degenerative disease. And that relentless journey may go faster or slower, depending on how you and oxygen mix.

Don't get us wrong. Oxygen is absolutely essential to health. You couldn't survive for more than a few minutes without it. And up to a point, more is better. Athletes and other fitness buffs strive to increase their bodies' oxygen-processing capacity as a measure of enhanced vigor. But unless you are properly protected, fats or lipids (which are abundant in all your cells) can combine with oxygen at an excessive rate in a chemical process known as oxidation.

Given favorable conditions, oxidation will turn a shiny metal wrench into an ugly rusted wrench very quickly. Our bodies, of course, don't rust. But under the right circumstances, oxidative damage produces the kind of accelerated wear and tear that may lead to premature aging, lowered resistance, cancer and heart disease.

The guilty party is believed to be a tiny molecular fragment called a free radical. Free radicals are extremely unstable substances which, in the presence of oxygen, combine at random with unsaturated fats to form peroxides. In butter and other highly perishable foods, free radical reactions lead to spoiling or rancidity. In human beings, free radical reactions cause irreparable damage to cells and the protective membrane linings that surround cells. And this damage accumulates over the years with telltale age spots, wrinkling and worse.

Putting the Brakes on Free Radicals

Fortunately, nature has provided us with a way of slowing down such reactions. "Cells and tissues are protected against oxidizing free radicals by a complexity of antioxidant mechanisms," explains T. L. Dormandy of the department of chemical pathology at London's Whittington Hospital. "So long as the supply of antioxidants lasts, these free radicals are instantly trapped" *(Lancet)*.

"But one antioxidant molecule can scavenge only one free radical," the author warns. So a constant "self-regenerating" supply is needed.

Luckily, the three most important natural antioxidants—vitamin E, the trace mineral selenium and vitamin C—are easily obtainable if we're willing to make the efforts.

To understand how antioxidants protect us, let's take a look at some scientific findings.

Antioxidants can block the formation of tumors. Thirty-three weeks after exposure to a powerful cancer-causing chemical, animals whose diets were supplemented with a mixture of four antioxidants—including vitamins E and C—developed only about half as many tumors as unprotected animals *(Experientia)*.

One of the researchers, Homer S. Black, Ph.D., told us that the same antioxidant mixture showed "very marked effects" protecting against tumors triggered by ultraviolet light. And it's likely that this protection occurs at the cellular level: In other trials, the same antioxidants tested separately prevented the usual cell-destroying effects of ultraviolet irradiation.

"We're primarily concerned with skin cancer," says Dr. Black, who is director of the photobiology laboratory at the Houston, Texas, Veterans Administration Hospital. "But while skin cancer affects the epidermis, many other cancers arise in the epithelial lining of internal organs—and that's similar to skin. So I think what we're finding about antioxidants may have implications for other cancers, as well."

In addition to protecting against cancer, antioxidants may also have a beneficial effect in extending the life of cells. When clusters of rat brain cells are cultured in a test tube, they normally show signs of severe structural degeneration within 40 days. But when similar cell clusters were held in a culture supplemented with vitamin E, the cells were still well preserved and structurally sound after 40 days (*Anatomical Record*).

"The difference was like night and day," Bruce D. Trapp, Ph.D., of the National Institute of Neurological and Communicative Disorders and Stroke, told us. Dr. Trapp explained that the cells lived longer because of vitamin E, which may help preserve the cell membrane, letting various metabolites into clusters of cells while letting wastes escape. "Otherwise, the cells will die," he said.

Helping the Body Help Itself

Antioxidants also appear to play a key role in fostering immunity, the body's natural ability to repel invading disease organisms. According to Werner A. Baumgartner, Ph.D., and coworkers of the nuclear medicine department at the Wadsworth Hospital Center in Los Angeles, body stores of vitamin E and selenium tend to fall sharply when there is a tumor. And this antioxidant deficiency may be responsible in part for the depressed immunity so common in cancer patients. They suggest that antioxidant supplementation might reverse this often fatal situation *(American Journal of Clinical Nutrition).*

"In fact," Dr. Baumgartner told us, "there is growing evidence that even in healthy people the immune processes require more antioxidants than we normally take in with our food. The immune system seems to require *more* antioxidants than other cells in the body. So even a slight stress, such as a marginal deficiency of vitamin E, could impair the immune response."

In still another new report, Los Angeles dermatologists Samuel Ayres, Jr., M.D., and Richard Mihan, M.D., have found vitamin E to be of great therapeutic value in many disabling and stubborn skin disorders. And they believe the reason is vitamin E's antioxidant properties *(Cutis).*

All the diseases they discuss—including scleroderma, vasculitis and other disfiguring inflammatory disorders—seem to involve a breakdown in which the body's normal defense mechanism goes haywire.

Drs. Ayres and Mihan theorize that these conditions, called autoimmune diseases—in which the immune mechanism literally attacks the body's own tissues—are the result of cell rupturing caused by free radicals. Large doses of vitamin E—up to 1,600 international units daily—have produced dramatic reversals.

The most spectacular case was a 45-year-old man suffering from Raynaud's phenomenon. In this condition, constriction of small arteries in the fingers and toes can choke off the blood supply, leading to a bluish discoloration. This man had six ulcerated fingers as a result, and in three, gangrene had set in. But within eight weeks of applying vitamin E directly to the skin and taking the supplement by mouth, as well, the man's fingers were completely healed. On a continuing maintenance dose of vitamin E, there was no recurrence during the next year.

Extending Life Spans

One of the most enthusiastic supporters of vitamin E's value as an antiaging factor is Denham Harman, M.D., Ph.D., of the

University of Nebraska college of medicine in Omaha. In his studies, Dr. Harman found that, when various antioxidants were added to the daily diets of mice shortly after weaning, their average life expectancy was increased by 15 to 44 percent. They also developed fewer breast tumors and fewer senile plaques—small areas of degeneration in the brain.

"Support is steadily growing for the possibility that seemingly haphazard free radical reactions play a significant role—possibly the major one—in the breakdown of the human body during the process of aging," Dr. Harman explains. "It is reasonable to expect that one or more free radical reaction inhibitors, added to a properly selected natural diet, may increase the functional human life span by five to ten years. Those would be extra years of active, enjoyable life."

Dr. Harman adds, "Many free radical reaction inhibitors are known. However, the most prominent in living things, and best known, is vitamin E. . . . Thus, increasing the weekly intake of vitamin E by 300 to 500 international units may possibly increase our prospects for a long and healthy life."

Although vitamin E and selenium are the most widely discussed natural antioxidants, vitamin C also has antioxidant properties in addition to its more publicized cold-fighting and antiviral capabilities.

That's why vitamin C (in the form of sodium ascorbate) is now being added to many processed meats such as frankfurters and bologna. According to Terence W. Anderson, M.D., Ph.D., professor of epidemiology at the University of Toronto, vitamin C's antioxidant properties block the oxidative transformation of nitrate additives into cancer-causing substances called nitrosamines *(Nutrition Today)*.

For the same reason, one large pharmaceutical firm urged that vitamin E (alpha tocopherol) also be added to nitrate-preserved meats. Hoffmann–La Roche researchers have found that together the two antioxidants—E and C—work more effectively than vitamin C alone *(Food Chemical News)*.

As scientists focus more on the health-sustaining role of antioxidants, it's possible that still other nutrients will come into the spotlight. We already know, for example, that vitamin A acts as an antioxidant in some situations. And even the trace element zinc, while not thought of as an antioxidant, has been shown to prevent some harmful effects of free radicals.

For now, though, the two antioxidants you should be paying attention to, in terms of your own diet, are vitamin E and selenium.

Unfortunately, there's evidence that our modern Western diet is dangerously deficient in antioxidant protection.

The problem can be traced to the refining of natural grains, oils and other foods that normally contain ample antioxidants. Dr. Anderson points out that "in the raw state, most fats and oils that are high in polyunsaturated fatty acids contain enough natural antioxidants (mainly tocopherols) to inhibit peroxidation . . . but this antioxidant 'umbrella' can itself be destroyed by oxidation during prolonged storage or processing" *(Lancet)*.

Wheat germ contains an unusually large amount of vitamin E, he says, "so that whole grain wheat products normally contribute a surplus of antioxidants to the diet. By the end of the 19th century this surplus had been reduced by the general change from whole meal to highly refined white bread, but it was the introduction of oxidizing agents [chlorine and other bleaches] that finally eliminated bread as a useful source of dietary antioxidants."

Eventually, Dr. Anderson reasons, there came a point when there was not enough antioxidant in the diet to prevent the formation of harmful peroxides—a kind of rancidification right inside our bodies. "I believe that this point was reached in the British and North American diets about 1920," he adds.

Dr. Anderson theorizes that this unfavorable dietary shift may have been largely responsible for the rapid surge in heart attack deaths over the last 50 years. In animals, at least, peroxide free radicals can fatally damage the heart muscle.

How much vitamin E do we need to tip the scales back in our favor? "At present, we believe the optimal level to be between 400 and 600 units a day," says Jeffrey Bland, Ph.D., a biochemist at the University of Puget Sound. "Situations which would lead to rapid utilization of vitamin E, such as exposure to photochemical oxidants (smog), ionizing radiation (sun or X rays), smoking or other factors which lead to increased cellular oxidation, should be met with somewhat greater intakes of vitamin E." Also, the more polyunsaturated oils we consume, the more vitamin E we need.

Given oxygen's penchant for mischief, it's important to ensure an adequate supply of protective antioxidants—so long as we live and breathe.

69

VITAMINS FOR LIVING LONGER

When you've reached that point in your life when some of your friends are starting to pack for the retirement home (if not the nursing home), it's time to do some serious thinking about how you're taking care of yourself. Because if you play it right, you can be packing for a camping trip in the mountains, or a summer in Europe, or a seashore holiday full of evening barbecues on the beach and early morning bicycling—instead of the nursing home.

But it's got to be *you* that takes care of yourself. You can't depend on your doctor to be much help in keeping you *really alive*—healthy, energetic, and clearheaded. Your doctor is trained to prescribe drugs and perform surgery. The problems of aging require a different approach. To make the years after middle age the best years of your life, you have to take charge of the underlying factors that determine your health. And one of the most important of these is your diet.

For example, a British study found that, out of 93 geriatric patients with acute problems, *none* had a normal nutritional profile. A. G. Morgan, M.D., consultant physician, Airedale General Hospital, Yorkshire, United Kingdom, and five colleagues tested patients for vitamin A, thiamine (B_1), riboflavin (B_2), niacin, vitamins C, D, E and K and protein. Twenty-two of the 93 actually had lower than normal levels of most of the nutrients. The most common deficiencies were in protein, niacin and vitamins C, E and A.

Dr. Morgan at first suspected "that an inadequate dietary intake, due to disease or to physical and mental deterioration, was the most likely cause of these multiple nutritional abnormalities." However, by the end of his study, Dr. Morgan concluded that "their present illness could not have significantly contributed to their nutritional status" *(International Journal for Vitamin and Nutrition Research).*

In other words, *the dietary deficiencies came before the health problems, and not the other way around.* That is a key point. Were these people in the hospital because their diets weren't providing them with enough of the right nutrients?

Impressed by Vitamin C

Olaf Mickelsen, Ph.D., formerly of the department of food science and human nutrition, Michigan State University, East Lansing, is in a good position to comment, since he has participated in a number of scientific studies designed to answer that very question. He has also authored a review of the subject, "The Possible Role of Vitamins in the Aging Process," which appears as a chapter in *Nutrition, Longevity, and Aging* (Academic Press, 1976).

During an interview, Dr. Mickelsen told us he was "impressed by the effects a reasonable intake of vitamin C seems to have. People who have been taking more vitamin C seem to have fewer problems when they enter the hospital." And, as he writes in the book, "the results of a number of studies imply that a higher than normal intake of [vitamin C] appears to reduce the aches and pains to which older persons are prone, to lower mortality when the aged are ill, and to increase their longevity."

Dr. Mickelsen went on to discuss a study led by a colleague of his, Eleanor D. Schlenker, Ph.D., chairperson of the department of human nutrition and foods at the University of Vermont, in which the average protein and vitamin C intakes were measured in a group of 100 women over the course of almost 25 years.

The women who had higher intakes of vitamin C and protein lived longer. So the beneficial effect of increased intake is undeniable in this case. Furthermore, Dr. Mickelsen points out that the women who did survive tended to *increase* their intake of vitamin C between 1948 and 1972.

A follow-up study two years later by Drs. Schlenker, Mickelsen and two colleagues revealed "a striking relationship between nutrient intake and physical health. Those women who on the basis of medical examinations appeared younger than their years consumed fewer calories and substantially less total fat, saturated fat, and fat as a percent of total calories."

In contrast, "lower intakes of thiamine, vitamin A, and ascorbic acid [vitamin C] were noted among women who appeared older" *(Federation of American Societies for Experimental Biology)*.

In simpler terms—eat better, feel younger.

A Classic Longevity Study

Another study mentioned by Dr. Mickelsen is probably the classic study in the field of nutrition and aging: the San Mateo County, California, survey of health and nutrition of 577 people over the age of 50. The study was begun in 1948, with very close measurements of the dietary intake of each subject, biochemical tests that are associated with health and disease (such as blood levels of cholesterol, vitamin C and sugar), and recording of diseases. Four years later, Harold D. Chope, M.D., reexamined 306 of the original 577 people and went into the record books to look for evidence that nutrition had played a part in their aging process.

He found it. *People with higher than average intakes of vitamins A and C and niacin tended to live longer* than those with lower intakes.

And the differences were quite remarkable. Among the people whose intakes of vitamin A were less than 5,000 international units per day, the death rate was 13.9 percent. For those whose daily intakes of vitamin A were 5,000 to 7,999 international units, the death rate was 6.9 percent. But among the people whose daily intakes were 8,000 or more international units, the death rate was only 4.3 percent—less than a third of the rate for the group getting under 5,000 international units.

The data on vitamin C was even more remarkable. Among those whose intakes were *less* than 50 milligrams per day, the death rate was 18.5 percent. For those whose daily intakes were *over* 50 milligrams, the death rate was 4.5 percent, less than a quarter of the rate for those whose diets provided less than 50 milligrams!

The difference adequate nutrition seems to have had on delaying death is impressive. But what about what doctors call *morbidity*—illness, suffering and general ill health? Did nutrition affect these important factors in the lives of the people in the study?

Again, the answer is *yes*. Dr. Chope writes in the report of his study, "In subjects with low intake of vitamin A (less than 5,000 I.U. [international units]), the incidence of nervous system, circulatory system, and respiratory system disease was high. . . . Low thiamine intake (less than 0.80 mg. a day) seemed to be associated with nervous system disease and circulatory disease; the higher the intake of thiamine, the lower the incidence of disease of these two systems. Diseases of the circulatory system and the digestive system were associated with low intake of ascorbic acid (less than 50 mg. per day). Among persons with a high intake of ascorbic acid (110 mg. and over), there was a low incidence of nervous system and circulatory system disease" (*California Medicine*).

Looking at Dr. Chope's results, you might be led to wonder how many of the people took nutritional supplements. Unfortunately, Dr. Chope did not determine which people did or didn't. But there have been some studies in which the effects of vitamin supplements on health in the later years of life have been documented.

The Value of Supplements

A British physician, Dr. G. F. Taylor, took part in one study in which 40 geriatric patients were given supplements containing 15 milligrams thiamine, 15 milligrams riboflavin, 50 milligrams nicotinamide (a form of niacin), 10 milligrams vitamin B_6 (pyridoxine) and 200 milligrams vitamin C. Another group of 40 received dummy tablets.

After a year, Dr. Taylor (who did not know which patients were getting supplements) was able to determine who was or wasn't receiving supplements merely by examining them for the signs of nutritional deficiencies and other illnesses.

Dr. Taylor describes his experience in these words: "At the start of the trial I recorded 13 of the 80 patients as having no marked signs of nutritional deficiencies. . . . After six months of the trial, I could not decide with certainty in more than half the cases whether they had had treatment or not. . . . But at the end of the year's trial, it was obvious which patients had received active tablets and [which ones received] dummy tablets. . . .

"In the treated group, the classical signs of malnutrition improved slowly. After 12 months' treatment, many signs had disappeared with a return to normal appearances. In some cases improvement was still continuing after 12 months' treatment. At the end of one year's treatment there was a striking improvement in the general physical and mental condition. In the untreated group clinical signs did not improve and in many cases deteriorated. Deterioration during infections, and when antibiotics, steroids, or diuretics were given, was especially marked. . . .

"One of the most dramatic and significant findings in this study arose after the trial had officially finished. All cases were observed clinically for six to nine months after stopping treatment, and signs of nutritional deficiencies reappeared in many previously treated cases. . . ." (*Vitamins in the Elderly*, John Wright and Sons, 1968).

This classic study not only underscores the importance of supplemental vitamins, but reveals that the good they do often takes time—close to a year of regular supplementation.

Further, the good they do is not some kind of "cure." Vitamins are concentrated foodstuffs. They nourish your body's innate desire to be healthy. As Dr. Taylor noted, when the added nourishment ceased, the benefits faded.

Do vitamins like A, the B complex and C extend your life, then?

Maybe—but maybe not. A more scientific view is that, rather than extending life, superior nutrition merely keeps life from being unnecessarily shortened—as is so often the case. But when you've worked hard all your life and you've finally reached the point where you can pack your suitcase and go anywhere you want, without worrying about job responsibilities or who will take care of the kids, that's really quite a bit.

CHAPTER
70

B VITAMINS CAN KEEP YOU ON THE BEAM

To a certain group of senior citizens in New Jersey and Maryland, it must have seemed the stuff of magic. Not that their wrinkles uncreased, their snowy hair turned black or their bodies reverted to supple specimens of youth.

No, their transformation from ailing oldsters to revitalized men and women was less dramatic but nonetheless striking. The signs of rejuvenation and vigor were unmistakable: renewed health, diminished aches and pains, fewer nervous disorders, improved coordination, softer skin and more attractive appearances.

The man who prompted these changes is no wizard, but Herman Baker, who holds a doctorate in metabolism and nutrition and teaches at the New Jersey Medical School in East Orange. In fact, it didn't require any sorcery at all for him and three colleagues to reverse what seemed to be the inevitable infirmities of the elderly.

Magic? Hardly. The secret to many so-called problems of old age, he discovered, was no more than a vitamin B deficiency that can impair one's health if left untreated.

As it happens, Dr. Baker, a professor of medicine and preventive medicine, is no stranger to the field. He first launched his studies on the effects of nutrient deficits 25 years ago as an important tool in diagnosing maladies of the aged.

Apparently, Dr. Baker's interest hasn't waned. His most recent project focused on 473 elderly people, ranging from 60 to 102 years old, in New Jersey and Maryland. Of this sample, 327 lived in nursing homes and the rest resided at home. At the study's onset in 1978, blood tests and physical examinations revealed 7 to 8 percent of the subjects had signs of anemia, skin dermatitis, cracked lips, nerve disorders, muscular aches and pains and poor visual coordination. However, evaluations also showed as many as 39 percent suffered from subclinical vitamin deficiencies that hadn't yet blossomed into noticeable symptoms or ailments.

What were the culprits responsible for this charade of "old age" in otherwise healthy, nonbedridden people? The critical ingredients turned out to be none other than absentee members of the vitamin B family—nutrients that not only affect the central nervous system and coordination, but are crucial to mental and emotional well-being. According to Dr. Baker, the elderly he studied exhibited strikingly depressed levels of B_6 (pyridoxine), niacin and B_{12}, as well as inadequate amounts of folate (folic acid) and thiamine, other components of the B complex.

To remedy those deficits, an injection of the entire B complex was given to the group once every three months during the year's experiment. After the first shot, Dr. Baker told us, symptoms began to disappear. In another 12 weeks, following the second injection, the investigators noted an increased level of circulating nutrients in the subjects' blood. At the study's conclusion, the elderly's physical woes had vanished along with their vitamin deficiencies. "They're all in good health now," says Dr. Baker.

"Vitamin deprivation may affect the young far less because they retain adequate reserves, thanks to sufficient vitamin-binding sites in the liver," he contends. Perhaps, then, increased nutrient needs in the elderly reflect, at least in part, decreased vitamin storage sites, Dr. Baker speculates. In addition, metabolism difficulties and medication may interfere with vitamin absorption in later life.

Dr. Baker isn't the first to recognize the need for vitamin supplementation to protect the elderly.

Back in 1968, senior citizens were the target of a British study designed to treat symptoms of malnutrition with vitamin preparations. The outcome? "There is evidence of chronic vitamin deficiencies in a large number of elderly people," concluded a hospital study, "which can be reversed by large doses of vitamin supplements for long periods" (*Vitamins in the Elderly*, John Wright and Sons, 1968).

The supplements in this case were four B vitamins—thiamine (15 milligrams), riboflavin (15 milligrams), B_6 (10 milligrams) and nicotinamide (a form of niacin—50 milligrams)—along with vitamin C (200 milligrams). The project divided 80 aged patients into two equal groups: 40 participants received one daily vitamin preparation; the other 40 were given identical-looking dummy tablets. The pills were distributed so that researchers had no idea which subjects were ingesting the vitamin supplements or swallowing the placebos.

Malnutrition Disappeared

At the experiment's onset, clinical workups disclosed "classic signs of malnutrition"—such as skin hemorrhages, a fissured red tongue, grayish white skin patches around the mouth—in all but four elderly patients.

However, after 12 months' treatment, the physicians found many of these symptoms disappeared with a "striking" improvement in patients' physical and mental conditions. "At the end of the year's trial," the report noted, "it was obvious which patients had received active and dummy tablets, except for a few marginal cases."

The vitamin-treated group showed marked progress, while the placebo-fed group manifested clinical evidence of deterioration in many cases.

After vitamin supplements were stopped, signs of the deficiencies reappeared in the treated group.

Dr. Baker believes immune response in the aged may be weakened because of persistent vitamin B_6 and folate deficits, increasing susceptibility to severe bacterial and viral infections. "The extensive degree of subclinical vitamin deficiencies may contribute to physical and mental dysfunction far more than previously recognized," Dr. Baker concludes in his report (*Journal of the American Geriatrics Society,* October, 1979).

In fact, in his next research project, Dr. Baker is focusing on the relationship between vitamin deficiencies and mental deterioration in the aged. It should come as no surprise, then, that he should be an enthusiastic advocate of vitamin preparations, especially for those 65 years and older. "For some vitamins, like the B complex," notes Dr. Baker, "continual supplementation may be needed to protect the elderly against hypovitaminosis."

Besides vitamin supplements, it's important to spike your diet with generous helpings of food rich in B vitamins, such as liver, whole grain cereals, nuts, yeast, dark leafy green vegetables, poultry and fish, for that extra ounce of protection.

After all, there's no need to grow old before your time. Remember, it doesn't require any magic to hold back the clock, especially if the signs of "aging" are something as preventable as a vitamin deficiency.

CHAPTER
71

AGE WITH EASE THROUGH WISE NUTRITION

Maggie looked at the doctor as if he were mad. After all, it was *her* birthday, and if she wanted to brood the day away it was *her* business. Turning 50 just isn't easy. But across from her sat the doctor, wearing a full grin and looking at Maggie as if she were the luckiest person alive.

"Fifty. It must feel wonderful," he glistened. "Today has got to be the best day of your life."

Maggie shot him a glance. She wasn't going to let this crazy talk get to her. "What's so wonderful about turning 50?" she snapped back. "Look at me. I'm getting *old*."

"Yes, and isn't it great," he answered. "It's a privilege not given to everyone."

Indeed. There's a lot to be said for getting older. Never before has such a large population of older Americans been living so long. Had Maggie been born 100 years ago, she wouldn't have been expected to live beyond 40. But today, at 50, she's considered to be only *middle-aged,* with the probability of another quarter century of living ahead of her. But how active and healthy those coming years will be will pretty much depend on how well Maggie treats herself.

411

Being in her 50s makes Maggie vulnerable to a malady that's all too common among our older generations—poor nutrition.

"Poor nutrition is a very big problem as we grow older," says Linda H. Chen, Ph.D., a University of Kentucky professor and nutrition researcher. "A lot of older people may think they're getting a proper diet but they're not.

"A 20-year-old woman can devour the exact same meal as her 65-year-old grandmother, but the older woman won't necessarily be getting the same nutritive value out of it."

Why? Simply because the older body can't assimilate vitamins and minerals the way it used to.

"Digestion and absorption get poorer as people get older. It's a natural part of aging," Dr. Chen explains. There are other things that naturally happen to the body as we age: Metabolism slows, kidney function decreases, muscle and fat balance changes, and our ability to metabolize sugar declines. Generally, activity levels slide with age.

"What it all boils down to," says Dr. Chen, "is that our need for calories lessens as we get older, but our need for nutrients does not." As Maggie said, getting old isn't easy.

Research studies show that as high as 50 percent of Americans over the age of 65 are consuming less than two-thirds of the Recommended Dietary Allowances of calcium, iron, thiamine, riboflavin, niacin and vitamins A and C. Zinc, folate (folic acid) and vitamins B_{12} and B_6 are also common deficiencies among the aged.

Dr. Chen concentrated her studies on riboflavin (vitamin B_2), vitamin B_6 and iron in a group of elderly people in central Kentucky.

"Deficiencies were significant," she told us. "I found one-quarter had iron deficiencies, one-third were deficient in riboflavin and half showed a vitamin B_6 deficiency. In studies of nursing-home populations, deficiencies were even more severe. This was probably due to the residents' poorer health and the fact that they were on medications, which can also hinder the absorption and/or increase excretion of some vitamins and minerals."

On the other hand, there is research indicating that getting less than the RDA is not as much of a problem among those who take vitamin and mineral supplements. That was illustrated in a study of an elderly population that included many supplement users.

"The population is unique in that all the people were in good health, lived in their own home or apartment, were more educated than the average for their age group and, for the most part, were considered to be health-conscious individuals," James S. Goodwin, M.D., one of the researchers on the project, told us. Sixty percent of both men and women, whose average age was 72, took one or more vitamin supplements, with vitamins C and E being the most popular.

For the group as a whole, food intake of vitamin C, niacin and vitamin A was well above the RDA for most of the people. However, through food alone, a substantial percentage of the population was receiving less than the RDA for vitamins B_6, B_{12}, D and E, folate, calcium and zinc. But the supplement users, thanks to their extra measure of protection, showed virtually no nutrient shortcomings.

For example, nonsupplementers got less than 50 percent of the RDA for vitamin B_6, but those taking a supplement got a whopping 275 percent of the RDA (*American Journal of Clinical Nutrition*, August, 1982).

The study points to the need for some kind of dietary supplementation for the elderly. "I feel everyone over the age of 65 should take a multivitamin pill," says Dr. Goodwin.

Of course, the ideal way to attain proper nutrition would be through diet alone. But doing so admittedly gets tougher as we get older simply because, at around the age of 40, we have to start worrying about middle-age spread. It's the time in our lives when maintaining weight no longer means just watching our calories. It means cutting them down.

The Expert Committee on Energy and Protein Requirements has made these recommendations: After age 40 we should cut calories by 5 percent and do so again after age 50. At age 60, calories should be sliced another 10 percent and again after 70.

"Maintaining nutrition on fewer calories isn't impossible to do," says Frank Beaudet, a nutrition expert at the Andrus Gerontology Center at the University of Southern California. "As you get older, quality of the food must count much more than quantity. Simply reducing starch, sugar and fats and switching to proteins, fruits, vegetables and whole grains can keep you in nutritional balance.''

Beaudet admits that getting people to change lifelong eating habits isn't always possible. Often, getting older people to eat at all can be the problem.

"There are a whole range of economic and social factors that can affect an older person's interest in eating," says Beaudet. "The death of a spouse, living alone, eating meals alone all can cause a disinterest in food. Poor nutrition can result, and in some cases, even malnutrition.

"When people aren't eating right, a vitamin supplement is one way to help solve the problem," he says.

Being on a sensible diet doesn't always guarantee that you're also in nutritional balance. "Elderly people take an awful lot of drugs, and there are many drugs that can adversely affect vitamin and mineral absorption and excretion," says Dr. Chen.

The most popular of these is probably aspirin, commonly used by many older people as a pain killer. It can block vitamin C from entering the blood. Aspirin, as well as phenobarbital and the diuretic triamterene, can also affect folate utilization.

Some drugs that can cause vitamin B_6 deficiency are hydralazine, used in the treatment of hypertension, and L-dopa, used in Parkinson's disease.

Mineral oil, a long-time favorite laxative, has adverse effects on the absorption of carotene and vitamins A, D and K. Antacids containing aluminum inhibit intestinal absorption of phosphorus and increase the excretion of calcium.

"Drug-related deficiencies are sometimes the hardest to pinpoint because older people take so many drugs and get them from so many sources," says Dr. Chen. "It's important that they don't just arbitrarily take them and not let their physicians know."

So take stock in what you eat. As the doctor told Maggie, getting old is "a privilege not given to everyone."

CHAPTER

72

THE ANTI-CANCER
VITAMIN
COMBINATION

Scientific breakthroughs do not obey the laws of supply and demand. Millions in research grants do not guarantee results. No matter how much society may need a particular cure or vaccine, sometimes it's just not available at any price.

By the same token, important advances may take place in the most underfunded, understaffed lab. Dedication and inspiration sometimes get results that money can't.

The work of Sister Mary Eymard Poydock, Ph.D., director of cancer research and former professor of biology at Mercyhurst College in Erie, Pennsylvania, is a case in point. The Mercyhurst labs are not large or well endowed. But 20 years of painstaking work by Sister Eymard and her associates have now produced results which indicate that a combination of vitamins C and B_{12} may have a powerful effect against cancer. While Sister Eymard's work has been confined to laboratory animals, the implications for further research are obvious.

For 20 years, Sister Eymard has been testing a substance that had been advanced as a possible anti-cancer agent. The first results were promising, and the name "mercytamin" (from the Sisters of Mercy) was applied to the substance. Mercytamin was

415

actually a combination of vitamins C, B_{12} and a variety of enzymes. Through scientific testing of the solution, the enzymes and other chemical additives were eliminated as possible active agents. Finally, only the vitamins remained, and in 1978 the name mercytamin was dropped.

Sister Eymard held back on publishing her findings until she was certain the results she was getting were true. "We've done enough experiments now, testing hundreds of mice, to establish that it works," Sister Eymard says. "We've got it down to a point now where, if you do it according to the 'recipe,' it will work everytime."

Sister Eymard and her research staff implanted three common types of cancer into laboratory mice—sarcomas (cancerous growths of connective tissues), carcinomas (cancers of skinlike tissues) and leukemias (cancers of the blood-forming organs). Those cancerous tissues were implanted both in the abdomens and under the skin of the mice. The mice were then injected with the mixture of vitamins C and B_{12} (in a ratio of one part B_{12} to two parts C) near the site of the tumor transplant.

Within four days, some of the tumors from the abdomens of the mice were removed, and the cells were examined under the microscope. There was a dramatic change in the tissue. *The cancerous cell division had stopped completely.*

Tumors Didn't Grow

The tumors growing under the skin were treated the day after implant with the C-B_{12} combination. The results were similar—no tumors would grow. In the control animals (those mice with transplanted tumors which were not given the C-B_{12} combination), the tumors continued to grow at a rapid rate.

Inhibiting tumor growth was only part of the results of Sister Eymard's experiments. She also wanted to see if the C-B_{12} mixture would prolong the lives of animals already suffering from cancer. To find out, Sister Eymard and her colleagues injected the mixture near the cancerous growths of diseased mice for seven successive days.

Treated animals lived longer than those mice not given C and B_{12}. In fact, *all* the treated mice outlived the control group. It appeared that the combination of C and B_{12} not only inhibits the growth of cancer cells, but also prolongs the lives of animals impregnated with cancer.

"There are few things presently on the market that will ensure a 100 percent survival rate with cancer," Sister Eymard says, "but we had a 100 percent survival rate after the controls were dead. Most of the treated mice outlived the controls two or three weeks."

To be sure that it was really the C-B_{12} concoction, and not an unknown factor present in mice, that was responsible for her results, Sister Eymard conducted experiments on free-living cancer cells growing on a culture medium. The vitamin C-B_{12} complex was used as a treatment on three types of cancer cells and on healthy cells, as well. The treated cells, the untreated control group and the healthy cells were left to incubate.

At the end of the incubation period, the untreated control group was infested with cancer cells. In the treated group, however, *not one cancer cell of any of the three types was to be found*. The healthy, noncancerous cells were unaffected by the C-B_{12} complex. It appeared that Sister Eymard had found a cancer-inhibiting agent that not only stopped many kinds of cancer, but did so with absolutely no side effects in healthy tissue.

Sister Eymard also tested each vitamin separately to determine if either was primarily responsible for the anti-cancer effects. The combination of the two vitamins, however, always performed much more effectively than either one alone.

Tests showed that the combination might be working by boosting the animals' immune systems to fight the cancer. Sister Eymard is confident that, with more experimentation, especially on larger mammals and humans, the vitamin C-B_{12} combination could prove to be a useful preventive weapon in the fight to eliminate the second leading cause of death in America.

The scientific community has taken note of Sister Eymard's findings.

A spokesman for the American Cancer Society, which helps fund Sister Eymard's research, told us, "The physicians on the committee which reviewed Sister Eymard's work were most impressed with the results she was getting. She has come forth with work of considerable promise."

Sister Eymard herself takes a modest stance.

"I'm glad you're looking into this," she told us. "Every bit of information helps to educate the public. It might give them some hope, and that's what they need most."

CHAPTER
73

VITAMIN C
AGAINST CANCER

When most health-conscious people think of extending their lives, they think in terms of *years*. You may tell yourself, "If I give up smoking now, I may reasonably expect to live 5, maybe 10 years longer." Or, "If I stick to a regular exercise program and watch my diet, I may be good for an extra 15 years." The emphasis is always on a long and healthy life of indefinite span, with several additional productive years tacked on the end as a bonus.

When the terminal cancer patient contemplates his future, he thinks in terms of *days*. In the final stages of that dread disease, when the battle has been lost and even the doctors have given up hope, time assumes a different dimension.

One study, however, holds out promise that even these patients can look forward to an extra round of life—thanks to vitamin C. For the evidence now points to the distinct possibility that daily supplementation with this nutrient in relatively large amounts can add many precious days to the lives of terminal cancer victims. In some cases, as we shall see, vitamin C has turned those remaining *days* back into *years*.

The study in question was done by Linus Pauling, Ph.D., and Ewan Cameron, M.D., a surgeon. Dr. Pauling, a Nobel prize–winning chemist, is associated with the Linus Pauling Institute of Science and Medicine, Menlo Park, California. Dr. Cameron practiced medicine at Vale of Leven District General Hospital, Loch Lomondside, Scotland.

In their clinical study, Drs. Cameron and Pauling compared the survival time of 100 terminal cancer patients, selected over a five-year period and given vitamin C, with 1,000 similar patients who did not receive the vitamin. All were patients at the Vale of Leven hospital, whose surgical unit treats most of the advanced cancer patients in the Loch Lomondside area. Each person receiving vitamin C was matched with 10 control patients of the same sex, close to the same age and suffering from the same type of tumor, who did not get vitamin C. (Patients in the non–vitamin C group were selected—some in retrospect—by a random search of the hospital's case records over the past ten years; most had died before the doctors began administering vitamin C.)

Vitamin C Gave Extra Days to the "Hopeless"

"For strong ethical reasons," the researchers point out, "every patient in the treated group was examined and assessed independently by at least two physicians or surgeons (often more than two) who all agreed that the situation was 'totally hopeless' and 'quite untreatable' before ascorbate [vitamin C] was commenced."

In other words, before turning to vitamin C as a last resort, all the people were first treated with surgery, radiation, chemotherapy or hormones—all the conventional forms of cancer treatment. In every case, such methods failed. For example, ten women with breast cancer had undergone mastectomy and subsequent radiation treatments, as well as receiving hormones.

They had improved for a while but then relapsed. Their tumors were running out of control. At that point, the patients were declared terminal, the decision to begin giving vitamin C was made and the doctors began counting *survival days*.

A similar point of no return was selected for each of the patients in the non–vitamin C group by examining their records. From that date when exploratory surgery revealed that a tumor was inoperable or conventional anti-cancer treatments were abandoned in despair, the patient was considered terminal, and the remaining survival days were totaled up for comparison purposes.

Those persons receiving vitamin C were started out with 10 grams (10,000 milligrams) a day intravenously. This was usually stopped after about ten days, and then the patient began taking the same dosage of vitamin C by mouth. As Drs. Cameron and Pauling describe it, the vitamin C approach was begun "cautiously" but was continued with new patients over the next five years because "it seemed to have some value."

In the light of their summarized findings, that would seem to be an understatement. For in every type of cancer treated, the people receiving vitamin C tended to live longer than those who did not receive the vitamin.

Lung cancer patients, for example, survived an average of 3.53 times longer after being declared untreatable than their controls. Those with stomach cancer lived 2.61 times longer. Bladder cancer victims survived 4.49 times longer. Patients with kidney tumors displayed a greater than fivefold increase in life expectancy. Those with breast cancer lived 5.75 times longer. And those with cancer of the colon managed to survive, on the average, 7.61 times longer on the vitamin C regimen!

Case Histories

Let's translate some of those findings into actual days, months and years. A 74-year-old man whose lung cancer was pronounced untreatable began taking vitamin C and lived for more than a year longer—427 days. The ten individuals in his control group (other men of about his own age with approximately the same degree of untreatable lung cancer) survived for an average of only 17 more days. Three died within 2 days; the longest any survived was 31 days. Could the lack of vitamin C have made such an incredible difference?

Another patient in the vitamin C group, a 69-year-old man with inoperable cancer of the colon, also received an unexpected new lease on life. Those in his control group survived for an average of 37.3 days—little more than a month. But this man's condition improved considerably after beginning the vitamin C. He lived for 1,267 days, almost 3½ years.

A 67-year-old woman with cancer of the ovary responded well to vitamin C. She was still alive at the time these results were tabulated, 240 days after commencing treatment. She had already survived almost six times longer than the average for her control group.

Another remarkable turnabout involved a man, age 62, suffering from bladder cancer. The men with bladder cancer in his comparison group lived an average of 63 days without vitamin C. But 669 days (almost two years) after starting with the vitamin, he was still alive at the time the paper went to press. He already had survived more than ten times longer than the average for the untreated bladder cancer victims in his grouping.

Overall, the 100 people in the vitamin C group enjoyed an average survival time 4.16 times greater than those 1,000 individuals in the control group.

"At the present time, we cannot conclude that ascorbate has less value for one kind of cancer than for others," Drs. Cameron and Pauling state. "Our conclusion is that the administration of ascorbic acid in amounts of about 10 grams per day to patients with advanced cancer leads to about a fourfold increase in their life expectancy, in addition to an apparent improvement in the quality of life" (*Proceedings of the National Academy of Sciences of the United States of America*).

That last point is especially important, since the final months or days of a terminal cancer patient's life are often filled with pain and despair. To prolong such a period of misery could hardly be interpreted as beneficial. But many of the people receiving vitamin C reported *less* pain. They were able to get by with less dependence on pain-killing drugs that numb the mind. In short, they not only lived longer, they found life more worthwhile.

When Drs. Cameron and Pauling proceeded to analyze their data further, they discovered an interesting breakdown in the way the vitamin C group benefited from treatment. They found that among those patients there were two distinct subgroups.

"The data indicated that deaths occur for about 90 percent of the ascorbate-treated patients at one-third the rate for the controls, so that for this fraction there is a threefold increase in survival time, measured from the date when the cancer was pronounced untreatable. For the other 10 percent of the ascorbate-treated patients, the survival time is not known with certainty, but it is indicated . . . to be more than 20 times the average for the untreated patients."

In other words, a small but significant proportion of the patients responded to the vitamin C treatment in what can only be termed a spectacular manner. In fact, at the time the final results were compiled, *18 people were still alive,* having survived an average of more than 970 days. Sixteen of those were considered clinically "well."

In one case, a woman, age 50, with breast cancer was still alive 4½ years (1,644 days) after starting with vitamin C. The untreatable cases in her control group had lingered for an average of just 83 days. Yet this woman was still alive, her cancer apparently brought under control.

Another success story: A 74-year-old man with an advanced, untreatable kidney tumor was still alive and well 1,554 days (more than four years) after he started taking vitamin C. Those in his control group had survived only an average of 169 days before succumbing to their cancers.

One of the most dramatic recoveries of all involved a 40-year-old long-distance truck driver suffering from cancer of the lymphatic system. The reversal was so remarkably clear-cut in this case that it rated a special report by Dr. Cameron and another

Scottish doctor, Allan Campbell, in the journal *Chemico-Biological Interactions*.

In the spring of 1973, the truck driver began complaining of spasmodic pains in the muscles between his ribs. He started to lose weight. Night after night he awoke shivering, bathed in sweat. Chest X rays revealed that the mass of tissues and organs separating the lungs was greatly enlarged. When doctors removed and examined one of the man's lymph glands, they found that cancer had spread throughout his entire lymphatic system.

Treatment with vitamin C—10 grams daily—was begun immediately. "The initial response to intravenous ascorbic acid was very dramatic indeed and far exceeded clinical expectations," Drs. Cameron and Campbell reported. "Within 10 days of commencing therapy, the patient claimed to feel quite fit and well, and had been transformed from a 'dying' into a 'recovering' situation."

The man appeared to make a full recovery. Chest X rays were normal. He returned to work. But when he discontinued the vitamin C, the cancer symptoms returned with new ferocity.

He was readmitted to the hospital, where he received intravenous infusions of 20 grams of vitamin C daily for two weeks. Then he was placed on a maintenance regimen of 12.5 grams of vitamin C a day by mouth. Once again, the cancer symptoms subsided, and the patient was declared "fit and well" with "no evidence of active disease."

As the latest report from Drs. Pauling and Cameron went to press, this patient was still alive and well, 1,106 days after his initial diagnosis of advanced cancer.

How can we explain such a favorable response? For that matter, how can we explain *any* prolongation of life, whether measured in days, months or years, in the patients who received vitamin C?

According to Drs. Pauling and Cameron, "A simple interpretation of these facts is that the administration of ascorbate to the patients with terminal cancer has two effects. First, it increases the effectiveness of the natural mechanisms of resistance to such an extent as to lead to an increase by a factor of 2.7 in the average survival time for most of the patients. . . . Second, it has another effect on about 10 percent of the patients, such as to cause them to live a much longer time. This effect might be such as to 'cure' them; that is, *to give them the life expectancy that they would have had if they had not developed cancer* [emphasis ours].

"On the other hand," the authors theorize, the vitamin C "might only set them back one or more steps in the development of the cancer. . . ." In any event, the immediate effect is the same: The patients receive a bonus of extra life.

How Could a Vitamin Help?

Why vitamin C? Drs. Cameron and Pauling note that "cancer patients have a much greater requirement for this substance than normal healthy individuals," apparently because all available vitamin C is mobilized by the body in a valiant effort to boost natural resistance and repel the invasive malignant growth.

One way that vitamin C conceivably works to strengthen the body's own immunity to cancer was explained to us by Robert Yonemoto, M.D., a surgeon and former director of the surgical laboratories at the City of Hope National Medical Center, Duarte, California. According to Dr. Yonemoto's own studies in conjunction with colleagues at the National Cancer Institute, vitamin C increases *lymphocyte blastogenesis* in healthy human volunteers.

Lymphocytes are white blood cells which gobble up and destroy foreign agents in the body. To divide and multiply, they must first undergo blastogenesis, which is a swelling process. The greater the blastogenic activity, then presumably the greater the effectiveness of the body's natural resistance against outside invaders.

When Dr. Yonemoto gave 5 grams (5,000 milligrams) of vitamin C daily to his five volunteers, they all showed a significant spurt in blastogenesis. When the intake was doubled to 10 grams—the same dosage used by Drs. Cameron and Pauling in treating cancer patients—the increase in lymphocyte blastogenesis was even greater.

"Vitamin C increases the general immunity of the individual," Dr. Yonemoto told us, "so we should be able to demonstrate that it is good for the cancer patient and that its intake should precede and immediately follow cancer surgery."

The new findings of Drs. Pauling and Cameron would certainly seem to confirm vitamin C's importance. As they say, their results "clearly indicate that this simple and safe form of medication is of definite value in the treatment of patients with advanced cancer."

Naturally, they would like to see vitamin C tried by other physicians, outside of Scotland: "It is our opinion that a similar effect would be found for untreatable cancer patients in other countries," they state.

In calling their promising findings to the attention of the worldwide scientific community, the two suggest that even larger dosages of vitamin C (above 10 grams daily) might be even more beneficial. And they stress that, in the future, patients should be given the benefit of vitamin C much earlier in the course of their disease, before the outlook has become so dim. In that way, they speculate, cancer patients might hope to live an additional 5 to 20 years.

Of course, any such results will need to be tested and retested in clinics and laboratories around the world before anyone can begin to breathe a sigh of relief about the menace of cancer. But in the meantime, based on the already quite substantial evidence that has accumulated, we suspect the wisest course of all would be to look to daily vitamin C supplementation as a potential *preventative* of tumor growth, rather than a cure.

Cancer is one battle that is best avoided completely.

CATARACTS

CHAPTER

74

NEW HOPE FOR CATARACT PREVENTION

What causes cataracts? Can they be prevented? The answers to those questions are not coming easily to medical investigators. In fact, the mystery surrounding the onset of these sight-robbing curtains on the eye has at times appeared as cloudy and impenetrable as the cataracts themselves.

But bit by bit, bright patches of knowledge are appearing, and none seems brighter than a report by three scientists at the National Eye Institute's laboratory of vision research in Bethesda, Maryland. For the trio has discovered that a commonly occurring natural family of nutrients, the bioflavonoids, exhibits a surprisingly potent blocking effect against certain types of cataracts.

Cataracts occur when the normally transparent lens of the eye gradually clouds over. Instead of focusing incoming rays of light into a sharp image on the retina, the impaired lens scatters the light, obscuring vision. If the clouding progresses far enough, sight can be completely lost. As a result, cataracts are a major cause of blindness all over the world.

Nearly 16 million people are severely disabled by this eye disease. More than 24½ million Americans alone, over age 60, suffer from cataracts (*British Journal of Nutrition,* May, 1982).

Viewed against such a backdrop, the work of National Eye Institute researchers S. D. Varma, A. Mizuno and J. H. Kinoshita takes on added importance. Writing in *Science*, the team described what happened when the bioflavonoid quercitrin was fed to laboratory animals especially prone to rapid cataract formation.

Quercitrin was chosen because, like other flavonoids, it has been shown to inhibit an enzyme, aldose reductase, which is normally present and almost inactive in the lens of the eye. Under normal circumstances, aldose reductase poses no problem, but when blood sugar levels rise (as in diabetes), the enzyme swings into action to convert the sugar into sorbitol. And sorbitol inside the lens is suspected as a cataract trigger. Scientists believe that's why diabetic individuals have a higher incidence of cataracts than other people.

The researchers found that supplementing diabetic animals' diets with quercitrin cut the sorbitol concentration inside the eye in half. And even more important, those animals receiving the bioflavonoid developed no cataracts during the course of the trial, while unsupplemented animals showed signs of lens clouding within ten days!

"This study," the authors concluded, "reveals for the first time that inhibition of aldose reductase not only leads to a decrease in the sorbitol accumulation in the lens but also impedes the cataractous process. The cataract formation in diabetes may thus be at least delayed, if not prevented. . . ."

Earlier tests by Varma, Kinoshita and another colleague *(Science)* revealed that all flavonoids tested—in addition to being relatively safe and nontoxic—"have significant inhibitory activity" against aldose reductase. However, the more widely known bioflavonoid rutin isn't as potent as quercitrin. Quercitrin, though, is not currently available as a food supplement. It is probably found in citrus fruits, but these amounts would not be enough to have a therapeutic effect, Dr. Kinoshita told us.

Eye researchers are quick to point out that there are many differences between animal lenses and human lenses, particularly with regard to cataract formation. But still the notion that the kinds of food we eat might have either a protective or detrimental effect with regard to cataracts isn't really so farfetched. The lens of the human eye "has a metabolism that is as finely tuned to its proper function as the metabolism of any other tissue," points out an authority on cataracts, English researcher Ruth van Heyningen of the University of Oxford's Nuffield Laboratory of Ophthalmology *(Scientific American)*. Conceivably, certain nutrients or their lack could profoundly alter that metabolism.

For example, simultaneous deficiencies of vitamin E and the amino acid tryptophan in pregnant rats result in cataract formation in their offspring. That was demonstrated by two scientists at Virginia Polytechnic Institute and State University. George E. Bunce and John L. Hess of the department of biochemistry and nutrition discovered that 33 percent of the young born to deficient rats developed cloudy spots in their lenses within 24 days *(Journal of Nutrition)*. That high incidence rate didn't show up, though, among other rats when only vitamin E or tryptophan alone was withheld.

Full Range of Vitamins Found Protective

In another study, by famed University of Texas biochemist Roger J. Williams and colleague James D. Heffley, several groups of young rats were placed on diets of varying quality and then fed high amounts of galactose, a type of simple sugar.

"By feeding galactose-containing diets to young rats, cataracts are regularly produced," the pair noted in *Proceedings of the National Academy of Sciences*. "When, however, we furnished galactose-fed animals with what may be considered a well balanced, full team of nutrients, cataract prevention was accomplished. On four galactose-containing diets supplied with a full team of nutrients, not a single cataract developed in 24 rats (48 eyes). On four diets using the same dietary galactose challenge, accompanied with inadequate nutritional teams, 47 out of 48 eyes developed cataracts.''

Next, the two scientists tried to reverse the cataracts in some animals by switching them to better diets. In more than half the cases, the condition of the eyes improved, although slowly and not completely.

The authors fortified the higher-quality diets for their animals with a nutritional team that included vitamins A, D and E, thiamine, riboflavin, niacin, folate (folic acid) and several other nutrients.

"It is evident that from our study no one could derive a precise list of the nutrients involved in protecting against cataract," they noted. "Our simple experiment shows that when we attempted to furnish enough of all the essentials, success was attained. . . .

"It seems possible that if the dietary challenge offered these rats had been less severe or if the change in diet had been instituted at the very first sign of cataract instead of waiting until the cataracts were well formed, the responses might have been more favorable."

The authors add that they would like to see the nutritional team approach tested for effectiveness in preventing human cataracts.

One might wonder about the sudden interest in preventing a condition that, once it has arisen, can be treated so readily. Modern surgery, which removes the affected lens or lenses, is a highly successful operation. However, cataract researcher van Heyningen, among others, considers surgery to be only "a partial remedy."

"Prevention would be much better than the present 'cure,' " she stresses, because once the natural lens has been removed, thick spectacles or contact lenses are then required to restore the eye's focusing ability.

So modern surgical methods notwithstanding, there appears to be a tremendous need for more research into cataract prevention and healing through the use of natural food substances.

COLDS, FLU AND
THE IMMUNE SYSTEM

CHAPTER

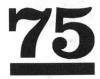

FIGHT OFF FLU AND COLDS THE NATURAL WAY

Every day, every hour, every minute of our lives there's a battle for survival going on inside our bodies. It's between us and them—those invisible germs and viruses that cause colds and flu and any number of other infections and diseases.

But silently and relentlessly our bodies fight back, keeping the invaders from taking over and making us sick. Our nifty immune system is the defense that does this for us automatically and, most of the time, perfectly.

Sometimes, our white blood cells track down germs and gobble them up. At other times, it's the antibodies produced by special cells that destroy the germs. There are even certain proteins called immunoglobulins, complement and interferon that our cells make just for fighting off viruses, bacteria and other foreign invaders. As if that's not enough, we are also stocked with fighters known as T cells, B cells and (believe it or not) killer cells.

Are you impressed? You should be because, if even one of these systems broke down, you'd be in serious trouble—healthwise.

"Each lack or deficiency presents itself clinically to the doctor . . . in its own particular way," says Ronald J. Glasser, M.D., author of *The Body Is the Hero* (Random House, 1976). "No antibodies, and the child has recurrent pneumonias and abscesses; no granulocytes [germ-gobbling white cells], and he has prolonged bacterial infections; no lymphocytes [T and B cells] and he has recurrent fungal infections and severe, recurrent, viral illness."

Luckily, most of us don't have to contend with that degree of immune dysfunction. On the other hand, you shouldn't take your immune system for granted. It needs the same TLC as the rest of your body in order to give you the best protection from disease.

That's where good nutrition comes in. "There is an intimate relationship between nutritional status, immune response and infection," says R. K. Chandra, M.D., professor of pediatric research at the Memorial University of Newfoundland. "When nutritional deficiency and infection coexist, the former is often chronic and precedes the latter acute process."

In other words, when your diet is inadequately supplying all the vitamins and minerals you need, your immune defenses go down, allowing germs to multiply and cause illness. And you don't have to be grossly undernourished either, adds Dr. Chandra, who is also the coauthor of *Nutrition, Immunity, and Infection* (Plenum Press, 1977). Deficiency of individual nutrients can undermine the immune system, too.

Robert Edelman, M.D., agrees. "Acquired immune dysfunctions in man occur with deficiencies of certain vitamins and minerals," says Dr. Edelman, who is chief of the clinical and epidemiological studies branch at the National Institute of Allergy and Infectious Diseases, in Bethesda, Maryland.

Actually, in animal studies, the most important immunological effects are produced by deficiencies of vitamin B_6, pantothenate (pantothenic acid) and folate (folic acid), according to Dr. Edelman. For example, a deficiency of B_6 alone depresses both cellular (T and B cells) and humoral (antibody production) immunity in animals. Other experiments have shown that T and B cells fail to multiply normally when tested against a foreign substance (like a germ). What's more, volunteers with short-term experimental B₆ deficiencies have shown reduced antibody responses to vaccines.

As for pantothenate, a deficiency of that nutrient appears to inhibit the stimulation of antibody-producing cells and their ability to produce the special proteins (immunoglobulins) that fight off foreign invaders.

Folate deficiency can cause its share of immune-system problems, too, adds Dr. Edelman. Animals lacking in folate show a shriveling of the tissues that produce lymphocytes, as well as diminished white blood cell numbers and impaired cell-mediated and humoral immunity (*Journal of the American Medical Association,* January 2, 1981).

"The good news," Dr. Edelman told us, "is that the immune system responds very quickly to adequate nutrition."

Of course, it responds in the opposite direction just as easily. "Experiments in animals have shown that a one-month deficiency in certain nutrients has negative effects on the immune system if the deficiency occurs during a period of rapid growth," says Kathleen Nauss, Ph.D., of the department of nutrition at the Massachusetts Institute of Technology, located in Cambridge.

"In our experiments, we fed animals diets that were marginally deficient in folate as well as choline and methionine [an amino acid]. These substances all play a role in cellular metabolism. Within a month, sometimes less, we found the animals' immune system to be depressed. It was particularly severe in young animals."

When it comes to people, both the very young and the elderly are especially susceptible to immune dysfunction: the young because their rapid growth rate creates an increased demand for nutrients, and the old because the immune system simply deteriorates with age.

What's more, the elderly often have an inadequate diet, compounding the problem. In fact, in one study, Dr. Chandra found that 41 percent of a group of people over the age of 60 had nutritional deficiencies that contributed to their immune dysfunctions.

Vitamin C and Colds

While good nutrition in general is important to a smoothly running defense system, several nutrients (besides those already mentioned) stand out as superstars in this area.

Vitamin C surely heads that list. After all, how many people do you know who swear by vitamin C for colds? Dr. Edelman does. "I don't get too many colds," he told us, "but when I do, I take large doses of vitamin C. It relieves the symptoms and shortens the duration of the cold. It seems to work well."

Kenneth Cooper, M.D., agrees. He's a fitness expert and author of *The Aerobics Program for Total Well-Being* (M. Evans and Company, 1982). "For many years, I have taken 1,000 milligrams of vitamin C daily, and during that time I've experienced almost complete protection from colds and other upper respiratory infections. Before I began to take this dosage, I regularly had two or three major colds each year. After I started taking some extra vitamin C each day, however, the number of colds declined dramatically. In my opinion, there is probably a causal connection between the vitamin C supplement and my good health," explains Dr. Cooper, "although it is impossible to draw a valid conclusion based on a study of one patient."

Other researchers, however, are working on proving just such a connection, and their studies have been centering on vitamin C's effect on the immune system.

"We became interested in vitamin C because of other studies we had seen on the relationship of immunity to this nutrient," says Richard Panush, M.D., chief of clinical immunology at the University of Florida college of medicine, in Gainesville. "We decided to carry out our own studies and see what we'd come up with. In the first experiment, we tested the effects of vitamin

C in the test tube and found that it boosted a wide array of immune responses.

"Our next study was done on a group of normal, healthy volunteers. We gave half of them vitamin C and the other half a placebo [harmless inactive pill] and then measured their immune response. Those taking the vitamin showed a measurable increase in their immunity," Dr. Panush told us.

"Now we're in the middle of an experiment that is testing the effects of vitamin C on the immune system of sick people to see if it will help them get better. We should have those results within the year."

In another study, researchers from Johannesburg, South Africa, tested the antibody response of two groups of guinea pigs. One group (the controls) received only a minimal amount of vitamin C while the other group received supplemental vitamin C. Antibody levels were then measured after the animals were injected with a foreign substance.

The animals receiving the supplemental C had significantly higher antibody levels than the control group. The researchers observed that vitamin C appears to stimulate the production of immunoglobulin M–type (Ig M) antibodies, in particular. And, say the researchers, "Ig M is a most effective first line of defense against invading organisms."

For the animals, the enhancement of the immune response was accomplished with 160 milligrams of vitamin C per day. A comparable stimulation of the humoral immune system in humans might require a daily vitamin C intake of 1.5 to 2 grams (1,500 to 2,000 milligrams), the researchers speculate (*International Journal for Vitamin and Nutrition Research,* vol. 50, no. 3, 1980).

For the elderly, who often have age-associated immune dysfunction, supplemental zinc may give them the boost they need. That's what doctors in Brussels have found out. In their experiment, the researchers gave zinc supplements (50 milligrams of zinc twice daily for a month) to 15 volunteers over 70 years of age. Meanwhile, another elderly group of 15 received no supplementation during that time. At the end of the experiment, the zinc group showed a significant improvement in the number of circulating T cells. "The data suggest that the addition of zinc to the diet of old persons could be an effective and simple way to improve their immune function" (*American Journal of Medicine,* May, 1981).

Another simple way to beef up your immune system might be to supplement your diet with arginine. That's an amino acid naturally found in meats, nuts, seeds, beans and sprouts.

Being able to fight off the germs that bombard you every day is a tough business. You win a few, you lose a few. But with good nutrition on your side, you can tip the scales in your favor.

CHAPTER
76

VITAMINS THAT PERK UP A SAGGING DEFENSE

A young brother and sister in South Africa have been in the medical limelight. The children had been plagued with frequent bacterial infections. Juvenile acne, pneumonia, recurring sinusitis, ear infections and upper respiratory tract infections were just some of the maladies their bodies seemed unable to battle. Both children also were allergic to animal hair, house dust, pollen and food, yet they apparently had no drug allergies.

The children were suffering from an unusual disorder called chronic granulomatous disease (CGD)—a severe immune deficiency disease in which part of a person's natural immune system defenses are impaired. It is an inherited disease whose victims are young people showing an abnormally high susceptibility to pus-producing infections. The infections are caused by certain species of bacteria against which the patient's body has no defense.

The youngsters were treated with drugs that lowered the frequency of infections, but they still had bouts with pneumonia, bronchiolitis and sinusitis. Finally, they began taking high doses of vitamin C.

After following a supplementation program with the nutrient, the two children experienced a "decrease in the frequency of infection and increased weight and growth rate," researchers noted. "Both children have remained free of infection for a 10-month period, which included the South African winter. In the previous two winters both children suffered from severe pneumonia and recurrent upper respiratory tract infections."

A brother, just over two years old and not included in the study, also had CGD. The boy developed an acute inflammation of the umbilicus shortly after birth. At the age of two weeks, he developed a serious abscess and complications. He was given 1 gram of vitamin C daily, and the problem cleared up. He has remained free of infection for nine months, the researchers reported.

They concluded that ". . . ascorbic acid [vitamin C] may be an important supplement to prophylactic antibiotics and chemotherapeutic agents in the treatment of CGD" (*South African Medical Journal,* September 15, 1979).

Why did vitamin C apparently help those children ward off infections? One clue appearing in blood samples of the older brother and sister was an increase in neutrophil activity after taking vitamin C.

"Neutrophils are a type of white blood cell and are the main killer cells that respond to bacteria in the body," explains Norbert J. Roberts, Jr., M.D., associate professor of medicine and a member of the infectious disease unit at the University of Rochester, in New York. "Vitamin C appears to be important for the migration of those killer cells. In the absence of vitamin C, the migration of these cells and phagocytosis—the eating—of bacteria can be depressed."

Dr. Roberts has been researching the effects of vitamin C and fever on the immune system. "There have been numerous speculations on vitamin C's role on immune function," says Dr. Roberts. "There also has been a lot of controversy and unknowns about hyperthermia [elevated body temperature]. Is fever good or bad? Should a person take aspirin to reduce fever or not?"

They decided to put both vitamin C and fever to the test, choosing to pit them against an influenza virus. "An infection with the influenza virus can depress a patient's immune function to other agents," Dr. Roberts told us.

First, they took some normal human white cells and stimulated them with a plant substance called PHA. "Normal cells should respond to PHA. If a person has an immune deficiency, his cell response to PHA will be less," explains Dr. Roberts.

After they observed how the normal cells responded to PHA, they exposed the cells to influenza. When the cells "came down with the flu," their immunity was lower, as shown by a lower than normal response to PHA. When the flu-infected cells were treated with vitamin C, however, they bounced back and exhibited a higher response to PHA. Infected cells which were raised to fever temperature also responded more favorabl to PHA.

"Both ascorbic acid and fever appear to enhance the response of the cells and to diminish the adverse effects of the virus, when examined in the test tube," Dr. Roberts says. "It remains open to question whether a person taking vitamin C and avoiding aspirin will find any benefit for the immune system, but our work suggests that it might. Repeated studies we have done show the same thing all over again. However, for certain individuals (a young child or a person with heart disease, for example), it might be important to lower fever" (*Journal of Immunology*, November 1979).

A Boost from Vitamin A

Vitamin C is not the only nutrient which may dramatically bolster the body's natural defenses. Benjamin E. Cohen, M.D., of Houston, Texas, has been studying vitamin A over the years and has found that it, too, may boost a person's immune response.

"While I was working at the National Institutes of Health in Bethesda, Maryland, I examined the effects of steroids and vitamin A on mice," he told us. "Steroids are chemical agents secreted by the adrenal glands. Among other things, high doses of steroids are known for their suppressive effect on a person's immune response. They are widely used drugs often given to transplant patients so that their immune systems will be less likely to reject the transplanted organ.

"When I gave high doses of steroids to mice, their immune systems were depressed. But when the mice were given vitamin A, the steroids were unable to depress the immune system. Vitamin A blocked the depression."

Dr. Cohen also discovered that vitamin A decreased the animals' susceptibility to a variety of bacterial infections. And when mice were given vitamin A in conjunction with a potent anti-cancer agent, the anti-cancer agent became 100 times more potent.

Dr. Cohen went to England on a fellowship from Harvard and began researching the effect of vitamin A on the immune system in humans.

"It has consistently been found that anesthesia and surgery result in a suppression of the immune response in patients," he says. "Whenever patients are anesthetized, it generally takes a few weeks for their immune response to recover."

Working with colleagues from Australia and England, Dr. Cohen conducted research with patients who were undergoing elective operations. The patients were divided into two groups. One group received vitamin A before, during and after surgery. The other group did not take vitamin A supplementation. Blood tests were performed immediately before and after surgery and one week later. A series of immune function tests was run on each sample.

"By and large, there was a tendency toward a depression of the immune function in patients not taking vitamin A," Dr. Cohen explains. "On the average, patients who *did* take vitamin A did not experience a depression of the immune response at all." Vitamin A seemed to keep the patients' immune defenses functioning normally despite their surgery (*Surgery, Gynecology and Obstetrics,* November, 1979).

Dr. Cohen theorizes that vitamin A's favorable effects on the immune system might prove to be beneficial in battling certain types of cancers. "The immune system has been implicated in the control of certain types of tumors," he told us. "If that is true, it may be possible to improve the immune system's work with vitamin A supplementation. That may be helpful in arresting or even eradicating the tumor.'' Dr. Cohen says vitamin A probably would be given to the patient as additional therapy. ''The nutrient might be used in conjunction with a more traditional approach.''

The immune system is a complex internal mechanism that still is not completely understood. But as researchers continue to investigate the ways in which certain cells in our bodies overwhelm and destroy dangerous bacteria and other foreign invaders, vitamins A and C are sure to receive even more attention.

CHAPTER

77

BOOST YOUR IMMUNITY WITH VITAMIN C

Interferon is a remarkable defensive substance that the body makes naturally when it's invaded by the likes of viruses and cancer. And extra vitamin C means extra interferon.

When an invader, such as a virus, enters the body, it attacks the cells that make up body tissues. Each individual virus attacks one cell and takes over the cell's reproductive cycle, making the cell turn out more viruses instead of more cells. Unless the body fights back in some way, it will quickly be overcome by the invaders.

Naturally, the body does fight back. According to Benjamin V. Siegel, Ph.D., a research professor at the University of Oregon health sciences center in Portland, interferon is the body's first line of defense. "Before the body is even producing any antibodies," Dr. Siegel told us, "interferon can just attack the disease. But the body has to be producing *enough* interferon."

Interferon does not work directly against the invaders. Instead, it is manufactured by the cell under attack and, like Paul Revere, is sent off to alert the surrounding cells. The other cells are stimulated into producing a substance which prevents the virus from reproducing any further. The invasion is stopped dead in its tracks—provided there's enough interferon.

"The beauty of interferon," according to Dr. Siegel, "is that it works against all viruses. A vaccine usually works against only one specific type of virus. And in the case of chemical virus killers, the viruses can develop mutant types that are resistant to the chemicals. But this doesn't happen with interferon."

What does happen with interferon, however, is that there are great variations in just how much interferon is available. Dr. Siegel offers this as a possible explanation of why some people are more resistant to viral infections than others.

Interferon Fights Cancer

The importance of interferon is not limited to fighting viral infections such as the common cold and influenza. These two items alone, of course, would guarantee that interferon would be a top priority for drug research. But interferon also stimulates another anti-invasion force, the macrophages. Dr. Siegel calls them the "angry" cells that seek out and destroy not only invading viruses, but any foreign intruder—including cancer cells.

In Sweden, persons with bone cancer were treated with large doses of interferon produced in a laboratory. The survival rate increased substantially. But the number of people treated with interferon was necessarily small, mainly because it is very difficult and costly to produce interferon in a laboratory. Nonetheless, the great promise of using interferon to fight cancer, as well as serious viral diseases such as hepatitis and influenza, is stimulating research to find a way of making the body produce more interferon.

According to Dr. Siegel, "pharmacological companies, which are interested in making money as well as helping people, have been trying for years to find an agent that will increase interferon production in the body. It is possible to produce interferon in the laboratory. But if interferon is produced like this, on the outside, it would cost thousands of dollars for enough interferon to cure a cold. So the trick is to produce it on the inside, to get the body to produce more of its own interferon. Vitamin C appears to do just that."

Dr. Siegel's first investigation into vitamin C's effect on interferon involved infecting mice with extremely lethal leukemia-causing viruses. One group of mice received large doses of vitamin C, one group did not. The mice that did get vitamin C developed milder cases of leukemia and produced more than *twice as much* interferon.

Vitamin C also boosts other defenses. The activity of macrophages, which is stimulated by interferon, is further heightened by vitamin C. White blood cells are also helped by vitamin C, as is the production of antibodies against specific diseases.

Double Evidence of Vitamin C's Power

Currently, Dr. Siegel is attempting to find out whether vitamin C can completely prevent or delay the onset of leukemia. In his earlier work, such large doses of the leukemia virus were used that there was never any doubt that all the mice would get the disease. The purpose was to measure the interferon production. But in his present investigation, lower doses of the leukemia virus are being used, in hopes of giving the vitamin C–interferon team a chance to show if it can stop leukemia before it gets started.

Of course, some of the questions medical skeptics are going to ask are whether Dr. Siegel's results can be duplicated and whether vitamin C can affect *human* interferon as well as it can that of a mouse. Other researchers have already begun to answer these questions—happily, in the affirmative.

Norwegian investigators recently published the results of their work with human cell cultures. Such cell cultures, grown in the laboratories, are often used in the early stages of research work when it is inconvenient to use volunteers or animals. The cells were *challenged* with viruses and supplemented with varying doses of vitamin C while interferon levels were measured. Vitamin C was found to increase the cells' production of interferon at all dose levels (*Acta Pathologica et Microbiologica Scandinvica*).

Dr. Siegel is pleased with the Norwegian reports, especially since these researchers set out to *disprove* his results. "But their results are almost the same as ours," he told us. "Our work is solid. It's established. What we've done is demonstrate, for the first time, what vitamin C does."

There is abundant evidence from still more researchers' work that vitamin C gives a significant boost to the body's ability to fight off invaders. Not all of them have considered the connection between vitamin C and interferon. But the husband-wife team of biochemists Carlton E. Schwerdt, Ph.D., and Patricia Schwerdt *did* in their work with human cell cultures and cold viruses. The Schwerdts set out to find if vitamin C could prevent or reduce common cold symptoms. The cells were treated with vitamin C for two days, then infected with a common cold virus.

The effect was described to us by Dr. Carlton Schwerdt: "The virus goes through one cycle of growth, but subsequent cycles seem to be inhibited." After the first cycle, 16 to 48 hours after the first infection, virus yield dropped gradually until it was one-twentieth that of the culture which was not treated with vitamin C. After 48 hours, the treated culture had a virus yield which was one-fortieth the size of the untreated cells.

If you think that sounds like the kind of population controlling effect interferon exerts on viruses, then you have that thought in common with the Schwerdts. At least one of their experiments demonstrated that vitamin C was increasing a form of antiviral activity similar to that of interferon.

As promising as all this research is for the battle against cancer and viral infections, there is one important thing to note. The drug industry is not going to spend much money trying to find out more about vitamin C's effect on interferon. They are spending their time and money trying to find a way to make *artificial* interferon or develop a drug which will do the same thing vitamin C does. The reason is simple. Everyone has access to vitamin C. No one can patent it and sell it for drug-high prices. Naturally, the drug companies won't promote something that won't make money for them.

CRAMPS

CHAPTER

78

VITAMIN E FOR THOSE PAINFUL CRAMPS

Cramps—they cramp your style.

A cramp in the calf can turn a pleasant walk into a forced march home. And did your community pool ever seem like the set of *Jaws*—only with your thigh muscles standing in for the shark? You could even hate writing a love letter if writer's cramp suddenly put on the squeeze.

There are over 100 muscles in your body. Any one of them could knot up. And few Boy Scouts could help you untie *these* knots. But you can be prepared for cramps—with vitamin E.

That's the news from Australia, where Dr. L. Lotzof is having "remarkable success" treating muscular cramps with vitamin E.

In a letter to *The Medical Journal of Australia,* Dr. Lotzof reported giving daily doses of about 300 milligrams of vitamin E to 50 patients suffering from muscular cramps. *In all 50 patients, almost all cramping stopped.*

As soon as Dr. Lotzof's patients stopped taking vitamin E, their cramps returned.

Dr. Lotzof was surprised by these excellent results. He asked other doctors to write to the journal and offer explanations as to why vitamin E controls muscle cramps. But it's unlikely he'll get much of a response. Modern medical science really has no clear idea what causes cramps. But scientific literature *is* full of reports by doctors like Lotzof who—without knowing the *why* behind their treatment—have cured muscle cramps with vitamin E.

Two such doctors are Samuel Ayres, Jr., M.D., and Richard Mihan, M.D. They treated 125 of their patients, who were suffering from nighttime leg and foot cramps, with vitamin E. "More than half of these patients had suffered from leg cramps longer than five years and many of these had had cramps for 20 to 30 years or longer," the doctors wrote in the *Southern Medical Journal*.

But vitamin E made short work of even these long-standing cramps. *Of the 125 patients, 123 found relief from their cramps after taking vitamin E.* One hundred three of these patients had "excellent" results: "complete or nearly complete control" of cramps.

A daily dose of either 300 or 400 international units of vitamin E cleared up most cramps. Some patients, however, needed more. So if you begin taking vitamin E for cramps and find a daily dose of 400 international units has little or no effect, don't hesitate to try a larger amount. "There are virtually no side effects from doses as high as 1,600 to 2,400 international units daily," the doctors assure us.

Also, if you find vitamin E does work, stick with it. "In a number of instances . . . it was learned that cramps recurred when treatment was stopped or greatly reduced, but promptly responded again when treatment was resumed," the doctors explain.

All in all, the doctors feel confident that vitamin E will do the job. "The response of nocturnal [nighttime] leg and foot cramps to adequate doses of vitamin E is prompt, usually becoming manifest within a week, and occurs in such an overwhelming number of cases that it appears almost specific for this ailment," they assert.

But not *only* nocturnal foot and leg cramps were healed by

vitamin E. Nocturnal rectal cramps, cramping of abdominal muscles and cramps from heavy exercise were also "relieved completely" with the vitamin.

Is Walking Painful?

Now, walking is *not* a heavy exercise. At least, not for most people. But if you have intermittent claudication—a painful cramping of the calf muscle that sneaks up on you after you've walked too far—a stroll around the block can have your calf muscle playing the "heavy" in a very unpleasant muscular melodrama. Well, help is on the way. No white hats or shining armor—just our old friend, vitamin E.

Knut Haeger, M.D., a Swedish surgeon, selected 47 men with severe intermittent claudication. He gave 32 of them vitamin E; the rest received drugs to improve circulation *(American Journal of Clinical Nutrition)*.

After about three months, the men were tested to see how far they could walk without pain. Fifty-four percent of the vitamin E group walked 1 kilometer (⅝ of a mile), the test's maximum distance. But only 23 percent of the second group could walk that far.

How did vitamin E help these men to walk? Vitamin E may stop intermittent claudication—and all cramps—by improving circulation. After about 1½ years of taking vitamin E, 29 out of 32 men in Dr. Haeger's study had an increase in the flow of blood to their calves. That's a big difference from those who took prescribed drugs. After 1½ years, 10 of 14 of those men had a *diminished* flow.

So even though scientists have yet to unravel the mystery of how vitamin E works to stop cramps, you don't have to wait to use it. You can unravel—now—twisted, tight and cramped muscles with vitamin E.

CRIME AND JUVENILE DELINQUENCY

CHAPTER

79

CRIME-BUSTER VITAMINS

Time was, convicts used files to escape from jail. Now they use knives and forks.

In Pitkin County, Colorado, 500 prisoners went on a diet free of sugar, white flour and coffee and ate dinners from a natural foods restaurant. A study showed that, from their release to the end of the study, not one prisoner has been in trouble with the law.

In Dougherty County, Georgia, every juvenile offender undergoes biochemical testing and is given nutritional supplements to help correct any chemical imbalance. The number of serious crimes by juveniles in Dougherty County is less than it was ten years ago—a pleasant exception to the trend in many American communities.

In Cuyahoga Falls, Ohio, 600 criminals have received nutritional education and gone on a diet emphasizing lean meats, whole grains and fresh fruits and vegetables. Eighty-nine percent of those people have not committed another crime.

That bad nutrition and bad behavior are closely linked is the truth, and nothing but the truth. But the people running America's multibillion-dollar criminal justice system are just beginning to wake up to the fact. They're being shaken awake by a small group of men and women who realize that no approach to criminal rehabilitation—social casework, psychotherapy, group therapy, psychiatry, academic and vocational training—can possibly work unless a good diet backs it up.

"Of the nearly two million criminals in jail, over 70 percent have been there before," Alex Schauss told us. "So *something* has to be wrong with the way most criminals are rehabilitated."

Schauss is a former state corrections training officer for the Washington State Criminal Justice Training Commission. He oversaw the training of parole and probation officers, the men who deal with criminals out of jail. To *keep* them out, Schauss put together a course called "body chemistry and offender behavior." Its many topics include diet, vitamins, minerals, stress, food allergy and exercise—detailed information about health that the probation officer passes on to the offender. But can this kind of approach really soften a hardened criminal?

"Not one single probation or parole officer has called me and said this approach doesn't work, and if it didn't, I would be hearing about it," says Schauss. Studies back up that claim.

Schauss chose 102 people who had committed a crime and were on probation. He had some of them receive nutritional counseling and others traditional counseling. (Traditional counseling advises an offender about his job, housing, clothing, family problems and other areas of daily life—except what he eats.) Schauss found that 34 percent of the people receiving traditional counseling committed another crime, compared with only 14 percent of the people receiving nutritional counseling.

In another study, Schauss again had probationers receive nutritional counseling. This time, he compared the probationers' arrest records before, during and after the counseling. Eight months after the counseling had ended, not one of the probationers had been rearrested while, statistically speaking, all of them *should* have been rearrested based on their previous arrest records.

Nutritional counseling works—beyond a shadow of a doubt. Schauss explains why: "Most people, criminals included, are extremely naïve about diet and how it affects their body and mind," he says. "Simply educating a criminal about nutrition, showing him that bad dietary habits ruin mental and physical health and keep him behind bars, helps him give up those habits." And of all bad habits, too much sugar may be the worst.

Most repeat offenders eat a glut of candy, soda and other goodies that add up to from 300 to 600 pounds a year, about two to four times more sweets than the average American eats. It's a crime they don't get away with. Eating that much sugar can cause a disorder in blood sugar metabolism called hypoglycemia, and studies show that almost 90 percent of all inmates have it. Many of the symptoms of hypoglycemia are psychological: irritability, paranoia, sudden violent behavior—*criminal* behavior. Educate a convict about sugar (and caffeine and alcohol, which can also cause hypoglycemia), help him cut it out of his diet and you can end up with John Doe instead of John Dillinger II. And most convicts, says Schauss, want that help.

"The one common denominator of inmates is to get out of jail. People don't like to be behind bars. About 70 percent of the convicts who receive nutritional counseling change their diet for the better and keep it changed."

And that change may include eliminating all the foods to which a convict is allergic.

Food allergy. It works just like hay fever except, for pollen, substitute eggs, chocolate, corn, citrus fruits, milk or wheat. (A person may become allergic to the foods he eats most often, and these foods, being so common, account for most food allergies.) But while hay fever and similar allergies attack the nose, a food allergy may attack the *brain*—and can make a good boy go bad.

"Aberrant social behavior can be directly caused by a food allergy," explains Ray Wunderlich, Jr., M.D., a St. Petersburg, Florida, physician and author of several publications on allergies.

"The brain is a target organ for food allergy," he told us. "Immediately after eating the offending food, a person's behavior changes for the worse. His brain can fog over, leaving him apathetic and sluggish, or he can go wildly hyperactive. In either case, he lacks good judgment. He doesn't see whole situations and reacts to fragments and details.

"If he becomes apathetic, he needs a severe and heightened thrill to interest him in life—being chased by police, being wanted by the law, being in danger. If he becomes hyperactive, he works on a different time clock than the rest of society, demanding things *now* and using violence to satisfy his urgent needs."

Dr. Wunderlich points out that not only can food trigger violence, but so can chemicals to which a person is allergic. Schauss illustrates the point with a story of "chemical warfare."

"A boy at school suddenly became ruthless and violent, beating up other kids and breaking furniture. Our staff investigated and found that he was allergic to fumes from the school's floor wax.

"How many convicts mired in the criminal justice system started going downhill after a few incidents like this? If someone's actions are socially unacceptable, people start to think of him as a misfit. If he repeats those actions often enough, he is labeled a misfit. Inevitably, he begins to think of himself as a misfit—and to act like one."

To break this cycle, which Schauss has named *biocriminogenesis,* a criminal must avoid the substances to which he is allergic and improve his diet. He also needs psychological counseling to restore his self-esteem. But before counseling, he needs nutritional supplements.

"Many delinquents and criminals do not have sufficient biochemical reserves to make positive mental changes," says Dan MacDougal, a lawyer from Atlanta, Georgia.

MacDougal is a consultant to the Judicial Service Agency in Dougherty County, an organization which works with juvenile delinquents. The agency, he says, "teaches them the proper use of will and new behavior patterns that are not based on fear or hostility, but are based on love."

Before psychological treatment starts, however, every delinquent undergoes biochemical testing and is then given nutritional supplements to correct any chemical imbalance. (The agency must be doing something right. Dougherty County has the lowest juvenile crime rate in the nation.)

"Vitamin B_6 lowers impulsivity and violent behavior," MacDougal told us. "Vitamins A, C and E aid in detoxifying a person whose violent behavior is being caused by heavy-metal poisoning."

Heavy metals—lead, cadmium, mercury, arsenic, to name a few. They pollute air, water and food. Most people aren't too bothered by the heavy metals in their bodies. Some are.

"I see lead poisoning contributing to an awful lot of criminal behavior," says Barbara Reed, former chief probation officer of the Municipal Court in Cuyahoga Falls, Ohio.

Mrs. Reed treated most of her probationers with diet, suggesting a steady fare of natural, unprocessed foods and the complete elimination of refined carbohydrates and caffeine. Of the 600 people who followed that diet, 89 percent never committed another crime. "But some need more help than a better diet," Mrs. Reed told us. "They need a vitamin-and-mineral regimen to cleanse their body of heavy metals.

"One man was referred to me after he had committed two felonies: trafficking in drugs and carrying loaded firearms. He was diagnosed as having lead and aluminum poisoning. After three months of special treatment and a good nutritional diet, he was eager to return to regular work."

Schauss also relates a case of a man with heavy-metal poisoning:

"A man was being held in the county jail who had been arrested for assaulting a policeman. During his arraignment, his behavior disrupted the court proceeding. Two psychiatrists and a mental health specialist interviewed him. One psychiatrist diagnosed him 'acutely schizophrenic.' The other two experts agreed he was a full-blown 'paranoid schizophrenic.' All three predicted that by the age of 30 he would become a vegetable.

"Well, our staff looked at him and noticed symptoms of lead poisoning. Tests were conducted and showed that he was suffering from toxic levels of arsenic, lead, mercury and cadmium in his system. Through vitamin and mineral supplementation, chelation therapy and counseling, he improved rapidly."

However, Schauss, Reed, MacDougal and many other professionals agree that nutrition is only one facet of biochemical treatment. Exercise, too, is very important, as are proper lighting, fresh air and sufficient sleep. "These are terrific tools," says Mrs. Reed. "By improving a criminal's health, we help him to perform better in the other rehabilitative services."

Good health. For thousands of criminals, it's the best accomplice for a *permanent* jailbreak—and a break with the past.

CHAPTER

80

NUTRITION: THE SILVER LINING

Mary sits slumped in a chair, her mascara smeared by an hour of crying, her thoughts black as the circles under her eyes . . . .

"Why did I bother putting on makeup this morning? I'm ugly and that's that. John must hate me. And what's the use of looking good, anyway? Life is so empty, so useless. If only I could run away."

But for Mary, and 50 million other Americans, there's no running away—from depression. Serious depression. Not just a day of the blues, but weeks, perhaps months, of symptoms like these: You hate yourself and everyone else. You speak hesitantly in a dull monotone. You can't concentrate or make decisions. Sex is a chore. Headaches are frequent. Sleep is restless, and during the day you move like a sloth. You feel frustrated, trapped, hopeless. And when you think of suicide (which is often), it's with relief.

Who gets depressed? Anyone can. But almost twice as many women as men do. Pregnant women. Women who've just had babies. Postmenopausal women. Women on the Pill.

But often the cause of their depression isn't psychological; it's physical—a nutritional deficiency.

In the week after they had given birth, 18 women were tested for severity of depression and blood levels of tryptophan, an essential amino acid. Doctors found that those with the most severe depression had the lowest levels of tryptophan *(British Medical Journal).*

A study of 15 depressed pregnant women showed that those with the deepest depression had the lowest blood levels of vitamin B_6 *(Acta Obstetricia et Gynecologica Scandinavica).*

Researchers discovered that postmenopausal women with depression have a disturbance in their tryptophan metabolism very similar to that found in patients hospitalized for depression *(British Medical Journal).*

Numerous studies show that women on the Pill who become depressed have low levels of vitamin B_6 *(Lancet).*

And a study shows that in the days before menstruation, a time of depression for many women, tryptophan metabolism is disturbed *(American Journal of Psychiatry).*

A Crucial Chain Reaction

Why tryptophan? Why B_6?

Because of serotonin.

Serotonin is a neurotransmitter, one of the chemicals in your brain that helps control moods. Some scientists theorize that low levels of serotonin cause depression. But to have enough serotonin, you need enough tryptophan, which is essential in its formation. And to have enough tryptophan, you need enough B_6, without which tryptophan can't be formed. B_6, tryptophan, serotonin: The chemical chain reaction that forms this neurotransmitter is more complex, but these links are crucial.

Estrogen can break them.

Estrogen, a female hormone, can block the activity of B_6, forcing it out of the body. And estrogen can speed up the metabolism of tryptophan, making less of it available to form serotonin. That doesn't happen every day. But if estrogen levels are high—if you're pregnant, taking the Pill or about to have your period—then you can have a shortage of tryptophan or B_6. And a long face.

The solution? Replace the nutrients.

When 250 "depression-prone" women received oral contraceptives supplemented with B_6, 90 percent remained free of severe depression *(Ob. Gyn. News)*.

In another study, doctors measured the blood levels of B_6 in 39 depressed women on the Pill and found that 19 had a severe deficiency. When they gave these women B_6, 16 improved in mood *(Lancet)*.

And those women probably got more than just an increase in their B_6 levels. Many women on the Pill suffer from a blood sugar disorder. When they take B_6, however, that disorder improves *(Contraception)*.

Not everyone suffering from depression is a woman, of course. But studies show that tryptophan and B_6 may help anyone who's depressed.

Doctors measured the severity of depression in patients hospitalized for the problem and then gave them tryptophan and B_6 for one month. After the month, they again measured their depression. It had decreased by 82 percent *(British Medical Journal)*.

Niacin Helps, Too

In another study lasting one month, doctors gave tryptophan and niacin to 11 depressed patients. (Ten of the patients were women, and their average age was 52. More than likely, they were in the throes of postmenopausal depression.) Why niacin? The doctors knew that, in some studies, depressed people took tryptophan but didn't get any better. They theorized that the tryptophan hadn't been metabolized properly and that niacin would correct this problem. They were right. After a month on tryptophan and niacin, the patients' blood levels of tryptophan rose almost 300 percent and their depression fell 38 percent *(Lancet).*

Research also shows tryptophan's superiority over a drug. For three weeks, doctors gave one group of depressed patients tryptophan and a second group the drug imipramine, an anti-depressant. Both groups did equally well, having "significant improvements." But the patients on the tryptophan, say the doctors, had fewer side effects *(Lancet).*

Researchers have also found they could give too much tryptophan. Depressed patients who received 6 grams of tryptophan and 1,500 milligrams of niacin (as nicotinamide) a day didn't improve, but those who received 4 grams of tryptophan and 1 gram of niacin did. The researchers theorize that there is an optimal range for blood levels of tryptophan in depressed patients, and that giving too much or too little of the nutrient is useless *(British Medical Journal).*

So if something is eating you—and taking a big bite—perhaps you should try increasing your intake of the nutrients we've discussed. Good nutrition and bad moods don't mix.

FATIGUE

CHAPTER

81

VITAMINS FOR PEAK ENERGY

Without mentioning any names, those television commercials about "iron-poor" and "tired" blood that we've been dunned with all these years gave us the wrong impression. Not only did they assault us nightly with something new to worry about and promise salvation in a relatively expensive, over-the-counter concoction, they also implanted the half-truth that our blood needs iron, and iron alone. They neglected to tell us that the blood also needs vitamins.

Now, no one doubts the importance of iron. It's the critical ingredient of hemoglobin, the molecule in red blood cells that carries oxygen from the lungs to the tissues. And no one doubts that many people, particularly preschool children, women of child-bearing age and the elderly, have a diet that's inadequate in iron. But iron is only one instrument in an orchestra of nutrients that helps pour forth a steady stream of new blood cells from our bone marrow. Iron may play first violin, but the French horns, oboes and timpanis are vitamins.

Folate, for instance. Without this B-complex vitamin, the body cannot manufacture some of the molecular building blocks of DNA. The DNA molecule, in turn, is the secret of cell division.

Less folate (folic acid) means less DNA, which means a slow-down in the creation of new cells, including red blood cells. (Folate deficiency also causes the production of abnormally large red blood cells.) Like iron, folate is a nutrient many people don't get enough of in their food. One physician called folate deficiency "the most common vitamin deficiency in man."

"Evidence is accumulating that folacin [folate] deficiency may be more widespread than previously suspected." That was the conclusion of a team of University of Florida and University of Miami researchers who studied blood samples from 193 elderly, low-income volunteers in the Coconut Grove section of Miami, Florida. Knowing that they would discover a high rate of nutrition-related anemia (an abnormally low concentraion of red blood cells or hemoglobin) in this group, the researchers hoped to single out the cause of the anemia. Surprisingly, the missing link wasn't iron. It was folate.

Based on the folate content of their red blood cells, 60 percent of the volunteers fell into the category of "high risk" for folate deficiency, and another 11 percent evidenced a "medium risk." Fourteen percent were frankly anemic. At the same time, "the iron status of these elderly people was normal and indicates that the anemia was not due to a dietary iron deficiency.

"These findings . . . point out the fallacy of the rather wide-spread assumption that anemia always reflects dietary iron deficiency," the Florida study noted. "It is important to reassess the true incidence of iron deficiency worldwide in view of mounting evidence of the extent of folacin deficiency" (*American Journal of Clinical Nutrition*, November, 1979).

A glance at the diets of the elderly volunteers revealed an absence of foods rich in folate. Only 17 percent of the group said they ate fresh vegetables and, in spite of the abundance of fresh oranges and grapefruit in Florida, only 30 percent reported eating citrus fruits. Some of these people also customarily boiled their vegetables for several hours, thereby destroying most of the folate.

Liver, actually, is the best source of folate. It's also, conveniently, a prime source of other nutrients that the blood thrives on, such as vitamin B_{12}, iron, riboflavin and vitamin A. Folate can also be found in lentils, other beans of various kinds and most vegetables. Whole grain bread, meat and eggs are moderately good sources of folate.

The elderly, with their tea-and-toast diets, aren't the only ones who risk folate deficiency. Teenagers, with their diet-cola-and-taco diets, need extra folate to keep up with their accelerated growth rate. But many of them aren't getting it.

In a study of 199 12-to-16-year-olds in the Liberty City section of Miami, the same group of researchers found approximately 50 percent of these low-income adolescents to be deficient in folate and about 10 percent deficient in iron.

Again, in a paper presented to the Federation of American Societies for Experimental Biology, the researchers stressed that folate shouldn't be eclipsed by an overemphasis on iron. "The incidence of folic acid [folate] deficiency during adolescence has not been widely studied." they said. "In fact, the potential for a folic acid deficiency is often ignored. If anemia is present, it is generally assumed to be due to an iron deficiency."

Researcher James Dinning, Ph.D., calls folate deficiency among teenagers a "high-priority area" and believes that it may affect more people than, for example, high cholesterol. "Folate deficiency could be the major problem in this country," Dr. Dinning said.

Of particular concern was the impact of low folate levels on adolescent girls, especially in light of the high rate of teenage pregnancies in the United States. "A long-term folic acid deficiency prior to pregnancy has been found . . . to adversely affect the outcome of pregnancy."

Depending on the severity, folate deficiency can trigger a wide range of symptoms. Sleeplessness, irritability, forgetfulness and depression are associated with acute deficiency. Lethargy, weakness and loss of color are symptoms of the megaloblastic anemia (a type characterized by oversized, incompletely formed red blood cells) that results from folate deficiency.

Besides anemia, folate deficiency has recently been linked to neurological problems. Researchers at the laboratory of neuroanatomy at McGill University in Montreal found that folate supplementation relieved mild depression, fatigue and abnormal intellectual or nerve function in certain people. These symptoms, significantly, appeared even before the folate deficiency was severe enough to show up on a routine blood test (*Nature,* March, 1979).

Serge Gauthier, M.D., one of the McGill researchers, told us that the neurological problems stemming from lack of folate are mild, "but since it's a common deficiency, it's worth looking into." His research group suggested that shortages of vitamins such as folate can influence behavior by decreasing the synthesis of neurotransmitters, the molecules that relay brain messages. Dr. Gauthier warned that older people are particularly vulnerable to the neurological effects of folate deficiency.

As mentioned before, it's not one or two but a constellation of nutrients that fuels the daily manufacture of blood cells in the bone marrow and keeps tham alive and functioning after they move into circulation. Here's a brief list of some other nutrients that work with folate in the process of blood formation.

Vitamin B$_{12}$: You can't talk about folate without mentioning B$_{12}$. Without B$_{12}$, the folate needed for DNA synthesis remains trapped in a form the body can't use.

This creates some confusion in diagnosing anemia, since a lack of either of these vitamins can cause anemia, and it's difficult to tell which one's missing. Meat, poultry, fish and eggs all supply B$_{12}$. Fruits, vegetables, grains and grain products do not contain it.

Riboflavin, or vitamin B$_2$: The complex mechanism of blood production relies partly on this vitamin.

In a study in Germany of pregnant women, supplementation with both iron and riboflavin was much more effective in raising the red blood cell count than iron alone (*Nutrition and Metabolism*). Researchers in London also found that even a marginal deficiency of riboflavin can shorten the life span of red blood cells (*Proceedings of the Nutrition Society,* February 1980). Foods rich in riboflavin are brewer's yeast, liver and beef heart, followed by milk, cheese, eggs, leafy green vegetables and grains.

Vitamins A and E: There's evidence that each of these vitamins plays a role in moving iron from the diet to the blood. In people deficient in vitamin A, iron supplementation did not raise their hemoglobin levels unless accompanied by therapy with vitamin A *(American Journal of Clinical Nutrition)*. And vitamin E, in combination with vitamin C, has been reported to enhance the uptake of iron into the process of blood formation.

So where the state of your blood is concerned, don't take you cues solely from ads about iron on the TV. Good nutrition is too complex for that, and putting energy back into "tired" blood means more than just pumping iron. It means making sure your diet provides the whole spectrum of nutrients necessary for healthy maintenance of the blood.

ENERGY VITAMINS TO MAKE LIFE A BREEZE

On your way to the "speedy mart" for a quart of milk, you drive by a tennis court. The white-toggged players are about your age, but their faces glow with a royal flush, and their backhands are youthfully crisp. As you realize that you just took the car instead of walking the mere half mile to the store, you wonder jealously, "Where do they get so much energy?"

Nutrients to keep your eye on are vitamin B_6, pantothenate (pantothenic acid) and vitamin C. Of course, we need all the essential vitamins and minerals, but those three are proven fatigue fighters. And they have been studied in depth.

"If a person feels fatigue, then taking certain vitamins and minerals, over and above what we get from our ordinary diet, should certainly decrease that fatigue."

So says John H. Richardson, M.D., a biology professor at Old Dominion University, in Norfolk, Virginia. About three years ago, Dr. Richardson, partly as a doctor and partly as an avid jogger, became interested in the relationship between different nutrients and stamina. So he set up a series of experiments to test the effects of vitamins and minerals on the endurance of lab animals. One of the vitamins was B_6.

Dr. Richardson assembled two groups of 20 rats each. He fed all of them a normal rat chow and conditioned each of them on an exercise wheel for 30 days. One group was supplemented with B_6 and the other wasn't. At the end of one month, he attached the rats' calf muscles to a spring and measured how many seconds they could maintain a contraction. In human terms, he told us, it was like timing how long you could hold yourself in the "up" position of a chin-up.

B_6 Increases Stamina

The supplemented rats were stronger. "Time to fatigue was measured for all animals. Results indicate that contraction time for B_6 animals was significantly longer than controls. This study suggests that vitamin B_6 given orally increases stamina," Dr. Richardson reported (*Journal of Sports Medicine and Physical Fitness*, June, 1981).

Dr. Richardson says he isn't sure why vitamin B_6 works. He only knows that it works consistently, and he believes it will work for people as well as animals. "In terms of performance or well-being," he told us, "I think we could feel better than we do if we took this nutrient. A lot of people walk around fatigued from lack of sleep or overwork or stress. I know I do. But with B_6, we might live closer to our potential. We wouldn't get tired so quickly, we would feel better, we could function at a higher level."

At Oregon State University, in Corvallis, James Leklem, Ph.D., has been intensively studying the blood of 15 male high-school cross-country runners and trained bicyclists. In all those young men, he found that the B_6 levels of their blood rose when they worked out.

That extra B_6 had to come from somewhere, Dr. Leklem reasoned. But there was no change in diet to explain the rise, and the body can't synthesize its own B_6. Apparently, the body met its needs by mobilizing the vitamin from tissues in the body.

"We have seen that vitamin B_6 levels in the blood go up during exercise," Dr. Leklem told us. Unfortunately, he adds, "our intake of B_6 isn't as good as it might be, and this all comes down to eating better, really."

Meanwhile, at the University of Oregon, in Eugene, an hour south of Corvallis, other scientists have also been investigating the link between B_6 and exercise. "There is always an increase in the need for B_6 during physical stress," Frantisek Bartos, Ph.D., told us. "People in general have a greater-than-RDA [Recommended Dietary Allowance] need for the vitamin, but in athletes the need is even more pronounced. We know that the amount of B_6 in a normal diet is not sufficient."

Dr. Bartos says that B_6 supplements have increased his own energy.

Unnecessary Fatigue

If those findings are valid, then there are many elderly people living in a state of unnessary fatigue. In a recent survey of men and women between 60 and 95 in central Kentucky, "aging was associated with a decline in . . . vitamin B_6 status."

The survey showed that 56.6 percent of the patients in nursing homes and 43.5 percent of the elderly living at home were deficient in B_6. More seriously, 27.3 percent of the institutionalized elderly were "severely deficient." Decreased digestive ability, use of diuretic medication, social isolation, limited income and lack of family support were among the reasons suggested for the widespread deficiency (*International Journal of Vitamin and Nutrition Research*, December, 1981).

There also seems to be a link between pantothenate and fatigue. It's known that from pantothenate the body builds coenzyme A (CoA), a catalyst necessary for the conversion of food to energy. Low levels of CoA can be dangerous. In one experiment at the University of Nebraska, Hazel Fox, Ph.D., and colleagues compared two groups of men—one group received the vitamin and the other was totally deprived of it. After ten weeks, the deprived men were listless and complained of fatigue *(Journal of Nutritional Science and Vitaminology).*

That was an extreme case, but Dr. Fox has found that most Americans consume barely as much as the lower end of the National Research Council's recommended daily intake of 4 to 7 milligrams. "The intake of pantothenic acid by Americans is decreasing," she told us. "In 1955, when I first measured the intake of the vitamin by college women here in Lincoln, the average was about 7 milligrams a day. We rarely get figures that high now. The average is 4 or 5. People just don't eat three square meals the way they used to. People aren't choosing the right foods. There are too many processed foods.

"Fatigue has been described as a symptom of pantothenic acid deficiency," she added, "and I would make a guarded statement that the evidence shows a relationship between fatigue and low pantothenic acid intake. It's something we need to look into."

Although the current recommended allowance for the vitamin is only 4 to 7 milligrams, it wasn't always that low. In 1963, a researcher in Hungary reported that "a healthy adult person requires about 15 milligrams of pantothenic acid daily," and he went on to say that physical work, surgery, injury and gastrointestinal infections can double the need for pantothenate. A deficiency can be caused by liver disease, allergies and sometimes as a side effect of drugs, he noted.

To avoid a pantothenate deficiency, avoid processed foods. Researchers at Utah State University studied a wide range of foods and found that products made from "refined grains, fruit products and extended meats and fish, such as frankfurters, sausages, and breaded fish fillets" are low in pantothenate. Also, pantothenate is water soluble, so part of it may be lost during cooking.

The elderly and others who eat lightly should make sure that they eat pantothenate-rich foods. Those foods are beef, chicken, potatoes, oat cereals, tomato products and whole grain products.

Vitamin C and Iron

Two other antifatigue nutrients are iron and vitamin C. Since vitamin C helps the body absorb iron, the two naturally go together.

In a study of fatigue among female garment factory workers in the Philippines, researchers discovered that iron and vitamin C supplements improved the output of workers who were moderately to severely anemic but didn't change the productivity of workers who were only mildly anemic (*Journal of Occupational Medicine*, October, 1981)

Also, a researcher in Switzerland has shown that an optimal dosage of vitamin C for nonsmokers should be 100 milligrams a day (compared to the U.S. RDA of 60 milligrams) and 140 milligrams for smokers and others under physical stress.

He noted that, when a deficient person was supplemented for 12 weeks with vitamin C, riboflavin and B_6, there was "a statistically significant improvement in working capacity" (*South African Medical Journal*, November, 1981).

Obviously, the nutrients mentioned here are only a few of those linked to overall fitness and energy. Good health depends on all of them, and the right blend might just enable you to better enjoy whatever you want to do—go swimming, play tennis, trim the hedge or just walk to the "speedy mart."

CHAPTER

83

GALLSTONES AND B$_6$

If you've been giving cheese omelets and gravy-laden hot roast beef sandwiches the cold shoulder, you're probably making it a point to avoid heart disease. But did you know that not eating fatty and cholesterol-ridden foods may be a good way to avoid gallstones, as well?

And that in itself could be worth your trouble, for developing gallstones could be the quickest date you'll ever make with a surgeon.

Gallbladder surgery has become one of America's favorite operations. No wonder! As one of the richest countries in the world, we boast one of the richest diets imaginable: lots of meat, lots of butter, lots of cream. And, consequently, we've got plenty of gallstones to show for it—some 20 million sufferers can attest to that.

Now, though, there is hope that some of those victims can avoid the trip from the dining room table to the operating table. One study from abroad suggests that, although surgery may be the best alternative in the management of chronic gallbladder disease, it isn't really the best answer to gallstones. Controlling the solubility of the bile cholesterol perhaps is.

The gallbladder is a pouch below the liver which stores a fat-emulsifying liquid, called bile, produced by the liver. A small amount of cholesterol in the bile is perfectly normal. Bile acids and lecithin help to keep it dissolved. But when there is more cholesterol than can be handled by bile salts and lecithin, supersaturation occurs and gallstones form. You'll get the picture of what's happening in your gallbladder if you toss a handful of sugar into a cup of tea. The cholesterol, like the sugar, will not completely dissolve and will clump together to form bigger crystals, or stones. In the gallbladder, these stones may be as small as peppercorns or as large as plums. As long as they are small enough to pass through the bile tracts, there's no problem. But once those nasty cholesterol stones have been fattened to the point where they're stuck in the gallbladder, there's one very effective—and very traumatic—way to combat the stabbing pain and burning irritation—surgery.

That's because, in advanced stages of the disease, the painful symptoms are as much a result of an inflamed gallbladder as they are of the stones themselves. There's no known way to treat an inflamed gallbladder. Nor will a grossly inflamed organ necessarily heal itself once the threat of stones has passed. Removal of the gallbladder is the only way out.

But don't expect surgery to provide a no-catch guarantee against future attacks. Even though the gallbladder may be adequately removed, stones lingering in the bile ducts are sometimes overlooked. Complete operative cleaning of the bile tracts helps. Nevertheless, gallstones may form again and lodge in the ducts if the bile remains supersaturated with cholesterol.

Attempts are often made to flush the bile tracts clean using an instrument which can help the physician peer into body cavities. But this technique, too, is galled with problems. For one thing, it is difficult to reach the portions of the bile tracts closest to the liver. And what's worse, the stones could be dislodged and pushed further up into the liver bile ducts. A stone blocking the bile duct leading from the liver can cause jaundice.

Obviously, getting rid of gallstones for good isn't easy. It would seem that the only logical solution might be altering the cholesterol saturation of the bile. Limiting your intake of saturated fats such as those found in meat and dairy products is the first step toward preventing supersaturation. Researchers are hard at work trying to uncover other ways.

How to Dissolve More Cholesterol

But, meanwhile, according to Dr. K. Holub of the Wilhelmina Hospital in Vienna, Austria, and associates, preventing gallstones may be as close as your nearest grocery and health foods stores. Based on their research, corn oil and vitamin B_6 (pyridoxine) taken together may provide a better and safer solution to cholesterol saturation (*Acta Chirurgica Austriaca*).

In a carefully controlled study, the bile from 22 gallbladder patients was evaluated three days after surgery. Then the same patients were given 1 tablespoon of corn oil and two 25-milligram tablets of vitamin B_6 at seven o'clock and midnight one night and at four o'clock the next morning. Bile samples were again taken and analyzed to determine whether there was any change in the cholesterol-dissolving capacity of the bile.

Indeed there was! Of course, the bile's ability to dissolve cholesterol differs greatly from individual to individual. But according to the Austrian research team, all patients were better able to keep their cholesterol in solution after treatment with corn oil and vitamin B_6. In fact, depending on the patient, the bile in the sample taken after the treatment was able to dissolve anywhere from 43 to 86 percent more cholesterol than before the administration of the corn oil–B_6 combination.

The effectiveness of this treatment may depend on long-term use. But never fear. There are no ill side effects associated with either the corn oil or the vitamin in the doses used, say the doctors.

And the treatment is easy to take. A tablespoon of corn oil can easily be added to a salad at lunch and again at supper. It may be a little more difficult to disguise the corn oil in your morning meal. So swallow your tablespoon's worth and follow it with a glass of orange juice. Vitamin B_6 tablets can be purchased in the health foods store in 25-milligram tablets. Just take two with each meal. Keep in mind that the oil and B_6 should be taken together and that this level of supplementation should be under the supervision of a doctor.

Now, corn oil and B_6 may not dissolve preexisting gallstones, but they might prevent small stones from becoming large stumbling blocks in your quest for good health. By decreasing cholesterol saturation in the bile, these natural substances may also shield you against the development of new stones. So if you've already undergone gallbladder surgery or know that you may be predisposed to developing gallstones, the above routine seems worth a try.

CHAPTER

84

KEEP YOUR GUMS IN THE PINK

You don't have to watch too many television commercials for toothpaste before your realize that teeth are the glamour items of the mouth. Shiny, white teeth are attractive, alluring, sexy— vying with the eyes as the focal point of a winning appearance.

Those same ads never extol the virtues of healthy pink gums. After all, what could be more unexciting than the soft, curving ridges which we take for granted and which, almost incidentally it seems, happen to be attached to those shiny white teeth?

But gums are the very foundation of a healthy mouth, the supporting structure upon which all else rests. Anything which weakens the gums must ultimately weaken the teeth because the latter, though they may be solid and cavity free, are actually no stronger than the fleshy mantle (the technical term is gingiva) that anchors them soundly to the bony sockets of the jaw itself.

And while each tooth is encased in a tough outer protective layer called the enamel, the gums lie exposed in all their supple softness. Each day they must face tremendous wear and tear, bathed almost constantly in bacteria, acids and the residue of decaying food particles. In such an environment, the gum tissue's ability to maintain, repair and defend itself is at least a minor miracle.

For all these reasons, it's important that you pay more attention to the health of your gums. Their appearance can tell you much about the overall state of the rest of your body, and trouble with the gums—if left unchecked—can lead to the loss of every tooth in your mouth.

According to Thomas L. McGuire, D.D.S., author of *The Tooth Trip* (Random House/Bookworks, 1973), there are several easily recognizable features of healthy gums. They are firm, pinkish in color, and they fill in all the spaces between the teeth. In addition, Dr. McGuire says, "Healthy gums have little dot-like indentations (stippling), especially found in the areas closest to the teeth. Your gum, in these areas, should look like the outside of an orange peel." There should also be an elevated roll or collar around the gum where it meets the tooth.

Unhealthy gums, on the other hand, may look smooth and puffy. They often bleed slightly after toothbrushing and show signs of inflammation—called gingivitis—around the gum line.

Because the gums can mirror deficiencies throughout the body, they have become a handy, though admittedly imprecise, dietary reference point. People suffering from scurvy, the vitamin C–deficiency disease, were found to have engorged, dark red gums that bled easily. And similar, though less severe, gingival inflammation has been associated with deficiencies of vitamins A and D, niacin, riboflavin and bioflavonoids. At the other extreme, excessively pale gums may be a sign of iron deficiency anemia.

Pregnancy can affect the gums, causing swelling and bleeding. And so can oral contraceptives and certain other drugs. Heavy smokers may develop a brown discoloration of the gums called "smokers' melanosis," which is more than just a stain from smoking.

The Tooth Destroyer

The most serious and widespread problem affecting the gums, however, is periodontal disease—a chronic, progressive inflammation and infection of the gum tissue and underlying alveolar bone (jawbone). Most medical researchers believe that the disease is caused by residual food, bacteria and tartar deposits that collect in the tiny crevices between the gums and the necks of the teeth. As the bacterial infection spreads deeper into the periodontal tissue surrounding the jaw-tooth connection, the jawbone itself begins to shrink around the sockets until teeth loosen and fall out. An estimated 75 percent of the adult U.S. population suffers from some degree of periodontal disease, and it is the leading tooth destroyer among the middle-aged and older.

Keeping the teeth and gums clean and free of the sticky plaque or film that can harbor harmful bacteria is essential. Careful, effective brushing (particularly at the gum line), along with daily between-teeth cleaning using dental floss, is the backbone of a preventive program. But sound nutritional habits can also play a critical role.

Writing in *Nutrition Today*, Dominick P. DePaola, D.D.S., Ph.D., and Michael C. Alfano, D.M.D., Ph.D., point out that the plaque which develops in the gum crevice "constitutes one of the most dense concentrations of bacteria to which man is exposed. It is, therefore, not surprising that the removal of this bacterial mass usually prevents the development of inflammatory periodontal disease, or arrests it once it has begun. The health of the periodontal tissues depends upon the balance between the virulence of the plaque and the resistance of the host."

Nutrition is one factor that can favorably influence that balance. Drs. DePaola and Alfano note that the cells lining the gum crevice have one of the highest turnover rates in the body—completely renewing themselves every three to seven days. This thin lining, or epithelial tissue, is in what they call "a continuous critical period."

"Nutritional stress during this period may impair the renewal of the epithelium and compromise its barrier function," they warn. "Animal studies from our laboratories have indicated that an acute deficiency of vitamin C almost doubles the ease with which bacterial toxins can penetrate the tissues of the mouth. More recently, we have noted similar effects on permeability caused by zinc and protein deficiencies."

C Provides the "Glue"

The need for vitamin C to cope with periodontal disease makes even more sense when we consider that the nutrient is essential to the formation of collagen, a kind of intercellular cement. Collagen is the glue that helps build and maintain all the connective tissue in our bodies, including the bones and gums.

Researcher Adrian Cowan of the Royal College of Surgeons faculty of dentistry in Ireland says that "collagen, although immensely strong, is completely inert . . . once it starts to break down under the influence of toxins spreading from the gingival crevice, it cannot repair itself."

To try to counteract this, Cowan gave a group of 69 patients vitamin C supplements ranging from 1 to 3 grams (1,000 to 3,000 milligrams) daily for one to five months. The subjects' periodontal membranes at the juncture between root, bone and gum were examined by X ray both before and after the trials. After supplementation, the periodontal pictures improved, indicating a strengthening of the collagen material (*Irish Journal of Medicine*).

As a result, researcher Cowan is "guardedly optimistic" that gum health can be improved or enhanced—even in relatively normal, healthy subjects—through high doses of vitamin C.

A classic nutrition experiment more than a quarter of a century old demonstrated a similar link between vitamin C intake and optimum gum health. The study, carried out by the New Mexico Agricultural Experiment Station, involved more than 200 schoolchildren at six schools scattered through the state.

The selected pupils had varying degrees of gum sponginess, and initial measurements showed that more than half had blood levels of vitamin C below the danger line. Eight of the youngsters had no detectable vitamin C at all in their blood serum!

When the children were given 100 milligrams of supplemental vitamin C over a period of six weeks or more, dramatic improvements were noted. The bleeding tendency of the gums was one of the first things to disappear. Soreness and discomfort also disappeared very rapidly. Redness faded more gradually, while over a period of weeks the gum surface became more firm instead of spongy. Infection was also reduced.

Except in cases where severe destruction of the gums had already occurred, the report concluded, "there was apparently complete reversal of all abnormal changes if vitamin C was given in adequate quantity for a sufficient length of time."

Folate Reduces Infection Rate

Vitamin C isn't the only nutrient that has been proven effective in resisting the ravages of gum disease. Folate (folic acid), one of the B vitamins, has also scored some impressive results.

In a study conducted by Richard I. Vogel, D.M.D., of the New Jersey Dental School in Newark, and several others, supplementary folate was given to one group of subjects for 30 days. Another group received a placebo, or dummy pill. The gum health of both groups was measured at the start and finish of the study.

Both groups scored the same at the beginning, but after 30 days those in the folate group had significantly lower levels of *gingival exudate*. That's the technical term for the fluid which flows from the gum margins and is associated with infection and inflammation. In fact, the subjects taking folate had 50 percent less exudate flow than those in the unsupplemented group (*Journal of Periodontology*). And this improvement took place even though plaque levels in the mouth stayed about the same.

Although blood tests indicated that none of the people had been suffering from an outright folate lack at the start of the trial, the authors state, "We can only conclude that there may be a deficiency at the end organ level" (in other words, in the gums).

The amounts of folate used in the study (4 milligrams daily) were far in excess of the Recommended Dietary Allowance (RDA) of 400 micrograms (0.4 milligrams) daily set by the federal government. And even that amount might be hard to obtain from some foods, since the authors note that from 50 to 95 percent of the folate in vegetables and other foods is destroyed in cooking, canning and other processing.

In another study, Dr. Vogel and several associates demonstrated that folate also may help protect the gums of women taking oral contraceptives. Pill users receiving 4 milligrams of folate daily had significantly less gingival inflammation after 60 days than others who took no extra folate *(Journal of Dental Research)*.

Preventing Bone Loss

It may turn out that part of vitamin C's beneficial effect may be traced to its influence on the jawbone. Animal studies at the Harvard school of dental medicine show that vitamin C inhibits bone resorption, or shrinkage, by 50 percent or more. The Harvard researchers suggest that vitamin C "plays a heretofore unrecognized but prominent role in the regulation of bone resorption as well as bone formation" *(Journal of Dental Research)*.

Another factor to keep in mind: Cigarette smoking apparently can intensify the periodontal disease process. Other researchers at Harvard found, after studying 684 healthy men, that smokers had greater bone loss in the jaw and a much higher percentage of loose teeth than nonsmokers *(Dental Survey)*.

So next time a toothpaste commercial tries to tell you that the key to happiness in life and love is whiter teeth, remember the real foundation of a healthy mouth. And take the necessary steps—including sound cleaning habits and an adequate intake of nutrients—to keep your gums firmly in the pink.

CHAPTER

85

NOURISHING (AND CHERISHING) YOUR HAIR

Want to do something nice for your hair and scalp? Let your organic vegetables go to your head. Literally. A glob of fresh, raw carrots applied to your noggin gives your scalp a fresh tingling feeling and your hair a nice luster, body and bounce.

So says hairdresser Monsieur Jacques, who grows vegetables in his back yard in Queens to use on the heads of his customers—after whirling in a blender (the vegetables, not the heads). Monsieur Jacques, whose New York shop carries his name, firmly believes that the fresh vitamins and minerals in fresh vegetables do almost as much good *externally* as internally. His convictions come not from laboratory studies on animals but from observations on humans, he told us. One good-size cut-up carrot goes into the blender with a little water and an herbal shampoo. The resulting foamy puree is massaged gently into the scalp and left on for a few minutes, then rinsed at least twice. This is great for oily hair, says Monsieur Jacques. For dry hair, he used a puree of avocado. And for normal hair, celery, string beans or cucumbers. And then there's invigorating mint, which is used to stimulate circulation. Customers like it so much that they bring their own bottles to take some vegetable shampoo home with them.

Monsieur Jacques got the idea for salads on the hair when he observed Arab women mashing fresh olives and wild green beans into a paste and combing it through their long, dark, beautiful hair.

Perhaps the most popular of all the foods that are applied to the hair is the egg. Whip two or three to a frothy foam and use as a shampoo for dry hair. This is a protein-rich cleansing shampoo that, with regular use, gives body and a lovely natural luster to your tresses, says Madame Reti, a New York hair specialist.

Panthenol Thickens Hair

Eggs are a rich source of panthothenate (pantothenic acid), which might explain the effectiveness of panthenol, a form of pantothenate, the anti-stress vitamin. Pantothenate is essential to the body's ability to utilize protein, which is what hair is all about. Panthenol thickens or swells the cuticle covering on the hair by up to 10 percent, whereas water alone under the same conditions swells hair by less than 1 percent. This was determined by examination under an electron microscope in a study conducted by an independent laboratory for Hoffmann–La Roche, Inc., of New Jersey (*Drug and Cosmetic Industry*).

The studies also demonstrate the ability of panthenol to repair hair damage like split ends, fly-away hair and general weakening of the hair shaft, conditions that are caused by chemicals, hot-air drying, vigorous brushing, combing and other environmental effects, a representative of Hoffman–La Roche told us.

Panthenol owes its effectiveness to more than the fact that it swells the hair. It also acts as a moisturizer, thus giving each hair the ability to retain moisture longer. It was determined, too, that panthenol penetrates into the hair shaft, leaving a thin elastic film which contributes to a thick, bouncy look. It also seems to make hair much easier to comb and set. This may be a boon for curly heads, for those with kinky hair and for children who hate to have their hair combed. Panthenol may not make you a double for Farrah Fawcett, but it can give your hair a nice luster and a healthy, vibrant look.

So if you would rather have your eggs sunny-side up on a plate and your vegetables and mayonnaise in your salad, you might enjoy the effects of panthenol on your hair. It comes in sprays, shampoos and conditioners. Scientists have found that it repairs damaged hair most effectively when applied as a leave-on conditioner. Every hair specialist we interviewed for this book stocks it.

While panthenol can do many nice things for the hair you have, don't expect it to grow hair on a bald head.

Other Nutritional Aids

Low serum iron may be a contributing factor to hair loss among women, says Irwin Lubowe, M.D., a New York dermatologist. Eat more liver or take iron tablets and folate (folic acid), which is also very important to healthy hair.

Some women lose their hair when they go on the Pill. Hair loss may continue for several weeks after the Pill is discontinued. Dr. Lubowe advises discontinuing the Pill when hair loss is associated with its use.

A. L. Leiby, M.D., a dermatologist in Akron, Ohio, finds that hair loss brought on by the Pill can sometimes be treated effectively with vitamin B_6. The hormones present in oral contraceptives have been associated with a deficiency of this vitamin, which is essential to the health of hair *(Skin and Allergy News)*.

Loss of hair is also known to occur following the use of methotrexate, an anti-cancer drug which has a damaging effect on the metabolism of folate, a B vitamin important to the blood.

It is recommended by Dr. Lubowe as an additional supplement which may favorably affect hair growth.

Dr. Lubowe, who believes that many factors affecting the health of the body can affect hair fall, gives his patients a complete blood and hair analysis and then prescribes accordingly.

A high-protein diet and large amounts of all the B vitamins, with special emphasis on inositol and folate, are important, he told us. He also suggests a daily zinc supplement along with other trace minerals.

CHAPTER

86

VITAMINS TO NEUTRALIZE HAY FEVER

He was recently out of college, tall and handsome. One would have thought he spent his summers chasing girls on the beach or tennis balls on the court. Instead, he weathered the fair season indoors, staring through a closed window at the revelers in the sun. He knew from experience that only the first frost would free him from his air-conditioned prison, for frost would kill the ragweed that caused his debilitating hay fever. Meanwhile, he took prescription antihistamines—eight a day, which was the most his doctor would allow. Still he suffered.

Finally, he took the advice of friends and went to see Brian Leibovitz, a nutritional consultant in Portland, Oregon. Leibovitz recommended a nutritional program that included taking 6 grams of citrus bioflavonoids every day.

A few weeks later—"during the height of the hay fever season that year," as Leibovitz recalls—the young man no longer required drugs to control his symptoms.

"That was two summers ago, and he's still doing well. He's probably outside right now, without an extra handkerchief or six in his pocket."

All of the symptoms of hay fever—the red, watery eyes, constantly runny nose, perpetual sneezing, intermittent congestion and even the asthma that characterizes the disease at its most severe—are caused by histamine. Histamine is a potent natural compound released when the immune system responds to an allergy-provoking substance. A relatively benign piece of ragweed pollen (or anything else) can set off an alarm in a sensitive person. Your body reacts as if you had a cold when there are no germs present.

Happily, hay fever has something else in common with the cold: Both respond to treatment with vitamin C. That's because vitamin C is a natural antihistamine.

A Natural Antihistamine

In a series of studies, researchers at the department of obstetrics and gynecology at Methodist Hospital, in Brooklyn, found that blood levels of vitamin C bore an inverse relationship to blood levels of histamine; as one went up, the other went down, and vice versa. "Persons with low plasma ascorbate [vitamin C] levels have high histamine levels," the researchers noted after processing blood samples from 400 healthy volunteers.

Next, the researchers took 11 with low levels of vitamin C or high levels of histamines and placed them on a program of vitamin C supplementation.

Improvement was rapid, occurring within three days. "It would seem that ascorbic acid [vitamin C] deficiency is one of the most common causes for an elevated blood histamine level, as all 11 of the volunteers given one gram of ascorbic acid daily for three days showed a reduction in blood histamine" (*Journal of Nutrition*, April, 1980).

"The need for vitamin C seems to be greater in some allergic patients," agrees clinical nutritionist Lynn Dart, a registered dietitian. In her work as manager of the nutrition department at the Environmental Healthy Center in Dallas, Ms. Dart has found that large doses of vitamin C are sometimes quite effective.

"The average allergy sufferer with a vitamin C deficiency usually responds to 4 to 8 grams a day when trying to either stave off a reaction or clear up a reaction in progress," she told us.

The responses of his own patients in Bennington, Vermont, have convinced Stuart Freyer, M.D., of the same thing.

"The hay fever season in Vermont can be pretty severe," says Dr. Freyer, who has emphasized nutritional therapy for 6 of the 12 years he's been a practicing otorhinolaryngologist (ear-nose-throat specialist). He gives his hay fever patients "relatively high amounts of vitamin C. Five grams or more is typical." But when advising his patients to take that much vitamin C, he cautions them to increase their calcium supplementation as well.

"High levels of vitamin C may bind with calcium and pull it out of the bones, then flush it out in the urine when the body discards any excess vitamin C. Vitamin C may also combine with calcium in the diet to interfere with absorption.

"There really should be no problem with calcium deficiency if a person either uses vitamin C in its calcium ascorbate form rather than its simple ascorbic acid form, or if the ascorbic acid is supplemented with adequate amounts of bone meal or dolomite. I usually recommend my patients take 400 to 600 milligrams of calcium a day during hay fever season."

Dr. Freyer has also found that vitamin C works better when his patients take B-complex vitamins, especially pantothenate, along with it.

"I recommend 200 to 500 milligrams of pantothenate, plus another 50 milligrams of B complex," he says. "Sometimes, when a patient has impaired absorption—and many people with allergies do—I also give them pancreatic enzymes. These help to break down the foods so vitamins can be absorbed better."

Vitamin C Works Best with Bioflavonoids

And if you really want to get the most out of your vitamin C during hay fever season, take it with citrus bioflavonoids, as well. Studies done on animals have shown that citrus bioflavonoids may favorably alter the body's metabolizing of vitamin C by raising the concentration of the nutrient in certain tissues and enhancing its bioavailability (*American Journal of Clinical Nutrition*, August, 1979).

In his own work, nutritionist Leibovitz has found citrus bioflavonoids are the answer to many a hay fever victim's prayers.

"More than once, I've had a hay fever patient who did not respond to vitamin C recover when given citrus bioflavonoids," he says. Early in his career as a nutritionist, Leibovitz worked with Linus Pauling, Ph.D., on studies with vitamin C. In his own research, done while a graduate student majoring in biology at the University of Oregon, Leibovitz found that large doses of vitamin C significantly reduced the mortality rate of mice with laboratory-induced anaphylaxis, a potentially fatal allergic response. In a paper delivered at the national meeting of the American Chemical Society, in Houston, in March, 1980, Leibovitz concluded that "these results suggest the possible use of ascorbic acid in human immediate-type hypersensitivities (allergy, asthma, anaphylaxis)."

Anaphylaxis isn't the only type of allergic reaction that may be fatal; a person could die from an asthma attack, too. And, "left untreated, hay fever can develop into asthma," according to a spokesman at the National Institute for Allergy and Infectious Diseases, in Bethesda, Maryland. "Actually, 'hay fever' is something of a misnomer because it isn't caused by hay and it isn't characterized by fever. Basically, when it occurs in the nose, it's called allergic rhinitis."

Asthma, Leibovitz notes, responds even better to citrus bioflavonoids than allergic rhinitis does. "In fact, a standard treatment for asthma, a drug called cromolyn sodium, is nothing more than a synthetic bioflavonoidlike molecule," he told us. "I found cirtus bioflavonoids work just as well for people with hay-fever-induced asthma.

Another thing that seems to help some patients is vitamin E, and findings by a Japanese researcher concur that vitamin E exhibits antihistamine properties.

After he injected 20 volunteers with histamine, Mitsuo Kamimura, of the department of dermatology at Sapporo Medical College, noted the skin around the injection site swelled up. However, when he gave the volunteers 300-milligram doses of vitamin E daily for five to seven days before injecting them with histamine, there was far less swelling than before (*Journal of Vitaminology*). Finally, Leibovitz rounds out his program by telling his patients to give up junk food and cigarettes. Dr. Freyer does the same.

"Smoking, in particular, increases the need for vitamin C," says Dr. Freyer. "Smoking is an irritant; it is also an allergen. Smoking is madness for anyone who suffers from hay fever."

But if you do smoke, Dr. Freyer cautions that hay fever season is, ironically, not the best time to quit. "Any change in your routine, your daily habits, is bound to cause stress—and stress will often aggravate an allergic reaction. I always advise my patients to go easy on themselves at this time of year."

So take it easy and breathe easy. A positive outlook, supplemented by vitamin C, bioflavonoids, pantothenate and vitamin E may be just what the doctor ordered. Just because there is pollen outside is no reason you can't be out there, too.

CHAPTER

87

NUTRIENTS THAT HELP YOUR BODY HEAL ITSELF

Imagine you were alive at the time of Homer's Greece, and in the heat of battle you caught a bronze-tipped arrow in the thigh. A valiant friend, carrying you on his back, managed to drag you off the battlefield and into the *klisia*, or medic's hut, before you passed out. What sort of first aid could you expect once you were there?

Well, if Homer's *Iliad* and *Odyssey* are any clues to ancient Grecian medical practice, you'd probably get: a seat, lots of storytelling, perhaps a cup of wine sprinkled with grated goat cheese and barley meal, served by a beautiful woman; and eventually your wound would be washed out with warm water. To stanch the blood, you'd receive their most popular remedy—someone would recite a charm or sing a song over the injury. So much for the Red Cross.

Considering the amount of fighting the ancients did—and their crude, if poetic, ways of treating deadly wounds—it's a wonder any of us are alive today. But (at least so far) the body's power of self-healing is greater than man's power of self-destruction. As one modern-day researcher has put it: "If the body were

488

not wise, man could not survive. Every cell, tissue, organ and system is programmed to heal. . . . The only reason we make it is that for every injury there is a healing response.''

The healing of wounds is a process so intricate and marvelous that much of it remains a mystery today. But one thing is becoming increasingly certain: When your body is on the mend, whether it be from major surgery or a nicked knuckle, good nutrition can do a whole lot to help it heal than telling a story or singing it a song.

''I do believe that everyone should know the beautiful deeds of which his or her tissues are capable,'' writes Guido Majno, M.D., describing the physiological wonders of wound healing in his delightful book *The Healing Hand: Man and Wound in the Ancient World* (Harvard University Press, 1975). Those beautiful deeds include the ability to clean up the terrible mess caused by a wound, to fight off the invading hordes of bacteria, and to set about building brand-new tissues and blood vessels.

Stepped-Up Demand

All this frantic activity at the site of the wound causes a stepped-up demand for carbohydrates, fats, minerals, vitamins, water, oxygen and—absolutely essential—amino acids, the famous building blocks of protein. And proteins are the bricks, boards and shingles of which the whole repair job is built.

In fact, ''even more or less minor wounds require a good nutritional state and normal protein metabolism for optimal wound healing to take place,'' says Sheldon V. Pollack, M.D., chief of dermatologic surgery at Duke University medical center. Besides slowing down the reconstruction of tissues, protein deficiency can also impair the body's ability to protect itself from infection, Dr. Pollack observes. So when you're recovering from injury, it's doubly important to make sure your diet includes plenty of protein-rich foods such as fish, milk, eggs, liver and wheat germ.

Injury also steps up the body's demand for certain nutrients, particularly vitamin C—a little hero of healing power. Researchers have shown many times that "a deficiency of vitamin C impairs wound healing in experimental lower animals and human beings and . . . an excess accelerates healing above the normal level," write W. M. Ringsdorf, Jr., D.M.D., and E. Cheraskin, M.D., of the University of Alabama school of dentistry.

Vitamin C is a star in the cellular dramas of wound healing because it regulates the formation of collagen. When the cat nips your hand, Dr. Majno explains, the wound is repaired "not with the original tissue, but with a material that is biologically simple, cheap and handy: connective tissue . . . a soft but tough kind of tissue, specialized for mechanical functions, primarily that of holding us together; it fills the spaces in and around all other tissues."

Because the creation of collagen depends on vitamin C, a deficiency can disturb the "architecture" of that connective-tissue repair job and delay the completion of the whole healing project. In one study, vitamin C deficiency in human cells decreased collagen production by 18 percent according to one biological measurement and by 75 percent according to another measurement (*American Journal of Clinical Nutrition*, March, 1981.)

In another experiment, designed by Drs. Cheraskin and Ringsdorf, two gallant dental students with normal vitamin C levels each allowed the dentists to remove a tiny plug of tissue from their gums. In order to precisely measure the speed of healing, the wound was painted with a blue dye and photographed each day until the blue dot (indicating unhealed tissue) disappeared. After a two-week rest, the students had another plug extracted from their gums—but this time, they also took 250 milligrams of vitamin C with each meal and at bedtime (for a total of 1 gram daily).

A comparison of the healing sequences in both cases showed that the vitamin C–supplemented wounds healed 40 percent faster than those made when the students were eating a "normal" diet. When the experiment was repeated using a daily dosage of 2 grams of vitamin C, the wounds healed 50 percent faster (*Oral Surgery, Oral Medicine, Oral Pathology*, March, 1982).

Actually, vitamin C's healing power has been recognized for decades. In the 1940s, A. H. Hunt reported that wound disruption or breakage had been reduced by 75 percent since doctors at St. Bartholomew's Hopital in London began routinely administering vitamin C to all patients having abdominal operations. Over a period of 30 months, Hunt observed that "leakage from suture lines has occurred in but one of a large number of operations."

In a British study, vitamin C's effect on the healing of bedsores was studied. Twenty surgical patients suffering from bedsores were divided into two groups: One group was given two 500-milligram vitamin C supplements daily, the other was given two placebos (or chemically worthless pills). After a month, precise measurements of the wounds showed that the bedsores in the vitamin C group had decreased in size by 84 percent; the placebo group showed only a 42.7 percent decrease. "It is well established that in scurvy [vitamin C–deficiency disease] wound healing is delayed and that the healing process may fail completely," the scientists observed (*Lancet*).

Injury Drains Vitamin C

When you're recovering from any kind of injury, it's also crucial to keep your diet vitamin C-rich because injury drains your body's supply. In one study, researchers found that vitamin C levels in the white blood cells of surgical patients had dropped by 42 percent three days after surgery (*Surgery, Gynecology and Obstetrics*). Drs. Ringsdorf and Cheraskin suggest that this and other studies showing a drop in vitamin C levels may indicate that "during postsurgical recovery the vitamin C in the body migrates toward and concentrates in the healing site."

Whatever the case, Duke's Dr. Pollack told us, "If you're recovering from injury and you're seriously ill, elderly, don't eat properly or otherwise have low vitamin C levels, it would be wise to take 1 or 2 grams of vitamin C a day.''

Although the details of its role in wound healing aren't very well understood, vitamin A is known to be a player in collagen formation, wound closure and infection fighting. A plentiful supply of vitamin A can also help ensure that the new tissue that forms across the wound is strong and resistant to breaking, according to studies at the University of Illinois department of food science.

The Illinois investigators explored the effects of beta-carotene (a substance that the body turns into vitamin A) and retinoic acid and retinyl acetate (two chemical forms of vitamin A) on the healing of wounds in rats with marginal vitamin A levels. The animals were fed a vitamin A–free diet for two weeks, then divided into groups: One received a basal diet, which provided a known amount of vitamin A, and the other received the basal diet plus one of the three vitamin A substances.

Five days later, when the animals were sacrificed and their wounds examined, it was discovered that the supplemental retinyl acetate and beta-carotene "resulted in increases of 35 percent and 70 percent, respectively, over the wound tensil strength [resistance to being torn open] of rats fed the basal level of vitamin A'' (*Federation Proceedings*, no. 3453, March 1, 1981).

Diabetics very often suffer from slowly healing wounds, a problem that can be worsened by another problem: They're also more apt to pick up infections. But in a study conducted by researchers at the Albert Einstein College of Medicine, in New York City, supplemental vitamin A was shown to increase wound strength in diabetic animals. The researchers also believe that vitamin A helps fight wound infections.

The researchers concluded that vitamin A works to strengthen wounds mainly by increasing the accumulation of collagen. "We believe that just as supplemental vitamin A improves immune responses of traumatized animals and surgical patients, it will be especially useful in preventing wound infection and promoting wound healing in surgical diabetic patients,'' they observed (*Annals of Surgery*, July, 1981).

Thiamine and Vitamin E: A Little Help from Your Friends

There is also growing evidence that at least some of the B-complex vitamins are involved in human wound healing. In one study, experimental animals fed diets rich in thiamine (vitamin B₁) were found to have heavier, denser granulation tissue (new tissue formed during wound repair) than those on deficient diets.

Based on thiamine's known biological activities in the body, the researchers concluded it probably aids healing by helping the body step up its energy metabolism at the healing site, where the furious breakdown and buildup of cells requires tremendous amounts of usable fuel (*Journal of Surgical Research*, January, 1982).

But no survey of nutrition and wound healing would be complete without mention of vitamin E.

Wilfrid E. Shute, M.D., a veteran vitamin E researcher, reported that vitamin E helps accelerate wound healing, is "the ideal treatment for burns" because of its ability to limit cell death to those cells that have been killed by the burning agent, and can even reduce old scar tissue when applied directly. Keloids, or progressively enlarging, raised scars caused by overproduction of collagen during the healing process, can be prevented by taking vitamin E orally and also applying it directly to the fresh wound, Dr. Shute says.

Not everyone agrees. Dr. Pollack, while observing that "there is some data to suggest that vitamin E can promote wound healing," told us that "the research is still kind of up in the air . . . we just don't know the precise role, if any, that vitamin E plays in wound healing."

But meanwhile, next time you peel your knuckle along with the potato—or catch a Grecian arrow in the thigh—you might give nutrition a try. It could just be your body knows some things your doctor doesn't.

CHAPTER

88.

PLATELETS—LITTLE LIFESAVERS THAT CAN KILL YOU

If you've ever seen a Western movie, you know the story. There are good guys and bad guys. The good guys—the sheriff and his men—are devoted to the law. They're always ready to go where needed, well organized and effective. They work well together.

The bad guys are dedicated, too—to mischief and mayhem. Any time they put *their* heads together, you know there's going to be trouble.

In real life, of course, things are rarely that simple. After rounding up the villains, on occasion, the sheriff and his posse just might spend a couple hours too many in the local saloon—and then set half the town on fire.

When you think about health and disease, it's all too easy to look for the same pattern: the bad guys (invading bacteria, harmful chemicals and similar sinister forces) against the good guys (strong drugs and the body's own defenses). But here, too, the truth appears to be that it's often the upright citizens who turn into the lawless mob.

Normally, those tiny, blank-faced blood cells called platelets are your body's way of keeping bloodshed to a minimum. After any injury, they pile on top of one another to form a living wall, the nucleus of a clot that brings bleeding under control. Were platelets not on the job, any minor mishap could turn into a major catastrophe. Properly functioning, they are lifesaving.

Functioning improperly, however,they can be life *threatening*. Time and again, when researchers investigate trouble in the heart and circulatory system, they find platelets in the midst of it. Strong evidence links platelet problems with heart attack and stroke and with blood clots that often follow surgery and that threaten women who use birth control pills.

When agonizing migraine headaches are about to strike, doctors have found, platelets begin acting strangely. Abnormal platelet activity has been associated with the complications of diabetes, too, and with the rejection of organ transplants. According to one theory, platelets play an important role in the development of atherosclerosis—clogging and hardening of the arteries.

The big question, obviously, is this: How can we keep platelets on the job but out of trouble?

Before we can attempt an answer, we need a better understanding of the problem. Which means asking another question. What are platelets supposed to do—and what makes them go wrong?

Ordinarily, platelets float peacefully and independently in the bloodstream, right alongside the red blood cells, which carry oxygen, and the white cells, which defend the body against invaders. A slip of the paring knife or a fall from your bike, however, lets blood out of the bloodstream—and sends platelets into action.

Instead of flowing freely out of the wound, platelets begin sticking to the injured blood vessel and to each other. This is called *platelet aggregation*, and it resembles the way logs and twigs swept down a river may start to pile up at a snag.

What happens next is very important and a bit more complicated. The platelets don't just lie there like a growing pile of logs; when they aggregate, they release a host of chemicals, including highly active enzymes and hormonelike substances called prostaglandins. Some of these chemicals make that loose bunch of platelets cling together much more firmly. That jumble of logs and twigs tightens up into a real dam. Soon other clotting materials are deposited by the blood; a safe, solid clot puts a stop to bleeding, and all is well.

All is not well, however, when platelets get carried away in the performance of their duties—when, without waiting for the proper occasion, they start to clump together on their own or congregate on the walls of veins and arteries.

Why does this happen? No one can say for sure, but a lot of recent attention has focused on the chemistry of the process. Some of the chemicals released by aggregating platelets, it seems, can go either of two ways. They can be converted into substances that promote clotting or substances that prevent it. When a platelet collides with the wall of an artery, for example, it releases its chemicals and an enzyme in the artery wall turns them into prostacyclin, which prevents platelets from clumping together—a natural protection against blood clots inside the vessels.

Normally, there's a balance between clot-promoting and clot-preventing chemicals, scientists speculate. It's an imbalance that causes dangerous, unnecessary clots.

The exact mechanism may be unclear, but there's nothing indefinite about the results when platelets clump together too easily. Often, this happens after surgery. Immobilized in bed, a patient may develop a blood clot in a vein of his leg. This is painful enough, but if the clot breaks off and travels up to his heart, lung or brain, it may threaten his life.

When platelets adhere to the artery wall, according to one widely held theory, it sets into motion the process that causes atherosclerosis. Less dramatic than a blood clot, but just as dangerous.

There's a connection between sticky platelets and strokes, according to a Kansas University medical center research team that tested the blood of 59 stroke victims and 15 healthy controls. They found that, in the younger group, platelets of stroke victims had a heightened tendency to aggregate.

"This leads us to suggest that the treatment of platelet hyperaggregability (the increased tendency to clump together) is a reasonable thing in the prevention of stroke," said researcher James R. Couch, M.D.

Clumps of platelets are a prime suspect when a heart attack takes place, too. Even if they are too small to block a vessel, according to one theory, they can fatally disrupt the electrical impulses that keep the heart functioning normally. The platelets of recent heart attack victims, studies have found, do show an increased tendency to stick together.

One recent study offers an especially ominous finding: 20 percent of people killed instantaneously in car accidents (whose death, that is, was not caused by bad health) had tiny clots forming in the veins of their legs. These *silent thrombi* (thrombi are blood clots; these are called silent because they give no sign of their presence) suggest that platelet problems are far from rare.

Obviously, there's a lot to be said for keeping platelets in line. But is it possible?

Doctors and scientists have long been intrigued by the question. For years, they have used anticoagulant drugs (drugs that keep the blood from clotting) to prevent strokes. Right now, two major studies are investigating whether aspirin, which inhibits platelet aggregation, can decrease the risk of heart attack and stroke.

But there are problems. Because they are so effective in preventing clotting, anticoagulants can cause dangerous bleeding. Aspirin often causes stomach bleeding, too. And, it has been suggested, as aspirin slows down platelet function, it also interferes with other aspects of body chemistry.

A long history of experimentation, however, suggests that it *is* possible to keep platelet activity under control without powerful drugs and their dangerous side effects—by natural, nutritional means. These can restore the chemical balance necessary for normal platelet activity and enhance the body's *own* protective mechanisms.

If you know your vitamins, it won't surprise you to hear vitamin E mentioned in this regard, first and foremost. More than a quarter of a century ago, Alton Ochsner, M.D., famed surgeon and teacher at the Tulane University school of medicine, started giving his patients large daily doses of vitamin E. The result: Blood clots, always a danger after surgery, became rare on his wards.

Since then, a lengthening series of experiments has been able to zero in on vitamin E's ability to cut down on blood clots: It works, they say, by discouraging platelets from clumping together.

In two young patients, a recent study found, a deficiency of vitamin E produced an abnormal tendency toward platelet aggregation. High doses of the vitamin brought platelet activity back to normal. In another study, researchers gave healthy volunteers daily doses of vitamin E. Here, too, the supplements kept platelet clumping to a minimum.

How does vitamin E keep platelets in their place? The process is not fully understood, but Manfred Steiner, M.D., a professor of medicine at Brown University, suggests it interrupts the chain of clotting events at the crucial point of the *release reaction*—the point at which the loose bunch of platelets hardens into a solid mass. Vitamin E "has a definite inhibitory action on the platelet release reaction," says Dr. Steiner. It steps in to prevent the formation of those potent chemicals that bond platelets to each other.

Another nutrient with the ability to prevent blood clots and protect against heart disease is vitamin C. And here, too, it seems that at least part of its power lies in its ability to regulate the reactions of platelets.

In England, Constance Leslie, M.D., gave 1 gram daily of vitamin C to 30 patients who had had operations that left them particularly vulnerable to clots. A similar group received no vitamin C. Patients in the vitamin C group, she reported, suffered only half as many incidents of deep-vein thrombosis as the unprotected patients. And when clots did form, they were less severe.

Powerful Protective Action

Elsewhere in her hospital, years of experience demonstrated that "vitamin C has a powerful protective action against thrombosis," Dr. Leslie added. The burn unit of the hospital had, as a routine practice, given all patients 1 gram daily of vitamin C since opening seven years earlier. "Only one death from pulmonary embolism (blood clot in the lung) has been recorded, and no cases of clinical deep-vein thrombosis have occurred for at least 5½ years," wrote Dr. Leslie *(Lancet)*.

While Dr. Leslie could offer no explanation of vitamin C's "powerful protective action against thrombosis," two recent experiments suggest that, as with vitamin E, control of platelets is the heart of the matter.

When a team of researchers led by Kay E. Sarji, Ph.D., and John A. Colwell, M.D., at the Veterans Administration Hospital at Charleston, South Carolina, tested the platelets of diabetics, they found two things. The platelets were abnormally sensitive to aggregating agents—they clumped together too easily—and they had low levels of vitamin C. This excessive stickiness, Dr. Sarji told us, may contribute to the development of complications of diabetes. "When platelets are more adhesive than normal, you may be more likely to develop thrombosis," she said, "and many of these complications are related to thrombosis."

When Dr. Sarji and her colleagues took plasma samples from normal subjects and added vitamin C to them, a striking change took place: The tendency of the platelets to clump together was much reduced.

To investigate further the effect of vitamin C on platelet clumping, Dr. Sarji gave oral doses to eight healthy nonsmoking men—2 grams daily for a week. Here, too, their platelets became significantly less sticky—less prone to clump together.

At the Louisiana State University school of medicine, in New Orleans, another study had similar results. A research team lead by Alfredo Lopez, M.D., Ph.D., added vitamin C to blood samples and gave oral doses of vitamin C to 12 healthy students.

In both cases, Dr. Lopez reported, there was a consistent increase in the lag time of platelet aggregation induced by collagen—a substance that normally makes platelets clump.

"The adherence of the platelets to the collagen is impaired," Dr. Lopez explained to us. "It takes longer for them to stick."

This could have very important implications. According to one theory, platelets clumping on artery walls is the first step in the formation of the dangerous blood clots that accompany atherosclerosis. The deterioration of the artery wall exposes collagen, which is in the connective tissue below the wall layer. When platelets adhere to the collagen, the process that leads to thrombosis is set in motion. Dr. Lopez's study indicates that vitamin C inhibits platelets' adherence to collagen.

"If that theory is correct, this inhibition could be highly significant," Dr. Lopez says.

How does vitamin C discourage platelets from aggregating too easily? One explanation, which Dr. Sarji cautions is "highly speculative," involves prostaglandins, those very potent chemicals that have a strong influence on platelet behavior.

"Platelets produce chemicals that can be turned into thromboxane, which *causes* aggregation, or prostacyclin, which *inhibits* aggregation. Possibly, vitamin C shifts the pathway, to favor the production of prostacyclin," she says. In other words, vitamin C may help your body produce its natural protective substances.

CHAPTER

89

VITAMINS FOR A HEALTHY HORMONAL SYSTEM

In the lakes near Mexico City lives a salamander called the axolotl. It looks rather like an overgrown tadpole and looks that way all its life, unless it's fed large amounts of the hormone thyroxine. That is the hormone responsible for the natural development of frogs from tadpoles. Thyroxine fed to the growing axolotl triggers the same action in that animal, and it sprouts legs. A comparable feat would be if humans could take pills to grow wings.

All of which seems more appropriate for a third-grade science unit than a health book unless, perhaps, you have a 13-year-old son or daughter. The enormous physical and emotional changes everyone experiences in the process of puberty and maturation are little less extraordinary than sprouting wings, if you think about it, and are entirely controlled by the secretion of hormones in the blood by the glands of the body.

The endocrine glands manufacture hormones which are involved in reproduction, in the body's physical reactions to danger, in the mechanisms that maintain a constant temperature in the body, in the process of growth and even, some scientists suspect, in the prevention of psychiatric disorders like depression.

Given such a central role, it's no surprise that a number of vitamins, and good nutrition in general, are vital to the healthy functioning of the endocrine glands.

Vitamins and the Adrenals

Many of the interactions between nutrients and the endocrine system have only recently been discovered, however, and many are not yet fully understood. Vitamin C, for example, is highly concentrated in the thyroid, but scientists don't know exactly what the vitamin C is doing there. It's clear, though, that the vitamin is necessary for the proper functioning of the glands.

The adrenal glands, perched atop the kidneys, are involved in the regulation of metabolism and the body's reactions to stress. When we are subjected to stress, the stores of vitamin C in the adrenals are depleted. When the glands are stimulated to produce hormones for an extended period of time, the stores of vitamin C can disappear completely, as if they had been used up. Many of the symptoms of scurvy (the classic vitamin C–deficiency disease), such as fatigue, weakness, impaired digestion and an inability to tolerate stress, are strikingly similar to the symptoms of adrenal failure. Researchers have found that a decline in the production of certain hormones by the adrenals in old age can be partially restored by vitamin C.

For whatever reason, vitamin C is obviously important. There is also evidence that both vitamin A and riboflavin deficiencies can disrupt the healthy functioning of the adrenal glands.

Vitamin A is closely associated with the health of the thymus. Scientists working at the Albert Einstein College of Medicine in New York found that mice under stress suffered a shrinking of the thymus gland. When the mice were fed vitamin A, the losses were not as severe, and vitamin A also sped the recovery of thymus weight after the stress was removed. Later studies showed that stress caused a loss of vitamin A in the thymus (*Federation Proceedings*).

And when the stress came in the form of cancer cells inoculated into the mice's bodies, vitamin A continued to boost the action of the thymus. Vitamin A minimized the degeneration of the thymus, which occurred with the development of cancer in the body, and speeded recovery of the gland when tumors were surgically removed. As part of a strong immune system, vitamin A seems a crucial factor in the whole anti-cancer defense structure.

That's just another example of an obvious pattern. Whether they act directly on a gland, boost the action of its hormones or operate in a way that we haven't yet figured out, vitamins A and C are indispensable to the health of the glandular system. It's up to us to make sure we get the right nutrients in the proper amounts to keep the system purring.

INFERTILITY

CHAPTER

90

VITAMINS FOR
WEAK SEED

Even men with normal amounts of sperm have their share of duds and weaklings. It's not uncommon for as much as 40 percent of their sperm to be slow swimmers or abnormally shaped. So while millions of sperm may start the journey to the egg, only a choice few actually reach their destination, and only one wins the prize.

Or—in more and more cases—none. Fertility specialists, who once concentrated mainly on the woman when pregnancy failed to occur, now are finding that male infertility is increasing in frequency. In fact, the number of sperm that men are producing has dropped by almost half during the last 30 years, according to several studies—from 107 million per measured unit (a milliliter, or one-thousandth of a liter) to 62 million per unit. Not that 62 million is bad. It'll do the job. But in this case, more is definitely better.

Because the implications of the sperm decline can have far-reaching effects for future generations, scientists are anxious to get to the bottom of it.

Some researchers now think toxic chemicals should be considered as one of the culprits. They point out that, during the same 30 years sperm counts have been declining, our use of these substances has steadily increased, with thousands entering the environment each year.

One researcher who agrees with that theory is Ralph C. Dougherty, Ph.D., professor of chemistry at Florida State University in Tallahassee. "We are much too casual about the chemicals we introduce into our environment," says Dr. Dougherty. And he should know.

Dr. Dougherty recently completed a study which found a correlation between lower sperm counts and the presence of polychlorinated biphenyl (PCB) in seminal fluid. The average sperm count of the 132 students tested was found to be 60 million per unit, but 23 percent of the group had counts of only 20 million per unit or less, the level often accepted as defining functional sterility. "More important," Dr. Dougherty told us, "every seminal fluid sample in the study showed amounts above background level of environmental contaminants such as PCB, hexachlorobenzene (a fungicide) and DDT metabolites. About 25 percent of the reduced sperm counts correlated with the presence of PCB," he added. "PCBs act by inhibiting cell divison through DNA damage—the material in genes. It takes eight cell divisions to get a mature sperm. If cell division is slowed by 10 percent, it can result in a 60 percent decrease in the number of sperm produced."

People become contaminated with these chemicals via the food chain, says Dr. Dougherty, where they usually accumulate in fatty tissue, resisting breakdown because of their built-in stability. PCBs above 1 part per million (1 part PCP per million parts something else) are in virtually every freshwater fish. And even though they've been banned by the government, there are still more than a billion pounds of PCB being used in industry or being discarded into land fills where they can leach out and contaminate the environment.

A Man's Job Can Put His Sperm Out of Work

Donald Whorton, M.D., a specialist in occupational medicine at the University of California at Berkeley, was asked to study a group of men who worked with the pesticide dibromochloropropane (DBCP) when the male employees began to notice that few of them had recently fathered children. Examination of the semen revealed a low sperm count in 14 of the 25 men tested. Nine of the men had no sperm at all, and 2 others had counts below 1 million per unit. Through questioning the men, it became apparent that infertility was associated with the length of time the men worked with the DBCP. "The relationship was striking," writes Dr. Whorton. "Workers with sperm counts below one million had been exposed at least three years. None with sperm counts above 40 million had been exposed for more than three months" *(Lancet)*.

"DBCP was the so-called eye-opener to the problem of male infertility due to occupational exposure," Dr. Whorton told us. "It's an emerging field which will require years of research. We do know that the damage caused by DBCP is dose dependent. And that goes for its reversibility, as well. Where the sperm count has been decreased, it takes three months to a year to return to normal. But where the sperm count has been reduced to zero, it may take up to six years to come back—if ever."

Occupational exposure to lead, kepone, microwaves, chloroprene—all have had documented effects on male reproduction.

Even something as seemingly innocuous as excessive heat in the work place can have adverse effects on male fertility. Marc S. Cohen, M.D., a urologist with the New York Fertility Research Foundation, noticed that men who worked as short-order cooks or pizza bakers were experiencing fertility problems. Dr. Cohen thought that their decreased sperm counts might be caused by the high temperatures to which they were routinely exposed. In an effort to help these particular men raise their sperm counts, Dr. Cohen has recommended cool baths and employed the use of a gadget that he refers to as "very experimental." His patients wear a scrotal pouch (developed by another doctor) during their hot working hours, which cools the testicles. "It's too soon to report results," says Dr. Cohen, "but it's worth a try."

Dr.Cohen routinely asks his patients with fertility problems about possible occuptional hazards. Unfortunately, he's in the minority.

According the Kenneth Bridbord, M.D., of the National Institute for Occupational Safety and Health (NIOSH) in Rockville, Maryland, "Right now the numbers of doctors who actually ask questions are few. Even those questions that do get asked only touch on a few areas like drugs and medications. The average physician doesn't know enough about occupational medicine to ask the right questions.

"But we're working hard to improve the situation," says Dr. Bridbord. Both NIOSH and the Health Resources Administration are funding programs to train professionals in the field of occupational health.

Sperm Enemies in Everyday Life

But there are more than environmental and occupational hazards that threaten male fertility. Some common medications prescribed by doctors have shown the same disastrous effects as toxic chemicals.

Cimetidine, a drug routinely used in the management of peptic ulcers, was administered to seven men in a study conducted at the Univeristy of Pittsburgh school of medicine. After nine weeks of therapy (1,200 milligrams per day), there was a 43 percent average reduction in sperm count. "This study suggests," write the researchers, "that caution be used in prescribing cimetidine for prolonged periods to young men who may wish to maintain their fertility" (*New England Journal of Medicine*, May 3, 1979).

Another drug, sulphasalazine, which is used to treat ulcerative colitis, was also shown to depress fertility (*Lancet*, August 11, 1979).

The list keeps growing. Add coffee, cigarettes, marijuana and alcohol, if you're keeping count.

While a controlled study comparing the amount of alcohol consumed to an actual decrease in sperm count has not been done, Jeanne Manson, Ph.D., says that the evidence strongly suggests a connection between the two.

Dr. Manson, of the Kettering Laboratory at the University of Cincinnati, did report, however, that there are studies which show a connection between smoking and sperm. It seems that the percentage of abnormally shaped sperm is directly related to the number of cigarettes smoked daily. And those smoking for more than ten years increased their disadvantage (*Work and the Health of Women*, CRC Press, 1979).

Marijuana smokers have abnormal sperm, too—what's left of them. Experiments showed that young men who smoked marijuana at least four times a week for six months had a decrease in sperm numbers in proportion to the amount smoked, falling to almost zero in some very heavy users (*Keep Off the Grass*, Pergamon Press, 1979).

Although the effect of caffeine on human sperm has not been studied, its effect on animals has. According to Paul S. Weathersbee, Ph.D., of the University of Washington's Alcoholism and Drug Abuse Institute in Seattle, both rats and roosters showed a complete absence of sperm three weeks after being fed caffeine.

That could be of some consequence to the man who normally consumes greater than 600 milligrams per day of caffeinated beverages, says Dr. Weathersbee—about six to eight cups of coffee a day.

Are we about to pollute ourselves out of existence? No, not in the immediate future. But the warning signs are there, and they shouldn't be ignored. Neither should the steps you can take to help yourself. Start by eliminating nicotine, caffeine and alcohol from your life. Already your sperm are breathing a sigh of relief. Now give them something to cheer about. Fortify yourself with nutrients like vitamins A and C as well as zinc, calcium, magnesium and manganese.

In one study, male rats were fed a diet low in vitamin A from three weeks to about four months of age. The vitamin A deficiency they developed caused degeneration and loss of sperm cells. The dependency of cells on vitamin A was supported by the appearance of new sperm within six weeks following vitamin A treatment (*Biology of Reproduction*, November, 1979).

In another study, Earl B. Dawson, Ph.D., of the University of Texas medical branch in Galveston, measured the effects of a vitamin C preparation (which also contained calcium, magnesium and manganese) on 20 men with spermagglutination, a condition in which sperm stick together in clumps and are unable to swim normally. Seven men were used as controls and received no vitamin C. All 27 men (ages 25 to 38) had been diagnosed as infertile; they had decreased motility (the ability of sperm to move in a forward direction) and relatively low sperm counts, the associated factors which make the clumping problem such bad news.

After 60 days, all 20 men taking the vitamin C preparation (1 gram per day) had impregnated their wives, while none of the men in the control group had. And not only had the vitamin C preparation reversed the spermagglutination, but it had also raised sperm *counts* by 54 percent (*Fertility and Sterility*, October, 1979).

"These results," says Dr. Dawson, "suggest the possibility of a cooperative action between the metabolism of vitamin C and the essential metals studied which are vital in sperm physiology."

Spermagglutination has, by some estimates, been implicated as a cause of male infertility in as many as 10 percent of all cases. Which means that over 150,000 men in the U.S. population could have a spermagglutination problem affecting their ability to father children.

"Perhaps," speculates Dr. Dawson, "supplements of vitamin C, calcium, magnesium or manganese can reverse spermagglutination routinely, eliminating the need to use a donor to impregnate the wife.''

So while you're waiting for the government to clean up the environment and train professionals in the field of occupational health, concentrate on the things you can do for yourself.

Avoid toxins that you can, be on the alert for possible pollutants in your work place, and be sure to give yourself the advantages of vitamins and minerals. Good nutrition *can* make a difference when you're trying to be reproductive—or just productive.

CHAPTER

91

PREVENTING KIDNEY STONES THE NATURAL WAY

Have you ever been stoned?

Kidney-stoned, that is. If you have, then you probably remember the experience. Kidney stone sufferers say that no pain, no torture, no desperation quite matches the jagged agony caused by the presence of a small chip of stone inside a human kidney.

Indeed, those whose composure has been rocked by one of those attacks—which hospitalize more than one million Americans each year—have left few stones unturned in their search for the right diet or drug or medical device that will prevent them from ever going through that kind of misery again.

Prevention of these stones (which have been called a "disease of affluence") is a must, because there is no easy way to remove a stone once it forms and lodges itself in the kidney. Open-kidney surgery is still the treatment of choice in the United States, but people sometimes lose kidneys, or parts of kidneys, as a result.

Difficult as they are to get out, most kidney stones get in by a simple biochemical process that anyone can understand. First, imagine a glass of water and a small cardboard drum of table salt. Start pouring salt into the water and it will dissolve and disappear. Pour in enough salt, however, and the water becomes saturated—it can't hold any more salt—and you'll start to see crystals of salt falling like snowflakes to the bottom of the glass.

Most kidney stones start the same way. The fluids that pass through your kidneys contain different kinds of minerals and molecules. One of those minerals is calcium and one of those molecules is oxalate, which combine to form calcium oxalate. Normally, it floats invisibly in the fluid, but when there's too much of it, or too little fluid, it starts to fall out of solution. Here or there a calcium oxalate crystal forms and attracts another and another until there are enough to make a nice little stone snowball, with sharp edges to torment its owner while defying almost every effort to get rid of it. This problem has stumped many people, including the inventive Benjamin Franklin, who tried and failed to shake loose his stone by eating blackberry jelly and standing on his head.

Results with Magnesium

One modern strategy for preventing kidney stones is to fight mineral with mineral. In other words, fight unwanted calcium crystals with crystals of a similar mineral, such as magnesium. Magnesium supplements seem to inhibit new kidney stones from forming in people who are prone to them. And magnesium is one of the oldest cures for kidney stones—its use has been documented as far back as 1697.

More recently, the Swedes have taken an interest in magnesium. In one study, Swedish researchers gave 200 milligrams of magnesium per day (in the form of magnesium hydroxide) to a group of 41 men and 14 women who individually had averaged about one stone per year (0.8 to be exact) and who, as a group, had passed a whopping 460 stones during the ten years before the experiment.

Magnesium's effects were excellent. After two to four years of the therapy, only 8 of the 55 patients reported new stones.

And as a group, their average rate of developing new stones fell by 90 percent, to only 0.08 stones per year per person.

For comparison, the researchers kept an eye on a group of 43 stone sufferers who did not use magnesium. They averaged a much higher formation rate. After four years, 59 percent of those tested had developed new stones.

Briefly, here's one theory explaining how magnesium works. Like calcium, magnesium can bind itself to oxalate and form a mineral compound. When calcium and magnesium are both present in the urine, they compete with each other to link up with oxalate, almost as if oxalate were a pretty girl they both wanted to dance with.

The critical difference is that magnesium oxalate is less likely to form crystals. It usually remains dissolved in the urine and passes out of the body—unstoned (*Journal of the American College of Nutrition*, vol. 1, no. 2, 1982).

A Role for Vitamin B_6

Another way to approach the prevention of kidney stones is to lower the amount of oxalate in the urine. You can do that by avoiding foods such as spinach, rhubarb, tea, chocolate, parsley and peanuts, all of which are high in oxalates. You can also do it by using more vitamin B_6. By a complicated chain of reactions that still isn't entirely understood, B_6 lowers the amount of oxalate in the urine of people who have a disposition toward kidney stones.

Researchers in India found that a supplement of only 10 milligrams of B_6 per day lowered the oxalate content of urine "significantly" in 12 stone-prone people, all of whom had developed at least one stone per year for the past few years (*International Journal of Clinical Pharmacology, Therapy and Toxicology*, 1982).

That was a discovery worth reporting. Why? Because the Indian researchers got results with only 10 milligrams of B_6 per day, while other scientists have prescribed as much as 100 to

1,000 milligrams per day. And they studied B_6's effects for six months—longer than anyone else.

But more important, they found that B_6 achieved better, faster effects than thiazides. Thiazides are a family of drugs commonly used to lower blood pressure and prevent kidney stones. They do it by increasing the output of urine from the body. But they also cause light-headedness, and they can elevate the amount of sugar and uric acid in the blood, which can promote diabetes and gout, respectively. Thiazides can also reduce the amount of potassium in the blood, which translates into muscle weakness and cramps.

Do magnesium and vitamin B_6 work as well at home as they do in controlled experiments? One doctor we know says they do. Jonathan Wright, M.D., a Kent, Washington, physician who stresses natural remedies, says he's put 25 to 30 kidney stone patients on the nutrients in the past eight to nine years and none has returned with a new stone.

CHAPTER

92

HOW VITAMINS
HELP MENOPAUSE

Anything that can make Edith Bunker talk back to Archie must be a very big deal, indeed. It was on the episode where Edith goes through the "change of life" and is suddenly no longer her normal, sweet self. Archies calls her a dingbat once too often, and she tells him where he can stuff it. Of course, this is television—Edith's "raging hormones" transform her into a *total* monster, she's that way for 30 short minutes (counting the commercials), and by the next show she's fine again.

Things are different in real life. Menopause is a complex, three-dimensional, serious, but altogether natural change that occurs in the life of every woman. Many of the changes that women experience at that time, the assumption of new roles in the family, the changes in self-image, are also experienced by men of the same age. Certainly more is going on than can be conveyed in a half-hour sitcom.

And as with every big change in the body's chemistry, good nutrition is essential for a smooth transition. What you eat can help you deal with some of the unpleasant side effects of menopause and protect you against ailments that commonly afflict women after the change is complete. As the body's chemical balance shifts, its nutritional needs change, as well.

Menopause is the cessation of menstrual periods, which occurs in most women sometime between the ages of 45 and 53. At that time, the body's reproductive machinery shuts down, though the shutdown is hardly an overnight thing. Some women may experience symptoms ten years before their periods actually cease. In some women, their periods stop abruptly, while in others the amount and duration of the menstrual flow tapers off gradually. The most common pattern, however, is irregular—there will be a heavy flow one month, a scant flow the next month, several months with no period at all, then another flow or two before the periods stop altogether.

In much the same way, the body's production of sex hormones slows down. The levels of estrogen, the main female hormone, and progesterone, the female hormone that plays a major part in menstruation, are reduced in the body. Often the reduction comes in fits and starts. The body's hormonal state is shifting into a new equilibrium, and sometimes the shift is jerky and uneven. The result can be a hormonal imbalance, the "raging hormone" syndrome that afflicted Edith Bunker.

There are estimates that 10 to 20 percent of American women suffer no symptoms at all at menopause. For the rest, the best-known symptom is hot flashes. Night sweats, irritability, depression, weight gain and osteoporosis (a loss of bone density) are other problems often encountered at menopause.

Medical science has an answer for those problems, but, as is often the case, the conventional remedy can cause more serious problems than those it is meant to relieve. For about 40 years, doctors have administered estrogen to women suffering the symptoms of menopause, including hot flashes and osteoporosis. Estrogen is now the fifth most prescribed drug in the country. Its use in menopause is designed to bring relief by dealing with the major change taking place in the body, the drop in the levels of naturally produced estrogen.

There is controversy over whether estrogen therapy really does everything it's claimed to do, but there is no question about its side effects.

Estrogen therapy increases the risk of cancer of the endometrium, the inner lining of the uterus. Furthermore, a study published in the *New England Journal of Medicine* found higher rates of breast cancer in women given estrogen during menopause. Estrogen therapy has also been associated with an increased risk of gallbladder disease and high blood pressure.

In most cases, you don't have to subject yourself to risks like that to get relief. Take hot flashes, for example. The phenomenon is essentially harmless, but uncomfortable and often embarrassing. Through some mechanism that is not really understood, the hormonal changes of menopause irritate the nerves controlling the blood vessels of the face and neck. If something sets the nerves off, the blood vessels widen and fill up with blood, causing a hot flash.

The flash lasts from 15 seconds up to a minute, characterized by a deep red color and a feeling of heat, kind of like a superblush. Some women report chills after a flash, and a few experience a tingling sensation in their fingers and toes.

Vitamin E Helped Many

Rosetta Reitz, the author of *Menopause: A Positive Approach* (Penguin, 1979), talked to hundreds of women about menopause in the course of putting her book together. She believes there is a simple, natural solution to hot flashes.

"Many women," she writes, "have found relief in two days from taking 800 I.U. of vitamin E complex, also known as mixed tocopherols. I have seen flashes disappear completely when the vitamin E is also accompanied by 2,000 to 3,000 milligrams of vitamin C (taken at intervals throughout the day) and with 1,000 mg. (also at intervals) of calcium from dolomite or bone meal. When the flashes have subsided, usually after a week, the women reduce the vitamin E intake to 400 I.U."

Ms. Reitz, in talking with women in workshops on menopause, found that hot flashes seemed to occur in many women at moments of high stress. One woman had taken vitamin E to relieve night sweats that would wake her in bed with drenched pajamas and sheets. The E worked against her night sweats and her hot flashes, but only up to a point.

"After three weeks without a flash," Ms. Reitz syas, "Priscilla went to see her doctor and told him about the miraculous change. He said it was nonsense. On the spot, that instant, Priscilla had a huge hot flash. She tells me her present condition is not as good as it was during the three weeks before she went to see the doctor, but that it is a lot better than it used to be."

Anxiety, irritability and depression are other symptoms of menopause for which the doctors have an easy fix. Tranquilizers like Valium and Librium are prescribed to many women to help them deal with the mood swings that often accompany menopause. Those emotional problems *should* be dealt with. Suicide and mental illness in general are prevalent during the menopausal years. It's just that you don't have to become a member of the drug culture to deal with those problems.

The B vitamins, particularly vitamin B_6, have been shown to be necessary for the healthy functioning of the central nervous system. Studies have shown that the essential amino acid tryptophan can be effective against depression. There may be a direct link between the depression some women suffer at menopause and a deficiency of tryptophan is in the body.

Vitamins for a Woman's Heart

The other big health threat that overtakes women at menopause is heart disease. A number of studies have reported an increase in the risk of heart disease in women after menopause. One of the most striking reports was a 1978 update of the "Framingham study." That study of residents of Framingham, Massachusetts, began in 1948, when women were enrolled, given a thorough heart examination and invited to return every two years for new evaluations.

By 1978, virtually all of the women in the study had ceased menstruating, and it was possible to look into the connections between heart disease and menopause. The results were striking.

Not one of the 2,873 women in the study had a heart attack or died of heart disease before menopause. After menopause, heart disease became a common occurrence. For women age 45 to 54, the incidence of heart disease during or after menopause was double the rate before menopause *(Annals of Internal Medicine)*.

There is a big jump in cholesterol in the blood at menopause, mostly due to a rise in the low-density lipoprotein (LDL) cholesterol, the kind of cholesterol particularly associated with heart disease. Japanese scientists have also found higher levels of triglycerides, another fat implicated in heart disease, in the blood of postmenopausal women (*American Journal of Epidemiology*, April, 1979).

Good nutrition can help you put the odds of developing heart trouble after menopause back in your favor. Vitamin C has been used to lower high cholesterol levels. Indeed, Emil Ginter, Ph.D., a noted Czech researcher, believes the recent drop in deaths from heart disease in the United States might be due, in part, to an increase in the consumption of vitamin C in this country.

And you should probably stick with the vitamin E you're taking for hot flashes even after you've licked that problem. Vitamin E apparently works against heart disease by lowering the tendency of platelets, special particles in the blood, to clump together. The clumping together of platelets can lead to a blood clot in arteries feeding the heart of brain, resulting in a heart attack or a stroke.

Good nutrition is obviously an important part of healthy living during and after menopause. Menopause is a natural development in the aging process, a change in women's lives that requires some special nutritional precautions, just as other life stages, like pregnancy, require special precautions.

It's by no means the end of the world. ''A women's life is not 'normal' for the 30 years she ovulates and 'abnormal' before and after,'' Rosetta Reitz says. Healthy living, with proper nutrition, goes on uninterrupted.

CHAPTER

93

CAN VITAMIN SUPPLEMENTS REVERSE MENTAL RETARDATION?

Out of sight for the slow of mind has been the standard operating procedure of treatment in medical history. And while admirable strides are being made to return some "slow" patients to the mainstream of society, for many the artificial life of the institution is all too real.

Conventional wisdom holds that there is only so much that can be done with limited abilities, unless . . .

Unless it were somehow possible to do the unthinkable and treat the retarded mind as an undeveloped flower in desperate need of richer soil.

What if proper nourishment could enable it to grow and blossom?

Farfetched?

Maybe not, according to a study conducted by Ruth F. Harrell, Ph.D., research professor at Old Dominion University in Norfolk, Virginia. She and her colleagues examined the intriguing possibility that retardation might be the result of nutritional deficiencies and therefore could be "amenable to treatment" with supplementary vitamins and minerals.

Their report, published in the *Proceedings of the National Academy of Sciences* (January, 1981), is cautiously optimistic.

Dramatic Rise in IQ

In the introduction to her study, Dr. Harrell relates the case of G.S., a severely retarded seven-year-old who, before being treated, was in diapers, could not speak and had an estimated IQ of 25 to 30.

After the boy's tissues and blood were analyzed, an appropriate nutritional supplement was devised. It took several weeks of trial and error to get the ingredients just right, but once Dr. Harrell had the correct dosage of vitamins and minerals, the boy's progress was remarkable.

"In a few days, he was talking a little. In a few weeks he was learning to read and write, and he began to act like a normal child. When G.S. was nine years old, he read and wrote on the elementary school level, was moderately advanced in arithmetic and, according to his teacher, was mischievous and active. He rode a bicycle and a skate board, played ball, played a flute, and had an IQ of about 90," she writes.

With that heartening result in mind (and earlier successes we'll be telling you about), Dr. Harrell enlisted the help of a team of biochemists and psychologists and recruited a group of 16 retarded children (including four with Down's syndrome, or "mongolism"), whose IQs ranged from 17 to 70, to participate in an eight-month study.

For the first four months, 11 children took a useless placebo while five received a six-tablet-daily regimen of 11 vitamins and eight minerals. The supplements included the B-complex vitamins (including folate and pantothenate), and vitamins A, C, D and E, along with calcium, zinc, manganese, copper, iron and other minerals.

In determining the strength of most of the nutrients, "we went far beyond the Recommended Dietary Allowance (RDA),"

Dr. Harrell told us. "It was 'mega' in size and went up and up and up until we got a mental response."

To give you an idea of just how "mega" the dosage was, the 15,000 international units of vitamin A represents approximately 3½ times the RDA. The B-complex supplements were over 100 times the RDA, while there was in excess of 25 times what is thought to be the body's normal requirement of C and E.

Most of the minerals, however, were closer to RDA levels.

Results Too Good to Believe

Following the initial segment of the study, *all* of the children took the supplements for an additional four months. And when all the data was collected and analyzed, and the progress of the children could be examined, "The results were such that I was afraid to believe them," Dr. Harrell admits.

"During the first four-month period . . . the five children who received supplements increased their average IQ by from 5.0 to 9.6 points, depending on the investigator, whereas the 11 subjects given placebos showed negligible change. The difference between these groups is statistically significant. During the second period, the subjects who had been given placebos in the first study received supplements; they showed an average IQ increase of at least 10.2, a highly significant gain," she writes.

"Several children improved greatly in school achievement. For example, J.B. (age five to six), who said only single words such as *mama* or *bye-bye* initially, could recite, without prompting, the 'Pledge of Allegiance' after eight months of supplementation and could read the first-grade primer. Two (T.C. and R.S.) have been transferred from programs for the mentally retarded to regular schools and grades, on the teacher's recommendations.

"They're not blockbusters—not superior, mind you—but I hope they can fend for themselves in an average sort of way," she notes.

From Slow to Normal

"All of our subjects who cooperated in taking the supplements showed improvement, sometimes dramatic and surprising to the teachers and other professionals who dealt with them. If our findings are confirmed by more extensive experiments, they bring new hope for improving the quality of life for the mentally retarded 3.2 percent of our population."

In essence, nutritional supplements were instrumental in reducing the mentally retarded portion of the study group by one-quarter. Translate that into the millions of members of the human family considered "slow"—IQs below 75—and the billions of dollars going into their special, and often custodial, care, and it's easy to see the far-reaching implications of Dr. Harrell's study.

If supplements are the key to unlocking the retarded mind—if they enable many of those so afflicated "to make their own way, to become hewers of wood and drawers of water," to use Dr. Harrell's words—we're clearly onto something major.

What is perhaps startling is that "everyone posted some kind of gain" across the entire spectrum of retardation, even those with Down's syndrome.

This condition—popularly known as mongolism because the facial features take on a distinctly Oriental appearance—is the result of too much of a necessary thing: an extra 21st chromosome.

This *trisomy 21*—its official medical designation—manifests itself in a number of unpleasant ways, the worst of them being severe retardation.

It has been thought that very little can be done for Down's syndrome children, and they often wind up in institutions.

Unexpectedly, the supplements helped.

Three of the four children with the condition "tended to lose the accumulated fluid in their faces and extremities. The large IQ gain observed (25 units) occurred in L.A. after eight months of supplementation."

Sushma Palmer, D.Sc., a biochemist-nutritionist at the National Academy of Sciences in Washington, D.C., and an expert on Down's, calls the results "suggestive" and gives at least one possible reason for the dramatic effects.

Early Diet Critical

"Children with Down's are characterized by a number of nutritionally related problems that may stem from a delay in feeding skills," she says. "It's frequently difficult for them to eat food. They may eat an insufficient variety and amount, and the outcome can be an unbalanced diet. If the nutritional status of the kids is inadequate, that will likely affect mental performance. The younger the child, the more severe the impact, because that's when the brain is developing faster."

If nutritional deficiencies play havoc with the mental development of these children, can supplements *reverse* the damage?

Dr. Harrell's work suggests that they can.

And interestingly enough, five decades earlier, she had inadvertently done something similar to her most recent experiment by "curing" a group of retarded boys.

The "poverty poor" diet of her first Southern students prompted her to personally undertake a voluntary starvation regimen of nothing more than white bread and water.

In short order, "I found I couldn't learn anything new."

Putting diet and dullness together, she came up with a plan for her teenage pupils.

If she could teach them something basic, like cooking, they might become employable, at least on a part-time basis. Her vocational education request for food to prepare was accepted by an incredulous school board, and before long, she was training budding chefs. But at the same time, she was encouraging them to eat the healthful meals they'd created.

"Remember, there was no free hot lunch back then," she explains. But this one good meal a day was enough of a nutritional boost to make an enormous difference in the boys' intellectual lives.

"My 20 boys made greater gains than any others in the school system. The following year, I lost 18 to normalcy!"

She's built on her work since then, with special emphasis on healthier minds through healthier mothers, and more complete recovery from brain surgery with nutritional supplements.

"You can't imagine what a cold shoulder I got," she relates.

The prevailing attitude toward the retarded was a strong "If God hadn't wanted kids to be idiots, He wouldn't have made 'em that way."

Her steadfast refusal to accept that has led to her breakthrough research.

The immediate question, of course is "How does it work?"

Born with Special Nutritional Needs

The road to an answer remains as trackless as Stanley's path to Livingstone, but there is an intriguing possibility that retardation is, in part, a *genetotrophic disease.*

Roger J. Williams, Ph.D., a University of Texas at Austin biochemist, conceived this concept more than 30 years ago when he suggested that "biochemical individuality" could cause problems.

"We're not born with the same genetics," he told us, "and we don't have the same nutritional needs."

If we don't get what we require, "metabolism can't go in the right direction, and one result could be mental retardation."

Those afflicted with a genetotrophic disease can't rely solely on the established RDAs of the various vitamins and minerals, either, for the very nature of this inborn error of metabolism demands an augmented supply of one or more specific nutrients.

As an example, a metabolic disorder called *homocystinuria* is known to cause retardation because of an excess of the toxic

substance *homocysteine*. Under normal circumstances, homocysteine is degraded into a nontoxic substance when vitamin B_6
is present. Because of a failure—a mutation—in the genes directing the entire operation, that doesn't happen.

The results are tragic—and often unnecessary.

"About half the patients with this condition are helped by
large levels of B_6," explains Willian Shive, Ph.D., of the Clayton
Foundation Biochemical Institute at the University of Texas,
Austin. Providing considerably more than the RDA is essential
to ensure there'll be enough B_6 floating around to keep homocysteine harmless.

By contrast with that one-vitamin genetotrophic disorder,
treating the many different metabolic causes of retardation with
nutrients demands a "shotgun approach."

"The real front in nutrition is to develop a diagnostic tool
that enables us to identify individual needs," Dr. Shive maintains. But he admits that, for now, researchers must simply try
a broad array of nutrients and hope for the best.

And while we've yet to learn the specifics, the nutritional
rehabilitation of the mind is an oasis in an otherwise drab landscape.

Brain's Metabolic Needs Are Surprisingly Large

"The brain is a metabolic hot spot," notes Donald R. Davis,
Ph.D., a member of the Harrell research team from the Clayton
Foundation Biochemical Institute.

"The organ comprises only 2 to 3 percent of our body weight,
yet it accounts for 25 percent of metabolism. And if it's not
functioning smoothly, it can lead to trouble."

When you consider all that could go wrong, it's a miracle
that, for so many of us, the mind runs with the precision of a
stationmaster's fine Swiss pocket watch. But if the "timepiece"
is slow, vitamin and mineral supplements may be the answer.

There's even the downright exciting possibility that they may prevent retardation from occurring in the first place.

"Everybody needs to care for his or her own internal environment," Dr. Williams advises. "And that's doubly true for the internal environment of unborn children. If all mothers were given appropriate supplements, there'd be a tremendous decrease in mental retardation!"

POLLUTION

94

BREATHE EASIER WITH VITAMINS A AND E

Is the air we breathe getting any cleaner? Some people, including many of the scientists whose job it is to monitor and record the levels of various pollutants, seem to think so. In fact, the results of a recent survey conducted by the National Wildlife Federation indicate that air quality is one of the areas where cleanup efforts have made progress over the last decade.

To the commuter who must drive to work each day in a backwash of auto and bus fumes, the statistics don't mean that much.

To the suburban family in the Los Angeles basin or any of the scores of other urbanized areas periodically bathed in a yellow-brown pall of smog, clean air is still a very precious— and elusive—commodity.

And the same can be said for the executive forced to sit for hours in smoke-filled conference rooms, the housewife exposed to the powerful fumes of cleaning agents, and the factory worker who spends 40 or more hours a week inhaling solvents.

In fact, if you're like most people, your lungs are probably being subjected to so many daily insults that any promise of a cleaner day coming is so far down the road it scarcely makes any difference. So what can you do in the meantime to protect your health and hopefully allow your lungs' hard-working natural defense mechanisms to rebuff environmental assaults?

One of the major threats to our respiratory health is ozone, an oxidant pollutant that is one of the main components of everyday smog. Evidence is mounting that daily supplements of vitamin E can help safeguard the lungs against the kind of destruction that occurs at the cellular level when ozone concentrations in the air rise too high.

Vitamin E's protective effect was clearly demonstrated in a study carried out by researcher Mohammad G. Mustafa, Ph.D., associate professor of public health and medicine, University of California at Los Angeles. Laboratory rats were divided into two groups and fed diets containing either 11 parts per million or 66 parts per million of vitamin E. After five weeks, the animals were exposed to various levels of ozone pollution for a seven-day period.

When the animals were later inspected for signs of oxidant damage, Dr. Mustafa found that, at higher levels of pollution, the lungs of rats receiving little vitamin E showed a greater level of abnormal change than those of better-supplemented rats. Vitamin E is believed to retard cellular damage, enhancing the animals' ability to withstand the stress of pollutants (*Nutrition Reports International*).

Interestingly enough, the rats on the low–vitamin E diet were actually receiving about the same concentration of the nutrient found in the average American diet, Dr. Mustafa pointed out. Yet, that wasn't enough to totally protect the animals' lungs. "The findings may be of relevance to human population exposed to photochemical smog," he concluded.

A researcher whose work supports these findings is Daniel B. Menzel, Ph.D., director of the laboratory of environmental pharmacology and toxicology at Duke University medical center. In fact, Dr. Menzel told the Eighth Annual Vitamin Information Bureau Seminar in Chicago that he favors daily supplementation with approximately 200 international units of vitamin E as "a wise precaution."

When Dr. Menzel exposed animals to doses of ozone equivalent to what large human populations are exposed to, those receiving vitamin E survived 50 percent longer than the E-deficient group.

In another study, Dr. Menzel found that animals exposed to lower levels of ozone tended to run out of body stores of the vitamin within a few weeks, while those breathing clean air did not. "We concluded that vitamin E is more rapidly used on ozone exposure than with pure air." he noted.

As Dr. Menzel told the Chicago conference, there has never been a large, long-term study to prove that vitamin E might prevent emphysema and other serious respiratory ailments, but given vitamin E's demonstrated safety, supplementation does seem to make good sense.

Another nutrient that now appears to play a critical role in lung health is vitamin A. In a five-year study of 8,278 men, Norwegian researcher E. Bjelke discovered a link between high lung cancer incidence and low dietary intake of vitamin A. And this relationship prevailed at all levels of cigarette smoking. On the other hand, those men whose diet included high or even moderate amounts of vitamin A were less likely to get lung cancer (*International Journal of Cancer*).

More Vitamin A in the Diet

According to Bjelke, who is associated with Norway's Cancer Registry in Oslo, one of the biggest factors in determining vitamin A intake was the amount of vegetables—particularly carrots—that the men consumed. (According to the U.S. Department of Agriculture's Handbook No. 456, a cup of cooked carrots supplies 16,280 international units of vitamin A—more than three times the Recommended Dietary Allowance for adults.)

Summarizing the study, Bjelke concludes, "The findings are in accordance with experimental results on animals and call for further exploration of the role of nutritional factors in the developing of human lung cancer." Perhaps, Bjelke suggests, heavy smokers who can't quit could be given preventive doses of vitamin A.

Further evidence that vitamin A is somehow involved in protecting against lung cancer comes from Dr. Alex Sakula of Redhill General Hospital in Surrey, England. Writing in the *British Medical Journal*, he notes that, among a group of 28 patients suffering from bronchial cancer, levels of vitamin A in the blood were significantly lower than in healthy persons or patients with nonmalignant bronchial disease.

A possible indication of just how vitamin A may exert its protective effect was provided by two researchers at the State University of New York in Stony Brook. In *Proceedings of the American Association for Cancer Research*, Bernard P. Lane, M.D., and his research associate described laboratory experiments in which 200 tracheal (windpipe) tissue samples were exposed to a potent cancer-causing chemical for two to three weeks. Cancer-associated changes were observed in many windpipe samples immediately following exposure to the carcinogen. But treatment with vitamin A was able to reverse those changes in many cases.

We are trying to tame ozone, industrial chemicals and other harmful pollutants, but the progress is slow. And new dangers have a way of popping up as old ones are eliminated. So until clean, fresh air once again becomes more of an everyday commodity than a sought-after luxury, we owe it to our lungs to give them the protection they deserve.

CHAPTER

95

A AND C: VITAMINS FOR A TOXIFIED WORLD

No one even knew the poison was there, locked away in a storage shed in Billings, Montana. But in June, 1979 it leaked—into 19 states, Canada and Japan. And wherever it turned up, destruction followed. Half a million contaminated chickens had to be slaughtered. Eighteen million eggs were smashed. And millions of dollars' worth of processed food was quarantined by health officials until they could test it. Test it for PCB.

PCB—polychlorinated biphenyl, a unique chemical formulated in 1927 that resists destruction even by super-high temperatures or corrosive acids. A chemical that can persist in the environment for decades—and has. It is *the* most widespread chemical pollutant, found everywhere from the polar ice caps to 11,000 feet under the ocean. And it's a chemical that, even in extremely low doses, can cause ill health—severe acne, cysts, skin discoloration, abdominal pain, nausea and loss of appetite, impotence, bloody urine and fatigue.

Industry has manufactured over 1 billion pounds of PCB, mainly for use as a liquid lubricant in electrical capacitors and transformers. Every year, 100 million capacitors are manufactured for air conditioners, refrigerators, television sets and other products, and each one contains PCB. Over 35 million transformers in the United States are filled with PCB.

One of them was in a storage shed in Billings, Montana.

It was an old transformer, out of use, and when a forklift accidentally hit it, a pipe on the bottom broke. Coolant—200 PCB-loaded gallons of it—leaked out and ran into a floor drain. That drain led to the waste-water collecting system of the Pierce Packing Company, a firm manufacturing meat meal for animal feed. It was a cost-conscious firm which *used* its waste water, gleaning it for solids, fats and grease.

They shipped 2 million pounds of contaminated meal. Eventually, over 1,000 companies were using or selling poisoned feed. And nobody knew.

In early July, a Department of Agriculture (USDA) inspector took a tissue sample from a laying hen in Provo, Utah. There was no special reason to take the sample. It was just a routine random check by the USDA, part of a program to locate chemicals in the food supply—not to stop them from reaching the public. A computer had decided on the time and the place. The sample sat for ten days in a freezer before it was even sent to the lab.

At the lab, technicians found PCB—*high* levels of PCB. But that didn't mean action; it meant forms, reports, red tape. From the time the sample was taken until the time the USDA told the Food and Drug Administration (FDA) about the problem, *six weeks* had passed.

Six weeks too many. From August to November, FDA personnel tracked down PCB. To a mayonnaise distributor in Washington. To frozen-food lockers in Pennsylvania. To chicken soup makers in Minnesota. but they couldn't catch up with all the contaminated food. It is possible that as many as 1,000 poisoned turkeys made it to dinner tables.

We don't mean to frighten you. In fact, we have good news. Two nutrients—vitamin A and C—may help protect your body against PCB. And that's protection you need. This PCB contamination wasn't an isolated incident. PCB is everywhere, and it's here to stay.

True, the government banned the manufacturing, processing and sale of PCB, a ban that took effect in 1979. What else could they do with such a dangerous chemical? One thing about the ban, though. There have been exemptions. A lot of exemptions.

The Environmental Protection Agency has approved almost 100 percent of the requests from industry to continue using PCB. Worse, industry still produces PCB as a by-product in the manufacture of other chemicals, such as silicone. Then there are the junked refrigerators, air conditioners and TV sets which, even if buried in land fills, will eventually leach out PCB. (There are 290 million pounds of PCB in land fills already). Add to that the more than 150 million pounds that now pollute the soil, air and water, pollute it with a chemical that will take years to degrade and disappear.

And because all of that PCB is odorless and colorless, it has a way of sneaking up on you (and into you).

In 1976, for instance, an estimated 800,000 pounds of PCB-contaminated trout from the Great Lakes were illegally caught and sold to food wholesalers. The trout were served in cities across America. (Large areas of the Great Lakes, as well as many of the nation's rivers, are polluted with PCB, and most of the fish caught in them are dangerous to eat.)

A few years ago, the FDA discovered lobsters from the Atlantic Ocean with PCB levels of 10 parts per million. Doesn't sound like much, does it? Well, the highest level permitted in shellfish by the FDA is 2 parts per million.

Before the government ban on PCB took effect, many municipalities and states used waste oil contaminated with PCB to control dust on roads and highways. During 1977, 10,000 gallons of such oil were about to be spread on Iowa's gravel roads. But, luckily, environmental officials discovered that the oil contained as much as 6 parts per *thousand* PCB—enough to kill.

The PCB-tainted waste oil illegally dumped along 211 miles of North Carolina road sides in 1978 didn't contain quite so much of the chemical. But it had enough to be dangerous. At first, the state planned to scrape up the poisoned soil and haul it to a rural land fill. That plan was vetoed as too costly. Instead, they plowed the oil into the ground, which was sprayed with activated charcoal. The *theory* is that the charcoal will neutralize that PCB. But nobody really knows.

You Contain PCB

Ever lick an envelope to seal it? The adhesive could have contained PCB. Ever buy packaged food? Food wrapping sometimes contains PCB that migrates into the food. Coatings for ironing-board covers can contain PCB. Certain types of carbon paper contain PCB. Some upholstery contains PCB. You contain PCB.

Over 90 percent of all Americans have detectable levels of PCB stored in their fatty tissues, levels often as high as 10 parts per million. And Lester Crawford, Ph.D., an FDA official who helped contain the recent PCB contamination, told us that the problem is getting worse.

"Since there is a low-level exposure to PCB all the time, and since the chemical accumulates in the body, body levels of PCB will go up in the future. I would project a level of 50 parts per million in human tissue. That shouldn't cause acute illness. But" Dr. Crawford warned, "*it may have a lot of chronic effects on health, effects we don't even know about yet.*"

Scientists, however, are beginning to discover one effect of long-term PCB intake—infertility.

In one study, researchers gave rats PCB and found that the animals delivered fewer young. In another study, chickens given PCB had a decrease in egg production.

But researchers didn't have to set up their own experiments to see PCB-caused infertility. They had a bigger laboratory already available—the world.

Several species of seals are dying out in the Baltic Sea, which is heavily polluted with PCB. A 1975 survey showed that among one of those species, ringed seals, only 27 percent of the females were pregnant compared to 90 percent in Baltic seal populations during the 1960s. Testing the seals, scientists found the PCB levels were far higher in nonpregnant than in pregnant animals.

Sperm Counts Declining

What about people? Well, scientists at the 1979 annual meeting of the American Chemical Society reported that sperm counts among U.S. men are declining—and the cause may be PCB. Measuring both the level of sperm and the level of PCB in seminal fluid, they found that the higher the amount of PCB, the lower the amount of sperm.

James R. Allen, Ph.D., a researcher at the University of Wisconsin who had conducted numerous studies on PCB, believes the chemical may affect "reproductive capabilities" by altering the normal functioning of hormones.

But, Dr. Allen told us, "even if chronic, low-level exposure to PCB has no effect in the adult, it still has an effect on the fetus and infant."

Unfortunately, Dr. Allen's statement was proven in Japan during 1968 when a machine containing PCB sprang a leak and contaminated rice oil. More than 1,000 people used that oil regularly for three months.

Cysts were the first symptom—on the fact, on the ears, all over the body. But cysts were the least of their problems. Those who used large quantities of the rice oil also suffered from severe fatigue, loss of appetite, impotence, bloody urine, numb limbs and painful joints. And the pregnant mothers who used the rice oil, even if they had no symptoms themselves, were slowly poisoning their unborn children.

Researchers later studied 13 women who used the rice oil while pregnant. Of their 13 babies, two were stillborn. Birth defects blighted all the the others.

A grayish, dark brown pigment colored their skin. Five also had dark nails. Nine had heavy eye discharges. Four had facial abnormalities such as protruding eyeballs.

After the incident, the Japanese government lowered the *tolerance level*—the upper limit of PCB permitted—for food.

America's tolerance levels remain much higher than Japan's.

They're lower than the 10 parts per million of a few years ago. But you can still buy poultry with 3 parts per million and fish with 2 parts per million. What's the reason for these high levels?

Although the FDA admits that there is no level "of PCB exposure that can be said to provide . . . safety," and that "it would be preferable not to have PCB in food at any level," it has set the tolerance levels to maintain a "proper balance of safety and economic criteria." In other words, better to put American lives on the line than American industry in the red.

Vitamins A and C Protect

That leaves protecting yourself up to you. You and vitamins A and C.

In a study of vitamin C and PCB, researchers fed young experimental animals high doses of the chemical. The animals grew poorly and had high levels of cholesterol. (PCB is known to interfere with fat metabolism.) The animals also excreted in their urine *44 times* the normal amount of vitamin C, a sign, say the researchers, that the animals' bodies were synthesizing large quantities of the vitamin in an attempt to detoxify PCB.

Next, the researchers fed another group of experimental animals PCB—but also gave them vitamin C. These animals grew normally and had normal cholesterol levels. They also had a "normal outward appearance," compared with the sickly appearance of the PCB animals who didn't get vitamin C *(Nutrition Reports International)*.

In a study of vitamin A and PCB, researchers fed two groups of rats PCB for six weeks but gave one group 3,400 international units of vitamin A. The vitamin A group "showed better growth" than the animals not on the vitamin *(Japanese Journal of Nutrition)*.

The researchers then fed another group of rats PCB and measured the vitamin A content of the rats' livers. They found a decrease in vitamin A "even at low PCB levels."

Citing these and other studies, the researchers concluded that "a large part of the symptoms" of the PCB poisoning "were based on a vitamin A deficiency" caused by PCB *(Journal of Nutritional Science and Vitaminology)*.

"PCB affects steroids and steroid-like compounds, one of which is vitamin A," Dr. Allen says. "I think there is a definite likelihood that vitamin A could be involved in PCB intoxication. Perhaps PCB blocks the vitamin A receptor sites in the cell. Believe me, scientists have yet to detect all the ways in which PCB causes ill health."

CHAPTER
96

CLEANSING INTERNAL POLLUTION WITH A VITAMIN BRUSH

Bound for New York City on the New Jersey Turnpike, you'll pass through the pits of pollution. But rolled-up windows and closed-off air vents can't stop the stench of petroleum refineries and chemical plants from seeping into your car. The acrid fumes make your skin crawl from the inside out.

Within the last 35 years, we have watched hundreds of chemical preservatives and pesticides sneak into our food supply. Dangerous minerals and other toxic substances run off the man-made wasteland into rivers, streams and springs, threatening our precious water supply.

We've become trapped in a murky mess. But, luckily, we don't have to surrender our health to the pollutants.

Countless studies suggest that vitamin supplementation—particularly with vitamins C and E—can protect the body against environmental pollution.

Scientists at the State University of Londrina, in Brazil, and at Kansas State University have tested the protective effect of various vitamins against the powerful cancer-causing substance aflatoxin B_1.

Aflatoxin is the product of a certain mold which can grow on peanuts, grains and other foods. It frequently shows up in samples of peanut butter. That worries public health authorities, because aflatoxins are known to cause liver cancer in man.

But in the latest study, the addition of vitamin C and the B vitamin choline to the diet of young Japanese quail protected the growing birds from the adverse effects of aflatoxin B_1. Birds generally suffer stunted growth as a result of mild aflatoxin poisoning. After 21 days on an aflatoxin diet, the quails supplemented with vitamin C and choline gained significantly more weight than those not receiving supplementation. In fact, in some instances, they gained even more weight than those on a nontoxic diet (*Veterinary and Human Toxicology*).

Whether we can translate the prevention of aflatoxin toxicity in quails to the prevention of aflatoxin-induced cancer in humans has yet to be determined. But we stand a pretty good chance of doing just that.

After all, vitamin C is being lauded as a natural pollution fighter. It seems to attack chemical pollutants in our bodies in a way similar to antibodies fighting off infections. But unlike antibodies, vitamin C cannot be synthesized by the human body, though it is made by various other animal species. Rats, for example, synthesize vitamin C at an accelerated rate when toxic chemicals are introduced into their bodies.

Liver Disease Linked to Vitamin C Shortage

Mounting evidence suggests that the human storehouse of vitamin C may make a difference in our survival in a polluted environment. One survey mentioned in the *British Medical Journal* links low tissue levels of vitamin C with environmentally induced disorders of the human liver. Of 138 patients, those with the liver disease called primary biliary cirrhosis (a rare form of cirrhosis sometimes brought on by tranquilizers and other drugs) had low concentrations of vitamin C in their tissue stores.

Apparently, vitamin C gives the liver a helping hand in its job of detoxifying harmful substances. According to Aniece A.

Yunice, Ph.D., of the medical service at the Oklahoma City Veterans Administration Hospital, and Robert D. Lindeman, M.D., now chief of staff, Louisville Veterans Administration Hospital, Kentucky, vitamin C may, for example, increase the activity of enzymes responsible for the detoxification of alcohol.

In the Oklahoma study, published in *Proceedings of the Society for Experimental Biology and Medicine,* five rats received toxic doses of alcohol over a four-week period, while another five received the same daily dose but were pretreated with large doses of vitamin C. By the end of the test period, all the rats on alcohol alone died. Four of the five on alcohol plus vitamin C were alive!

Vitamin C also seems to exert a protective effect against the wrath of nitrates. Most of us are already aware of the cancer-causing potential of nitrate preservatives in meats like bacon, bologna and ham. But even if we stop bringing home the bacon, we've only begun to reduce our cancer risk. Nitrates have infiltrated our well water and streams as a result of chemical fertilizers and animal wastes which have run off into our water supplies. And they've gotten a hold on some vegetables and fish.

Try as we might, we can't avoid them. But researchers suggest that, if we stock up on vitamin C, we may be able to divert nitrate from forming a cancer-causing substance. Nitrates pose a problem only when they combine in the stomach with certain substances known as amines. And when introduced into a simulated stomach environment with nitrates, the vitamin C has been found to effectively compete for bonding positions.

It's no wonder, then, that large doses of vitamin C are being used with great success in Hungary for the treatment of methemoglobinemia. That disease, in which the red blood cells (responsible for oxygen transport) lose their ability to carry oxygen, is caused by nitrate poisoning *(Archives of Environmental Health).*

Fighting the Poison Metals

But what's a body to do about the various toxic heavy metals such as cadmium, mercury and lead that are leaking into our environment and threatening our health? Well, here again, we can begin by looking to vitamin C, which has been shown to counteract the toxicity of cadmium.

Unfortunately, when it comes to detoxifying mercury and lead, vitamin C is of no use. But according to evidence cited in *Federation Proceedings,* vitamin E is. This vitamin, which just happens to be your best insurance against the ravages of air pollution and the onslaught of X-ray irradiation, has also been found to decrease the toxicity of methyl mercury in quail.

Since 1967, scientists have concentrated on the protective effect of the trace element selenium against mercury poisoning. However, according to vitamin E researchers Dr. S. O. Welsh and Professor J. H. Soares, Jr., the protective effect of vitamin E against mercury occurs independently of the selenium status of their animal subjects *(Nutrition Reports International).*

Calcium has been known to get the lead out of our systems. But, again, vitamin E can help. Orville A. Levander and colleagues at the U.S. Agricultural Research Center in Beltsville, Maryland, explain that lead increases the brittleness of red cell membranes so that they disintegrate easily. But with the addition of large doses of vitamin E to the diet of rats receiving lead, the red blood cells remained normally flexible *(Journal of Nutrition).*

In a separate study conducted by David S. Klauder and Harold G. Petering from the department of environmental health at the University of Cincinnati medical center, lead depressed the hemoglobin levels in rats whose diets were deficient in iron or copper or both *(Environmental Health Perspective).*

Of course, maintaining an adequate level of iron in your diet is fairly easy with iron supplements. For copper, turn to liver—which is also a superb source of iron.

Of course, if you've been doing your homework, you're probably already taking your share of vitamins C and E. In that case, it's still nice to know that your efforts are paying off with added dividends.

CHAPTER

97

HEALING SICK MINDS WITH VITAMINS

Peter: In the hospital, they serve me meat from the morgue and poisoned food. My medicine is really LSD. If I smoke a cigarette, a friend will die.

Martha: God told me I was going to have Christ's baby. He told me to walk with a cane. Then He told me to swim in the ocean; I fought with a monster for eight hours.

Mitch: They say my grandfather died two years ago, but I know better. I talk to him every night. He comes into my room and floats above the bed. Someone turned him into a purple ball.

Three schizophrenics. Three out of two million.

There are more people hospitalized for schizophrenia than for any other illness, mental or physical. In schizophrenia, *thought* and *perception* are diseased.

You hallucinate, seeing what isn't there and hearing voices when no one speaks. In a moderate case, you know you're hallucinating. But when it's worse, you can't tell the difference between what's real and what's not. Your thoughts are bizarre and illogical, perhaps paranoid, and you act on them. You might think there's a plot against you. You might think you're God. You could talk of suicide and, very possibly, commit it. Schizophrenics have a suicide rate about 20 times higher than the rest of the population.

A psychiatrist tries to keep a schizophrenic out of a coffin by putting him on a couch. He wants the schizophrenic to talk things over—and over, and over. Only in this way, he says, will the schizophrenic recognize and root out the cause of his disease: emotional trauma during childhood. But mommy and daddy aren't always the villains the psychiatrist thinks. Studies show that psychoanalysis almost never cures a schizophrenic.

Instead, some are helped by having their brains stunned by electroshock therapy. Many others live somewhat normal lives by taking powerful drugs. Those treatments have drawbacks, of course. But they work because they affect a schizophrenic's body. They work because schizophrenia is more than a mental illness.

Helped by Niacin

The weird thoughts and strange perceptions of schizophrenia are often the symptoms of *physical* disorders. Disorders that can be healed with nutrition. Unlike the psychiatric approach, that's not a theory. Thousands of schizophrenics have already been cured with a nutrient—niacin.

Niacin is one of the B-complex vitamins—and one of the most important. A lack of niacin can cause severe skin rashes and digestive problems. It can also cause madness. Soon after processors of white flour began fortifying it with niacin, 10 percent of all state hospital patients in the South were "cured." They had been diagnosed as schizophrenics, but they actually had pellagra, the niacin-deficiency disease. Some of the mental symptoms of pellagra—hallucinations and paranoia—perfectly mimic schizophrenia.

"If all the niacin were removed from our food, everyone would be psychotic in one year," says Abram Hoffer, M.D., a psychiatrist in British Columbia.

Dr. Hoffer was a pioneer in the nutritional treatment of schizophrenia. In 1952, he and a colleague gave niacin to eight schizophrenic patients. They immediately improved. Continuing the study, the doctors checked their patients' progress for the next 15 years. All were well 15 years later—and all were still taking niacin (*Orthomolecular Psychiatry*).

Schizophrenia can last a lifetime or a few weeks. Many patients walk out of state hospitals only to return. To see if niacin could keep schizophrenics permanently out of hospitals, Dr. Hoffer gave 73 hospitalized schizophrenics niacin and compared them to 98 who were not taking niacin. During the next three years, only 7 of the niacin patients had to be readmitted to a hospital, while 47 of the non-niacin patients were readmitted (*Lancet*).

The patients Dr. Hoffer treated did *not* have pellagra. They had what he calls a *vitamin dependency*.

A vitamin dependency, Dr. Hoffer explained to us, is the need for a larger amount of a vitamin than most people require. If you don't get that amount, you can suffer from a variety of physical and mental ills. Schizophrenia is one of them.

The dependency could be inherited. Or if you were deprived of the nutrient over a long period of time, you might need more of it to function normally. Many of the mental patients with pellagra, for instance, had to take 600 milligrams of niacin every day for the rest of their lives. Most people need only 5 milligrams.

Extra Vitamin C

Niacin isn't the only nutrient involved, however. Vitamin C is another.

When a normal person is given 5 grams of vitamin C, his tissues are saturated—he can't absorb any more. But studies show that it takes from *20 to 40 grams* of vitamin C to saturate the tissues of a schizophrenic. They don't need that much to get better, though. A doctor gave 1 gram of vitamin C a day to 40 schizophrenics, all of whom had had the disease for years. Many of them showed significant improvement.

Why vitamin C and niacin?

"Nobody knows for sure," Dr. Hoffer told us. "The scientific community is only beginning to look at the relationship of these substances to mental functioning. But even if the role of nutrition in schizophrenia isn't completely understood, there's no doubt in my mind that the disease is caused by a biochemical imbalance in the body that can be corrected with proper nutrition. I've treated 4,000 cases of schizophrenia, and I haven't ever seen one caused by psychological factors."

Another doctor who believes that schizophrenia is caused by a biochemical imbalance in the body is Carl Pfeiffer, M.D., Ph.D., director of the Brain Bio Center in Princeton, New Jersey.

Dr. Pfeiffer calls schizophrenia a "biochemical wastebasket" into which, he says, have been thrown ten diseases, all of which were once thought to be schizophrenia (because their symptoms are identical to those of schizophrenia) but which are now classified as separate diseases with separate causes. Among them are brain syphilis, as well as a thyroid disorder and a type of epilepsy.

Dr. Pfeiffer has turned that wastebasket into a filing cabinet. He believes that he has isolated the remaining biochemical abnormalities that cause schizophrenia. There are five, and nutrition can treat them all.

One of them is pyroluria. In this disease, a person eliminates abnormally large amounts of the chemical kryptopyrrole. Unfortunately, on its way out, kryptopyrrole grabs onto zinc and vitamin B_6, both of which are crucial to normal brain function. The result is very low body levels of those nutrients—and schizophrenia. The treatment, however, is simple: Replace B_6 and zinc. And the cure is almost automatic—95 percent recover. Unless they're taken off the nutrients. Then schizophrenia returns in two days.

Thirty percent of all schizophrenics have pyroluria, says Dr. Pfeiffer. And most of them are under 20. "Stress increases the amount of kryptopyrrole that is excreted," he explained, "and people from the ages 15 to 20 face the greatest level of stress."

Another 60 percent of schizophrenics suffer from a histamine disorder, according to Dr. Pfeiffer. Histamine, as any hay fever victim who takes antihistamines can tell you, is involved in allergic reactions. But that's not all it's involved in. "It would take a half an hour to explain all of histamine's functions in the body," says Dr. Pfeiffer. And one of those functions is as a neurotransmitter, a chemical that relays information in the brain. But when histamine levels rise too high or dip too low, the brain can relay the wrong information: Your deceased uncle is standing in the corner; there's a plot against you; you're the savior of the world. In short, schizophrenia.

For schizophrenics with high histamine, Dr. Pfeiffer prescribes calcium, which lowers histamine levels and relieves the constant or frequent headaches that accompany the disorder. Along with calcium, he gives the minerals zinc and manganese. The treatment also includes the amino acid methionine. "This helps to lower blood histamine by a process known as methylation," says Dr. Pfeiffer.

"For patients with low histamine, large doses of niacin and vitamin C are usually effective," he explains.

Proper nutrition seems to be the best way to treat schizophrenia. Yet, the American Psychiatric Association and the government's National Institute of Mental Health have been powerful opponents of treating schizophrenia with nutrition. Why?

"Resistance is the typical medical reaction to all ideas that strike out on new therapeutic ground," says Dr. Hoffer. "The attack on nutritional treatment is illogical, unjustified, extreme, emotional and not backed up by scientific evidence."

The scientific jury is still out on the megavitamin approach to schizophrenia. At present, it appears to be a promising alternative.

CHAPTER

98

VITAMIN RELIEF FOR SHINGLES

Remember when you had chicken pox as a child? You were pretty miserable (not to mention unsightly) for about two or three weeks. But finally the last scab fell off and you went skipping back to school feeling incredibly happy to be rid of the disease once and for all.

Or so you thought. Fact is, the same nasty little bug that gave you chicken pox as a child can come back to haunt you decades later as an aging adult, only worse. The bug is herpes, the disease—shingles.

It's true. The pox may be gone but the germs linger on. After your bout with chicken pox, herpes zoster (the official name of this virus) may take up residence in your spinal nerves, where it promptly goes into hibernation. You think it's gone forever, but it can wake up at any time and start multiplying.

When that happens, the affected nerve becomes inflamed, and pain radiates all along its path. The herpes virus then passes down the nerve and multiplies again in the skin, causing clusters of sores to erupt.

For four or five days before the expected rash, however, you may feel anything from numbness and superficial tingling, itching or burning sensations to severe, deep pain. Discomfort may be intermittent or constant. At its worst, the pain may even be mistaken for appendicitis, gallbladder attack or pleurisy. As if that's not enough, you may also run a fever for days and feel generally out of sorts, too. All this before eruption!

When the rash does make its appearance, it starts out as small reddened areas which quickly puff up with fluid to the size of a quarter, or larger in some cases. The skin over the blisters becomes increasingly rigid until, finally, by about the fifth day after eruption, the blisters burst. During the next week or two, crusts develop, but a total of two to four weeks may elapse before you see the last scab fall off.

The sores are not randomly distributed on the body as with chicken pox. The affected areas are always along the course of one or more of the spinal nerves beneath the skin.

Most typically, the rash progresses in a band around one side of the chest (55 percent of the cases), the neck (20 percent), the lower back (15 percent) or the forehead and eyes (15 percent), and all the while you may be feeling extreme discomfort.

The distribution and appearance of the sores is so characteristic of herpes zoster that no testing is necessary to confirm diagnosis. And with a million new cases each year, it's not long before even new doctors recognize this distinctive disease.

True, its appearance is similar to chicken pox, but shingles is not a youngster's disease. On the contrary, it's those over age 50 who are most susceptible. In fact, it's been estimated that half the people reaching 85 years of age have suffered from at least one attack of herpes zoster.

Shingles Often Affects Healthy Older People

And these are not necessarily sickly folks, either. Believe it or not, shingles often occurs in otherwise healthy older people. Sometimes it's a physical injury which precipitates a bout with zoster; one investigation found that 38 percent of their herpes zoster patients had had an injury to the shingles-infected area two weeks before the appearance of sores *(British Medical Journal).*

That finding, coupled with the decreased natural immunity that often accompanies old age, may help explain the prevalence of shingles in older people. Of course, anything which lowers your resistance may also trigger an outbreak of shingles. That means you may be more susceptible in times of physical or emotional stress or when your natural immunity has been compromised by another illness.

One thing's for sure, though; you can't catch shingles like you do chicken pox. Most patients with zoster have had no recent exposure to others infected with it or chicken pox. That's why the incidence of zoster does not increase during seasonal chicken pox epidemics. On the other hand, a person susceptible to chicken pox can catch it from someone suffering from shingles.

What's more, shingles is not a once-and-done disease like chicken pox. That means you can come down with a second or third outbreak, and it can affect the same nerve as it did the first time or a different one completely.

But no matter how or why the eruptions occur, each person is affected to a different degree. As with most diseases, some people get off with only a mild sentence while others wonder if they'll ever be set free.

Let us reassure you right now. Complications can be severe and quite serious, but they are rarely fatal or even permanent.

Still, you should know that herpes zoster is occasionally associated with paralysis of the arms, legs and chest muscles. Even when that occurs, however, adequate functioning returns in over 75 percent of cases. Eye involvement, on the other hand, may result in permanent visual impairment due to scarring of the cornea. Skin, too, may be permanently scarred if the sores are very deep.

But the most common and troublesome part of shingles is pain which lingers long after the obvious infection has gone. Doctors call this *postherpetic neuralgia* and believe it is caused by scarring of the damaged nerves.

It doesn't afflict everyone, fortunately, but once again, it's the older folks who suffer the most. As many as 70 percent of those over 60 years of age can expect moderate to severe pain for more than two months or, in some cases, for years.

While there doesn't appear to be any definite way to ward off an attack of shingles (except to boost your own natural immunities with good health habits), there are numerous ways to help relieve the discomforts of zoster, if it should strike.

First of all, while the sores are erupting, wear loose-fitting clothes. "And, especially, stay away from fuzzy garments," says Richard Mihan, M.D., from the University of Southern California school of medicine. As a dermatologist practicing with Samuel Ayres, M.D., Dr. Mihan has treated numerous cases of herpes zoster and the often accompanying postherpetic neuralgia. "The pain may be severe at times, requiring sedation and causing almost unbearable discomfort and loss of sleep," says Dr. Mihan. Rather than resort to drastic measures like cutting out the root of the affected nerve or repeatedly injecting local anesthetics into the area (which causes other negative side effects), Drs. Ayres and Mihan found a better, safer way to relieve the prolonged suffering—vitamin E.

Over a period of four years, they treated 13 patients with chronic postherpetic neuralgia with vitamin E, administered both orally (400 to 1,600 international units daily) and topically (directly to the sores).

Eleven of the patients had had moderate to severe pain for over six months. Seven of those had suffered for over one year— one for 13 years and one for 19 years! Yet, after taking vitamin E, nine patients reported complete or almost complete control of pain. The two patients who had had postherpetic neuralgia the longest were in this group. Of the remaining four patients, two were moderately improved and two were slightly improved *(Archives of Dermatology)*.

"The mechanism by which vitamin E relieves the persistent pain of postherpes zoster neuralgia is not known," concluded Drs. Mihan and Ayres, "but in view of its long duration in many of our cases, we do not believe it is coincidence."

And they still don't. "Vitamin E may not be 100 percent

effective," Dr. Mihan told us, "but many of my patients get relief from persistent pain."

But vitamin E doesn't just relieve pain. It also helps stop the rash from spreading. One woman told us, "Last August, I noticed a sore about the size of a silver dollar on my back. When I touched the spot, it burst as if it were a blister. I thought nothing of it until late that same evening, when I felt a rash very rapidly spreading all over my back. It was annoying and felt as though ants were crawling on my skin.

"Not knowing how to stop it from spreading, I wondered if vitamin E might help. I cut the tips of three vitamin E capsules (each 400 international units) with scissors, let the oil drip into a saucer and applied it to the reddish, tender sores. Vitamin E stopped the rash from spreading instantly and gave me so much relief that I was able to sleep well that night. By morning, my husband was amazed to notice how the sores had begun to heal and were already forming scabs.

"I paid a visit to our family doctor that afternoon, and he confirmed my own suspicions: It was shingles. Healing progressed quickly and completely as I continued applying vitamin E oil to the infected area, and during that time I was never laid up and was able to do all of my housework. It's no wonder that vitamin E is called the 'miracle vitamin.' "

Vitamin C Helps

Still, vitamin E doesn't work for everyone. But don't despair. Vitamin C may be the vitamin that'll do the job for you.

Juan N. Dizon, M.D., of New York, has treated herpes zoster with oral vitamin C and gotten excellent results.

"I have treated three cases of shingles with 10 grams (10,000 milligrams) of vitamin C daily (1 gram every hour) until the lesions dry up," says Dr. Dizon. "In each case, the lesions dried up within two to five days.

"I told another physician of these findings. When he tried the same on his patients, he had similar results.

"I am aware that this is all anecdotal and nonscientific, but considering that there is no good scientific treatment for herpes and that vitamin C is virtually harmless, I would hope that others will try this method on their patients and report their results. After enough anecdotal cases have been submitted, maybe somebody will do double-blind controlled studies."

An outbreak of shingles is not the end of the world, but it can certainly change your outlook on it for a while.

Keep yours bright with vitamins E and C and, hopefully, shingles will be just a short lapse in an otherwise healthy life.

CHAPTER

99

VITAMINS THAT TEAM UP FOR CLEAR SKIN

Several years ago, a 26-year-old man walked into the office of Samuel Ayres, Jr., M.D., looking for help. Patches of crusting, scaling, itching, wartlike growths covered most of his torso. Scattered outbreaks appeared on his scalp, arms and legs. The young man was suffering from Darier's disease (keratosis follicularis). He had battled the rare, hereditary skin condition for 13 years with little success.

"He was certainly a mess," recalls Dr. Ayres, who maintains a private dermatology practice in Los Angeles. The skin disease had been persistently severe and extensive. On three occasions, it had been serious enough to put the young man in a hospital. Corticosteroid drugs used to treat the problem provided only temporary relief. Hot weather, sun exposure and nervous tension made the condition worse.

"He couldn't even go out and play tennis," says Dr. Ayres. "His skin was extremely sensitive to sunlight, and he would break out disastrously whenever he went out in the sun."

Since vitamin A supplements had been used with some success for a variety of skin problems involving defects of the skin's outer layer, his doctors had placed him on an average daily dose of 200,000 international units. He had been taking the high dosages of vitamin A for about five years. During that time, he was monitored closely for any adverse reactions, since the dose was considerably higher than the Recommended Dietary Allowance and not recommended for normal use. Although he showed no signs of toxicity, there were no signs of improvement, either. "It was a baffling situation," says Dr. Ayres. "His doctors observed that, while the doses of A were not making him better, his skin condition worsened without it."

After reviewing the case, Dr. Ayres advised the patient to reduce his intake of vitamin A to 150,000 international units daily. At the same time, he was instructed to begin taking 1,200 international units of vitamin E each day. Eventually, the vitamin A dosage was reduced to 100,000 international units and the vitamin E was elevated to 1,600 international units. After 11 months, his back was entirely clear and all other areas were greatly improved (*Archives of Dermatology*).

Today his skin tans normally when he spends an afternoon outside playing tennis. "Since taking vitamin A with vitamin E, he has been able to live a reasonably satisfactory life. He has experienced slight relapses only when he has attempted to markedly reduce his maintenance doses of vitamins," Dr. Ayres told us.

What had prompted the doctor to try that particular combination of nutrients when other treatments had failed? As Dr. Ayres told us, "I was familiar with the work of S. R. Ames, who had lectured at a symposium at the Massachusetts Institute of Technology. Dr. Ames spoke on the metabolic function of vitamin A and emphasized the important role vitamin E plays in the absorption, transport and storage of vitamin A in the body. He reported experiments which indicated that vitamin A absorption was severely impaired in animals that were on an E-deficient diet."

In those experiments, Dr. Ames discovered that the body's ability to use vitamin A increased sixfold when oral supplements of vitamin E were also taken. When he took vitamin E-deficient mice and gave them shots of vitamin A, the vitamin A levels within their bodies remained low. But after Dr. Ames injected the mice with vitamin E, the vitamin A levels of the mice increased markedly *(American Journal of Clinical Nutrition).*

Those laboratory findings led Dr. Ayres and his colleagues, Richard Mihan, M.D., and Morton D. Scribner, M.D., to see if vitamin E would work together with vitamin A to treat several skin diseases involving defects in the upper layer of the skin in their patients. In addition to Darier's disease, they've made encouraging progress in treating two other skin conditions over the past several years *(Cutis,* May, 1979).

And Dr. Ayres believes that people with those particular skin problems may have a physiological defect which raises their requirements for certain nutrients. "We may be born with different vitamin and mineral requirements just as much as we're born with different looks," he says.

Although Dr. Ayres warns people against taking unnecessarily high doses of vitamin A, he believes that some individuals with chronic skin disease may need large doses. "Some of those columnists in the newspapers will try to tell people they get all the nutrients they need from the average American diet," he says. "That is just not true. Some individuals may need 10 times more of a certain vitamin than other people. Or a person's requirement may be 100 times greater."

He also suggests that the so-called average American diet may not deserve much homage. Patients on the vitamin A and E program are advised that there's a lot more to good nutrition. "The average American diet consists of eating enriched white bread," says Dr. Ayres. "Enriched bread contains inorganic iron, which combines with vitamin E and destroys it. So people taking vitamin E for therapeutic purposes should avoid eating enriched white breads and cereals. They also should not take mineral supplements containing inorganic iron unless they take the vitamin E and the mineral supplement eight hours apart." (Ferrous gluconate, ferrous fumarate, peptonized iron and iron lactate are preferable sources since they are organic.)

Dr. Scribner has witnessed that phenomenon in his own practice. A 12-year-old boy once came to him with pityriasis rubra pilaris, a skin condition the youth had had since infancy. The condition is a rare, chronic, inflammatory skin disease in children and adults, characterized by pink, scaling areas and prominent hair follicles.

Under Dr. Scribner's supervision, the child was given 100,000 international units of vitamin A and 800 international units of vitamin E daily. No change was observed during the first six months of treatment. Then the condition began to clear up, and there was a 50 percent improvement. During that period, it was discovered that, contrary to instruction, the boy was taking an inorganic iron supplement daily in the form of ferrous sulfate. He discontinued the iron, which apparently was combining with and inactivating the vitamin E. After another two months of treatment, his skin was almost totally clear. He presently takes a maintenance dose of 30,000 international units of vitamin A and 400 international units of vitamin E daily. His skin remains virtually clear.

Acne vulgaris, or common acne, is another skin disorder that seems to respond well to the combined therapy. Acne is probably one of the most common diseases of the skin. It usually occurs on the face, with pimples and blackheads being the most obvious symptoms. While acne has been treatable, it has remained incurable.

"Vitamin A has been used by itself to treat acne, but with little success," says Dr. Ayres. What about combining A and E? He and his colleague, Dr. Mihan, have their acne patients taking an average daily dose of 100,000 international units of vitamin A and 800 international units of vitamin E daily. "We've had very good results with this treatment," says Dr. Ayres. And the doses of vitamins can usually be reduced after a few months.

The patients also use a topical medication—benzoyl peroxide gel—and are told what foods to avoid. "Extra iodine can aggravate acne, so we advise our patients to avoid iodized salt. Excess milk, fats and sweets also can cause acne to flare up. Many commercial soft drinks contain brominated vegetable oils as stabilizers, which may irritate acne conditions, too. We tell our patients to drink fresh fruit juices."

While nutrition is a very important factor in maintaining healthy skin, problems can erupt at any stage of life for a variety of reasons. "The skin is a complicated organ," Dr. Ayres explains. "There are external irritants like overbathing, using too much soap and water or cosmetics. Internal malignancies or internal infections will sometimes reflect themselves through skin problems. Chronic infections of the teeth, bladder or other organs, and malfunction of organs such as the liver may cause skin eruptions, too. Some external causes of allergy, and internal causes like reactions to certain drugs, also can create skin trouble."

Although he has observed progress in his own practice and in the work of his colleagues, Dr. Ayres says research on the combined A and E therapy still needs to be conducted in laboratory settings. And despite the high dosages prescribed, he has observed no ill effects in his patients.

"Dosages taken at those levels should be monitored by a physician, though," Dr. Ayres stresses. "And people with high blood pressure, heart disease or diabetes should not take high levels of vitamin E at first. Vitamin E improves the tone of the heart muscle, and a large dose too soon can make the blood pressure rise. Vitamin E also improves glycogen storage, so diabetics on insulin could develop an insulin shock reaction if they took too much vitamin E too soon. People with these conditions should not begin with any more than 100 international units of vitamin E a day. The dose may gradually be increased under a doctor's supervision."

Dr. Ayres thinks the combined vitamin therapy may be helpful in treating other chronic skin conditions. "There is room for further investigation. We just see unusual conditions occasionally, and we try different things that seem to work. I don't know how far the vitamin A and E therapy will go. But it's certainly given relief to some."

CHAPTER

100

LOOK TO VITAMINS FOR SHARPER VISION

"Eyes without speaking confess the secrets of the heart," observed St. Jerome about 15 centuries ago. And he was right, as generations of lovers (and liars) can attest. Only in fairly recent times, though, has medicine begun to realize that the eyes reveal other kinds of secrets, as well.

"The eye is an extremely sensitive barometer of faulty diet," says Ben Lane, O.D., a New Jersey optometrist. "When the eye's dimension changes a single millimeter, it makes an enormous difference in vision. Poor nutrition, in the eye, is exquisitely measurable."

The connection between good eyesight and a sound diet—or poor eyesight and a bad one—may not be terribly obvious. But consider this: Helen Keller International, an American voluntary agency working to prevent blindness overseas, has estimated that 250,000 Asian children go blind from malnutrition every year.

Xerophthalmia, the leading cause of child blindness, is brought on by general malnutrition and, particularly, lack of vitamin A. For this reason, the agency has conducted massive efforts to administer vitamin A to children at risk and to encourage their parents to include vitamin A-rich fruits and green leafy vegetables in the youngsters' diets. Fortunately, the disease is now on the retreat worldwide.

Few Americans are in any real danger of losing their eyesight due to diet. But the human eye is a device of such wondrous complexity that it requires a whole smorgasbord of different nutrients to keep all its parts in working order. And shortages of some of them may be more common than you think.

One of the classic signs of vitamin A deficiency, for example, is night blindness. That's because in dim light the remarkable process we call seeing—actually chemical changes turning to electrical impulses turning to mental pictures—requires, at one point, a light-sensitive pigment known as rhodopsin, or visual purple. And the primary source of rhodopsin is vitamin A.

When a Florida optometrist randomly tested 100 patients for night vision, 26 of them failed some portion of the test. As optometrists, "we have been content with measuring our patients' ability to see only under daylight conditions," he observed, "and overlooking the possibility that as many as one in four may become visually impaired when the sun goes down."

Actually, the link between vitamin A and night blindess is hardly a fresh revelation. Way back in the sixteenth century, a Dutch poet noted, "He who cannot see at night / Must eat the liver of the goat. / Then he see all right." Liver, of course, is a rich source of vitamin A. But it's also a good source of many other nutrients, which may have had something to do with the effectiveness of the poet's prescription.

Zinc Helps Vitamin A Help You See

One of those nutrients, it now appears, is the dietary mineral zinc. In a recent study at Johns Hopkins Hospital and the University of Maryland school of medicine, in Baltimore, researchers demonstrated that both vitamin A and zinc are key ingredients in the chemistry of night vision.

The study involved 11 patients suffering from a type of cirrhosis of the liver not caused by drinking. In 9 of the patients, the researchers found blood serum vitamin A deficiencies along with poor night vision; 4 of them were also low in zinc. Seven of the 9 were treated with oral vitamin A (25,000 to 50,000 international units daily) for 4 to 12 weeks.

(One patient died of liver failure before the treatment was completed; another didn't return for follow-up studies.)

All seven patients who completed the course of treatment showed normal serum vitamin A levels at the end of the study. But in three of these patients, normalization of serum vitamin A didn't fully correct their poor night vision. After it was discovered that these three were also zinc deficient, oral zinc supplementation brought their night vision back to normal.

"Zinc," the researchers explain, "is important in conversion of vitamin A to its active form, retinaldehyde, in the retina. . . . Thus, despite a normal serum vitamin A level, impaired dark adaptation can result from inadequate synthesis of retinaldehyde from vitamin A due to zinc deficiency" (*Hepatology*, vol. 1, no. 4, 1981).

Vegetables for Vision

But zinc and vitamin A aren't the only nutrients that can affect your vision, by night or by day. A researcher at Johns Hopkins Hospital, David L. Knox, M.D., associate professor of ophthalmology, has been exploring the effects of folate, vitamin B_{12} and other nutrients on an unusual eye problem called *nutritional amblyopia*.

He told us, "I've been studying the possibility that folic acid [folate] or some other unknown vitamin from green and yellow vegetables may be essential to the maintenance of normal vision and optic nerve funtion." It is, he says, "extremely important for people to eat enough green and yellow vegetables to maintain normal vision."

Some food additives, particularly monosodium glutamate (MSG), may have a less than wholesome effect on the eye, according to John Olney, M.D., Professor of psychiatry and neuropathology at Washington University, in St. Louis. Glutamate is a naturally occurring substance that is harmless when it's part of a protein molecule, he told us. But when it's added to commercial foods in large amounts (as a flavor enhancer), it may damage nerves in the retina and parts of the brain by "exciting them to death."

Though Dr. Olney's animal studies have involved the ingestion of massive doses of MSG, well beyond the amounts the average adult would ingest, he told us, "I would definitely go out of my way to avoid feeding MSG to children." While adults have well-developed barriers to the toxic effects of glutamate, he explained, a child's system is less fully developed and thus more vulnerable to visual and brain-cell damage.

Ordinary nearsightedness (myopia), a problem so common that nearly one in three Americans wears lenses to correct for it, is another eye condition that may have a dietary link. Though the old theory that eye-focusing strain causes myopia still seems to hold up, Dr. Ben Lane has data that indicate poor diet may worsen its effects. In particular, he reports in one study, people with increasing myopia statistically eat too much sugar and flesh protein, are deficient in chromium and do not metabolize calcium properly (*Documenta Ophthalmologica*, vol. 28, 1981). "The wealth of new nutrition studies relating to vision is staggering," Dr. Lane adds.

Vitamin E as Protector

Among those studies are a considerable number exploring the effects of vitamin E, or the lack of it, on the health of the eye. W. Gerald Robison, Jr., Ph.D., chief of the experimental anatomy section, laboratory of vision research of the National Eye Institute, has been examining the effects on animal retinas of diets deficient in vitamins E and A. Results? "A highly E-deficient animal will go blind in time," he told us.

Although he cautions that his work so far has been with animals only, and that it's unlikely a human would develop vitamin E deficiencies as extreme as those he's produced in the lab, Dr. Robison's studies have produced some intriguing clues into the nourishment of the eye.

The retina is a sheet of nerve cells at the back of the eye that changes light (via chemistry) into electrical impulses, the language of the nervous system. The cells it's made of, Dr. Robison explains, especially the light-sensitive or photoreceptor nerve cells—the things we see with—contain large amounts of unsaturated fatty acids. Because these fatty acids are readily oxidized (broken down by oxygen, or "rusted out") "we can suspect that the retina is quite susceptible to oxidation unless it's protected by an antioxidant," he says.

Because vitamin E is a potent antioxidant, or protective agent against organic "rust," Dr. Robison decided to test the effect of a grossly E-deficient diet on the retinas of rats. He also tested the effects of diets deficient in *both* vitamin E and vitamin A.

After five months, he told us, a diet low in E but adequate in A "produced a significant degeneration of photoreceptor cells and an accumulation of aging pigments [highly oxidized, insoluble fatty acids] that was five times greater than normal." Because the visual cells were damaged but not killed, he says, "the damage may be reversible." A diet deficient in both A and E, on the other hand, resulted in the permanent destruction of nearly half the visual cells in eight months. "Vitamin A," he concludes, "appears to protect against this cell loss."

In another study, at Cornell University, dogs fed diets deficient only in vitamin A were also found to develop retinopathy, or damaged retinas. The damage first showed up on the retina after as little as three months. Next came night blindness and finally "severe day visual impairment" (*American Journal of Veterinary Research,* January, 1981).

Help for Cataracts?

The possibility that vitamin E may also help prevent cataracts in diabetics, one of the groups most likely to develop them, is currently under study in a Canadian laboratory. A cataract—a clouding or opacity of the eye's crystalline lens—can result in partial or total blindness.

But John Trevithick, Ph.D., professor of biochemistry at the University of Western Ontario, has shown that massive doses of vitamin E may prevent the formation of cataracts in rat lenses. Five years ago, he and his co-workers began their studies by placing rat lenses in test tubes containing a high glucose concentration, to simulate the conditions in a diabetic's body. Vitamin E appeared to prevent the formation of cataracts in those lenses.

Then, in live rats who had been artifically induced to develop diabetes, vitamin E was also shown to protect against cataract formation. Rats not given vitamin E always developed cataracts; those given vitamin E did not. However, these results were obtained only with injections of E in extremely large amounts.

Dr. Trevithick told us he has administered vitamin E orally to animals in equally large amounts. The oral administration, he found, results in serum levels approximately three times higher than normal, and "the preliminary evidence is that vitamin E can almost totally prevent cataracts in diabetic rats."

What's more, in preliminary experiments with rat lenses in test tubes (known as *in vitro* studies), Dr. Trevithick has been able to partially reverse existing cataracts with vitamin E, rather than merely prevent their formation. Does the same thing work in live animals *(in vivo)?* "So far, our preliminary in vivo work does seem to confirm the in vitro work in some respects," he told us.

Though much about cataracts remains a mystery—no "cure" is known, so thousands of cataract-removal operations are performed each year—one study may shed some light on their development.

As part of a national health program in Australia, doctors examined the eyes of over 100,000 people from remote rural areas scattered all across the country. By comparing the incidence of cataracts with zones of average daily sunshine (ultraviolet radiation) the examiners were able to demonstrate convincingly that "cataract develops earlier in life and also has more severe visual consequences in areas of high UV [ultraviolet] radiation" (*Lancet,* December 5, 1981). This was especially true of the aborigines, apparently because they spend most of their lives outdoors or under inadequate shelter in the bright sun.

The researchers pointed out that UV light has been shown to produce a clouding of the lens in other studies but that this effect "is inhibited by physiological levels of ascorbate [vitamin C] and glutathione [a substance that carries oxygen]." This, they added, "provides an enticing clue to the specific function of these two substances in the lens."

In research labs around the country, medical detectives are on the trail of many an enticing clue to the mysteries of sight. In the meantime, while we await the final unraveling, we'd do well to think of our eyes as we do the rest of our bodies— marvelous, irreplaceable and happiest when they're well fed.

CHAPTER

101

AVOID LOW-LEVEL VITAMIN DEFICIENCY

For years, the elderly gentleman had been leading the sort of life Ebenezer Scrooge would have found delightful. A lifelong bachelor, he lived alone and took all his meals alone in restaurants. He despised fruits and vegetables. Instead, his diet consisted almost entirely of fried eggs, bread and boiled potatoes, a suitably cheap, unappetizing, Scrooge-style bill of fare.

He was 83 when his gloomy habits began to produce alarming side effects: His chronic exhaustion reached the point where he became breathless with the least exertion, and his legs had become painfully swollen and covered with discolored, purplish spots. Dismayed, he sought medical help at the Thomas Jefferson University hospital in Philadelphia.

The examining physicians found a weak, toothless, apathetic old man who showed many of the signs of scurvy, the vitamin C-deficiency disease that was once a killer of epidemic proportions but today is relatively rare. Still, the doctors reported later, even though full-blown scurvy is uncommon, at least one study has shown that some 40 percent of elderly people admitted to hospitals have subnormal body levels of vitamin C. And the old man's dreadful eating habits made it seem all the more likely.

But the doctors were perplexed. At one point, they almost abandoned their diagnosis of scurvy because several symptoms so common they're considered hallmarks of the disease just weren't there. For example, swollen, scaly, raised areas around the hair follicles with coiled or looped hair shafts, surrounded by a red halo of inflammation, are among the most well-recognized symptoms of advanced vitamin C deficiency. But this triad of signs was absent in the bachelor's case, as were bleeding gums and frequent nosebleeds.

Yet, laboratory tests confirmed the doctors' original suspicions. The man was started on 250 milligrams of vitamin C daily, and later on iron, folate (folic acid) and vitamin B_{12} supplements. Within four days, the swelling had gone down and the purplish patches were beginning to fade. After eight days, they'd vanished and the old gentleman was discharged "in good spirits . . . feeling quite well and free of fatigue" (*International Journal of Dermatology,* May, 1982).

The lesson to be learned from his case, the doctors advised their colleagues, was that "physicians should suspect scurvy in patients who present with ecchymoses [purple spots] and painful swelling of the lower extremities. Absence of swollen, bleeding gums . . . congested follicles, coiled hairs, and perifollicular hemorrhages [red inflammations around the follicles] should not dissuade one from the diagnosis of scurvy."

That the bachelor's nutritional deficiencies showed up *without* some of the classic signs may not be all that unusual. "Roger J. Williams [the pioneering nutrition researcher] speaks of metabolic differences among individuals of up to a thousand times— so, certainly, there are also great differences among individuals in the way they show deficiencies," says John Gaul, D.O., Ph.D., an osteopathic physician in Davie, Florida.

Just as there is variation of faces in a crowd, each of us has our personalized version of what it means to be healthy—or to be sick. We may show symptoms of nutritional shortcomings in the known, expected ways—or we may not.

One problem with identifying deficits of specific nutrients is that, at least in the early stages, the symptoms all tend to look the same. "Fatigue, malaise, insomnia, susceptibility to colds, bleeding gums, just a poor feeling in general—most deficiencies tend to produce those symptoms," Edward O. Shaner, D.D.S., a preventive-dentistry specialist, told us.

It's also important to remember that, in real life, deficiencies of a single nutrient, all by itself, rarely occur. "Every one of the 40 or more nutrients is related to every other one," explains W. Marshall Ringsdorf, Jr., D.M.D., of the University of Alabama school of dentistry. "So it's almost impossible to develop an isolated, single deficit, especially among the B vitamins."

It's also rare (at least in this country) for a physician to be faced with a bona fide case of deficiency disease like scurvy or pellagra, Dr. Ringsdorf told us. "If scurvy is a condition in which the body is 100 percent free of vitamin C, then we see cases of 30 and 40 percent depletion—just enough for subclinical problems to appear. We deal in shades of gray."

Still, taking all those qualifiers into account, there *are* certain telltale signs to point to deficits of specific nutrients, Dr. Gaul told us. Among the most common are gum disease, "the number one reason why people lose their teeth," associated with vitamin C deficiency; night-vision deficiency, linked to lack of vitamin A; chilosis, or cracking around the corners of the mouth, and swelling of the ankles in women taking oral contraceptives, both tied to vitamin B_6 deficiency; poor wound healing, in zinc deficiency; and brittle, breakage-prone bones due to a loss of calcium from the bones.

Nutritional shortcomings may manifest themselves in other ways, as well—some common, some not so common. Here are a few of them.

The Philadelphia doctors may have better understood the elderly bachelor's case if they'd seen the results of a study conducted at the Iowa State Penitentiary, in which clinical scurvy was induced in five inmates. The five men, ranging in age from 26 to 52, agreed to consume a diet totally free of vitamin C for as long as it took to produce genuine scurvy, while researchers made careful note of the changes that took place as the inmates' health began to fail. It took the men from 84 to 97 days on the C-free diet to reach full-blown scurvy.

The first signs the researchers noted were psychological: The inmates became increasingly depressed, withdrawn and (ironically) neurotically concerned about their health. They also reported feeling tired, weak and listless. "These changes are characteristic of individuals who are physically ill, as the subjects were," the doctors noted.

Then came the parade of physical symptoms, which made their debut in one man on the 29th day. Tiny, pinpoint, purplish spots called petechiae, caused by bleeding under the skin, were the first symptoms to show up (though they never did appear in one of the men). Larger purplish patches on the legs came next. Then came coiled hairs (in two of the inmates) and congested hair follicles (in all five). Other symptoms included swollen, bleeding gums, shortness of breath, swelling and pain in the joints, edema (water retention) and muscular aches and pains— though, once again many of these symptoms appeared in some men and not in others (*American Journal of Clinical Nutrition*).

Vitamin A Problems

The classic sign of vitamin A deficiency is night blindness— when you see poorly or not at all in dim light and your eyes are slow to adjust from brightness to dimness, as when you step into a darkened movie theater.

But your eyes aren't the only place an A shortage can show up. A condition called hyperkeratosis, or dry, scaly skin, has been linked to vitamin A deficiency, and forms of vitamin A are being used with great success in the treatment of acne. The chronic fatigue of anemia can also sometimes be traced to vitamin A deficits because, even if your iron levels are up to par, vitamin A is needed to help your body make use of the iron.

Unhealthy teeth and gums, stomach upsets and increased susceptibility to infection of the respiratory, intestinal and urinary tracts, as well as the mucous membranes, can also point to vitamin A deficiency. It's even been reported that low vitamin A may be a "significant factor" in middle-ear inflammation, called otitis media, which usually occurs in infants or young children after an upper respiratory infection (*Western Journal of Medicine,* vol. 133, no. 4, 1980).

Vitamin B Problems

Although pellagra, the niacin-deficiency disease, is almost unheard of in Western countries today, we've learned a lot from the days when it was frightfully common among the rural, Southern poor and in prisons. A quartet of symptoms, known as "the four Ds," tended to follow one another in this order: dermatitis in areas exposed to the sun, diarrhea, dementia and then death.

Today niacin deficiencies don't usually progress much beyond the early stages, but they can be very unpleasant just the same. Canadian doctors have described dermatitis caused by marginal niacin deficiency: It begins with a burning redness and puffiness in areas exposed to the sun, heat or friction, most often on the backs of the hands but sometimes the backs of the feet, arms or legs. Sometimes a "necklace" of irritated skin, which turns a scaly, reddish purple in time, appears on the front of the neck *(Canadian Medical Association Journal).*

More advanced niacin deficits can produce the personality changes formerly known as dementia, including depression, apathy, confusion, suspicion and hostility. In fact, writes Canadian researcher Abram Hoffer, Ph.D., M.D., "For many years it was debated whether subclinical pellagra should be classified among the neuroses. Just as fully developed pellagra resembles a number of psychoses, so does subclinical pellagra resemble any one of the typical neuroses." With colleague Humphry Osmond, D.P.M., Dr. Hoffer has pioneered in the use of forms of niacin in the treatment of schizophrenia.

A Lack of Thiamine

Complaining of severe shortness of breath that had steadily worsened over the preceding 30 hours, a 40-year-old Kansas City, Kansas, man was admitted to the Veterans Administration Medical Center there. His hands, feet and the area around his mouth had turned blue, his heart was racing and his blood pressure had fallen dramatically. The doctors who treated him learning that he was a heavy beer drinker, made a shrewd diagnosis and injected the B vitamin thiamine.

His blood pressure began rising almost immediately, and he eventually completely recovered *(Chest).*

The man was a victim of what the doctors called "acute pernicious beri-beri heart disease," caused by chronic thiamine deficiency due to drinking. Over the long haul, thiamine shortages can cause a weakening of the heart muscle and, eventually, cardiac failure.

Deficiencies also show up in the gastrointestinal system, in the form of indigestion, severe constipation and loss of appetite, and—worst of all—in the central nervous system. Problems may develop in the peripheral nerves—such as a tingling or burning sensation in the toes, burning feet (especially at night), sore calf muscles and even irritability, depression and confusion.

Quite similar symptoms have been attributed to deficiencies of vitamin B_{12}: unsteady gait, lack of coordination and a burning, tingling ache in the feet and legs, more pronounced in the feet at night and in the legs by day. An electric-shock-like sensation when the neck is bent, called Lhermitte's sign, may also be caused by B_{12} deficiency, which does its damage, like an absence of thiamine, by affecting the central nervous system.

Precisely how a deficiency will manifest itself in your body is, at least to a certain degree, an individual matter.

But by taking care to eat right and stay fit, you can spare yourself the pain of finding that out.

BOOK IV

The
Nutritional
Healers

INTRODUCTION

There are plenty of specialists around. In fact, when you're being shuttled from doc to doc—the kidney man doesn't know a whit about your bones, and the bone man thinks you need an appointment with a neurologist—it seems like there are too many. But even with a specialist on every block, where do you go when you want to see a doctor who's an expert on your medical problem *and* a specialist in that all-important field most doctors ignore: the drugless therapy of *nutrition?* Well, that doctor has office hours in book 4: The Nutritional Healers.

In the pages that follow, you'll be able to consult with experts in various health fields—but experts who also realize the *prime* importance of proper diet and nutritional supplements. A pediatrician will tell you how kids with learning disabilities can be helped with food supplements. An eye doctor will describe his vitamin recipe for better vision. You'll meet a pharmacist who advises patients on which vitamins to take to mute the side effects of prescription drugs; a psychologist who uses nutrition to relieve stress. In all, two dozen doctors and health professionals share with you their tips for a healthier, happier life. So turn the page—the doctor is in!

CHAPTER

102

MUFFLE THOSE BELLS IN YOUR EARS

A 53-year-old auto mechanic has been totally deaf for 20 years. Yet, he still suffers from loud buzzing in his ears—sometimes as loud as a chain saw. The noise is so annoying that he can't relax or sleep. He has consulted several ear specialists, but they could offer him no hope of a cure. "Try to live with it" was their advice. But often he feels so frustrated and anxious that life scarcely seems worth living.

Over 7 million Americans suffer from the auto mechanic's problem, while over 36 million more suffer from it in a less severe form. It's called tinnitus: ringing, hissing, buzzing or roaring in the ears. You don't have to be deaf to have it; most tinnitus sufferers aren't. In fact, everybody has probably suffered from a temporary form of tinnitus—when, for example, you've stood too close to a gunshot or a backfire or banged your head on a low-hanging plant, and usually it's no big deal. But for those who suffer from tinnitus for prolonged periods, it can be anything from a persistent annoyance to an unbearable affliction.

The fact that most doctors can suggest only that the majority of tinnitus sufferers try to live with their problem doesn't help. Though ear specialists have tried various treatments for tinnitus, including surgery and drugs, they have had few successes. Even *tinnitus maskers,* hearing-aid-like devices that drown out the noise with other sounds, only cover up the symptom without helping the underlying problem. And tinnitus is always a symptom of an underlying hearing disorder, which often leads to some form of hearing loss.

But now a new approach, developed in the last six years, offers hope to tinnitus sufferers. Paul Yanick, Jr., Ph.D., a clinical audiologist and adjunct assistant professor at Monmouth College in New Jersey, believes that tinnitus, as well as many other hearing problems, can be traced to metabolic disturbances. And in partnership with several physicians, he has developed this theory into a successful clinical therapy.

For instance, the auto mechanic we mentioned was eventually referred to Dr. Yanick. Dr. Yanick began with a battery of very precise hearing and metabolic tests that are the first step in his holistic approach. "It's important," he told us, "that the tests be precise enough to detect each patient's special hearing difficulty and metabolic makeup. Everybody is a biochemical individual, and both hearing and metabolic problems vary critically in each person. Neglecting to take account of that individuality easily leads to misdiagnosis."

The mechanic's deafness was so profound that Dr. Yanick had to communicate with him through written messages. Examination revealed that he had hypoglycemia—a condition of abnormally low concentration of sugar in the blood—and suffered from a variety of vitamin and trace mineral deficiencies.

Hypoglycemia a Culprit

Hypoglycemia, Dr. Yanick is convinced, is the most commonly underrated cause of tinnitus and other hearing problems, including the progressive deafness that the mechanic also suffered from.

"A diet high in refined carbohydrates raises the blood sugar level too high and too fast," he explains. "The pancreas overreacts to these dangerously high sugar levels by producing too much insulin. Then the insulin drops the sugar level down too low and too fast. Since the inner ear has the highest energy requirement of any organ in the body, the drop in blood sugar puts a lot of stress on it. Finally, the body's stress reaction floods the system with adrenaline, which constricts the highly sensitive vascular network in the ears—this is often what causes the ringing of tinnitus. As a result, the ear is starved of energy and oxygen and can't get the nutrients it needs to function.''

So the next step was to remove from the mechanic's diet all refined, processed and chemically treated foods and to take him off cigarettes and caffeine. The man was also placed on a natural high-protein diet with supplements of vitamin A and B complex (three times daily) as well as zinc and chromium.

"Hearing improvements with vitamin A are well documented," Dr. Yanick told us. "A laboratory study on animals found ten times more vitamin A in the inner ear than in other tissues of the body. Probably all sensory receptor cells, such as those in the inner ear, are functionally dependent on vitamin A. The B vitamins, too, are important for nerve functions. And they also play a major part in glucose metabolism."

The results were dramatic. Although there is little hope of recovery after 20 years of deafness, within only a month and a half the elated mechanic showed a 30 percent improvement of hearing and no tinnitus. And since then, he has had continued improvement of hearing.

Not surprisingly, Dr. Yanick's approach has been effective also in less severe cases of tinnitus.

Dr. Yanick told us of a 33-year-old contractor who consulted him about fluctuating tinnitus, a variety that seems to come and go. The ringing was worst in the quiet of the night. Soon its distraction and his worrying made it difficult for the man to sleep. He resorted to drugs—aspirin at first and then Valium. But the tinnitus remained. Hearing tests revealed that the contractor was already suffering from a slight, undetected hearing loss. Observation and questioning further revealed that the hearing loss, which was not evident to the patient, put great strain on him in social situations. "The person with a hearing problem," Dr. Yanick explained, "is under great stress. He's concentrating, trying to grasp every word."

Dr. Yanick further discovered that, in the course of his patient's work as a contractor, he was sometimes exposed to loud noises.

Metabolic and biochemical tests revealed that the contractor was hypoglycemic and deficient in magnesium, chromium and especially zinc.

First: A Pair of Ear Plugs

The first thing Dr. Yanick did was to prescribe a pair of ear plugs. "Exposure to loud noise is dangerous," he explains. "It constricts the blood vessels in the inner ear and deprives it of oxygen and essential nutrients." Then Dr. Yanick equipped his patient with a carefully fitted hearing aid. By correcting his slight hearing loss, this immediately relieved much of the stress he felt in social situations. "And," Dr. Yanick pointed out, "better hearing can itself drown out moderate tinnitus."

The patient's nutritional problems were also tackled. Dietary reforms were suggested, as well as a program of fast walking. Proper exercise makes the heart and blood vessels more efficient, helping to provide enough nourishment for the ear.

After two months of treatment, the contractor showed a 20 percent improvement of hearing and no more tinnitus. He was now also able to get on happily without tranquilizers and sleeping pills.

He Reversed His Own Hearing Loss

Dr. Yanick told us about another successful case: himself. At 19, doctors told him he was going deaf. Six years later, he couldn't hear people talking across a room. His case, he was told, was hopeless, but refusing to give up, he traveled the country to consult with leading endocrinologists and internists. Learning that he was hypoglycemic, he started to improvise the treatment he now shares successfully with others. At 30, Dr. Yanick has halted the progression of his deafness and improved his hearing.

Dr. Yanick started to develop his theory that tinnitus and other hearing problems are caused by metabolic imbalances in 1974, when he and E. J. Gosselin, M.D., studied the metabolism of 90 patients with hearing loss. They found an extremely high correlation between metabolic and hearing disorders *(Journal of the American Audiology Society)*.

Hypoglycemia isn't the only metabolic abnormality related to hearing problems; high blood levels of fat are, also. "High blood levels of fats," Dr. Yanick explains, "cause red blood cells to stick together, reducing the flow of oxygen to the inner ear. When tests reveal that a patient has this problem, we recommend supplements of lecithin, iron and potassium, along with a diet high in grains, fruits and vegetables. That regimen has been very helpful in lowering fat levels and increasing the supply of oxygen."

Stress-reducing techniques (such as exercise, meditation and biofeedback) and a hearing aid that is scientifically tuned to deliver maximum clarity and comfort are also important in Dr. Yanick's holistic program.

"For some people, tinnitus gets louder just by worrying about it," Dr. Yanick says. "Stress is both a cause as well as a result of metabolic disturbances and plays a major part in hearing problems, especially tinnitus. I've found that, with my patients, fast walking or jogging usually helps to relieve ordinary stress."

Diet, nutrition, exercise, relaxation. "It's obvious that the ear is part of the body," Dr. Yanick concludes, "and it makes no sense to treat hearing problems in isolation from the body's general well-being."

CHIROPRACTOR

CHAPTER

103

DR. HATFIELD-McCOY

When we heard about Milton Fried, M.D., D.C., we didn't know much about him other than the fact that he was both a medical doctor and a chiropractor.

But that was enough to arouse our curiosity. We knew there was no love lost between the M.D.s and the chiropractors. Medical doctors charge that "chiropractic theory has about the same medical validity as voodoo or witchcraft" (*At Your Own Risk: The Case against Chiropractic,* Trident Press, 1969). Chiropractors fire back that "the American Medical Association is an extremist organization that is attempting to use political power to maintain a monopolistic health care situation here in the United States" (*Chiropractic Speaks Out,* Wilk Publishing, 1973).

We wondered how long someone caught in the middle of such caustic rhetoric could survive professionally.

So when we visited Dr. Fried at his busy office in suburban Atlanta, Georgia, we were happy to learn of the emphasis he put on nutrition in his practice and the importance he saw in treating the whole person. But what we wanted to hear about most was what it was like to be the man in the middle.

Question: How does it feel to be both a chiropractor and an M.D.?

Dr. Fried: It's like being a Protestant and a Catholic at the same time in Northern Ireland. The M.D.s love the fact that I'm an M.D., but they don't like the fact that I've been a chiropractor, and the chiropractors love that I've been a chiropractor, but some of them hate the fact that I'm practicing as an M.D. The more things you know how to do, the more chance you have of offending somebody. It's a paradox.

Q: What about your patients?

Dr. Fried: Oh, they love me! At least *someone* does!

Q: Why is there so much animosity between doctors and chiropractors?

Dr. Fried: I think that ignorance and bigotry are things that you find in all walks of life. You find it among some members of the AMA (American Medical Association), and you find it among chiropractors, too. You find the sort of bigotry that's involved in being ignorant of what the other person does and of being afraid of economic competition.

I think that the average chiropractor is a sincere person trying to help sick people, and I think the average M.D. is, too. One of the things I try to do is bridge the gap of trust between the two sides.

Q: How did you get yourself in this strange position?

Dr. Fried: When I finished my bachelor's degree at New York University, I wanted to be a physician, but I didn't think I had enough money, so I got a diploma in physical therapy and rehabilitation. In my work in that field, I began to see patients who were getting really good results by going to chiropractors, and it didn't jibe with anything I knew.

I wanted to learn this art, to use it in my own work. So I went to the Chiropractic Institute of New York, and I became a chiropractor.

I practiced chiropractic for several years, but I still wanted to be an M.D. I wanted to know more. Basically, I considered myself—and I still do—to be a healer who was learning whatever

ways I could to help patients. So I went back to school and I
studied medicine. I graduated from UCLA (University of California at Los Angeles) medical school.

Q: Do you still use chiropractic techniques, like adjustment of the spinal column, in your practice?

Dr. Fried: Yes, but especially I use a lot of the philosophy
that I learned—for example, the idea that the body has the innate
ability to heal itself, given the correct circumstances. That is a
tremendous thing if you really put it to use with patients.

It frees you from the fear of taking on a sick person. Also,
you don't think in terms of treating a disease; you think in terms
of taking care of a human being. It's not just words, it's actually
a different way of practicing that flows from that.

When I see a patient, what I think of is not if I can cure
him, but how to arrange to give him the proper substances and
circumstances so that the innate healing ability of his body can
do its work. I frequently will take on patients who otherwise I'd
be afraid to take on, and they reward me by getting well.

Q: Does your interest in nutrition tie in with that?

Dr. Fried: Absolutely. If there's anything that's the center
of what I do, it's nutrition. Nutrition is the one thing that I
wouldn't want to do without.

If a person is taking a lot of garbage into his body, sooner
or later he's going to be sick, no matter what else you do with
him. Anyone who takes care of people and who observes them,
who really watches them, will come to that conclusion. Anyone
who takes care of any living things knows that what you feed
them has a tremendous effect on them.

To me it seems strange that the orthodox medical profession
doesn't take that much into account. Very strange, actually.

Q: Do you pay much attention to nutrition in your personal
life?

Dr. Fried: Yes, I do. Our family is very conscious of diet,
and I think it's done us a lot of good. There have been times
when we have gone away from that. I've noticed the difference,
and so has my family—what happens to us when we stop taking

our supplements and stop eating properly. We are very health conscious in my family.

As a general rule, we stay away from sugar completely. We try to give the children fruit, nuts and other wholesome snacks, whole grains, and they do very well that way. I'm very proud of them.

Q: Have you ever tried a vegetarian diet?

Dr. Fried: I have and I like it. I personally lean toward vegetarianism myself. I don't think that you must be a vegetarian to be a healthy person, but I feel very good on a vegetarian diet. I can't get my wife to stay on one, though. She doesn't want to, and I don't intend to change wives over it.

Q: Do you eat a lot of raw foods?

Dr. Fried: Yes, we eat a lot of raw vegetables and fruit. Raw things have enzymes in them, and also vitamins, that are destroyed by heat.

One of the exciting things in nutrition, that I'm writing about is an enzyme called superoxide dismutase. It's found in raw vegetables. It helps prevent damage to the cell membrane. It's a very exciting nutritional find and, like all enzymes found in raw food, it is destroyed by heat.

We also take raw milk in our house. We have a dairy in Atlanta that has a certified herd and produces a really good raw milk.

Q: You mentioned food supplements. What supplements do you take?

Dr. Fried: I take brewer's yeast, bone meal, desiccated raw liver. I take vitamin C. I take rutin. I take para-aminobenzoic acid (PABA) and pantothenic acid (pantothenate). I take some kelp. I take some alfalfa. I drink ginseng tea. . . .

Shall I continue?

Q: By all means.

Dr. Fried: I take niacin in a long-acting form. I think niacin is remarkable. The first time I ever took it, I had such a feeling of well-being that I knew I always needed more niacin. It has done me a lot of good.

I also take vitamin B_6. I take a very balanced B complex, but with additional amounts of B_6, niacin, para-aminobenzoic acid and pantothenic acid.

Q: How does your interest in nutrition carry over into your practice? How does it affect the things you do with patients?

Dr. Fried: Well, I practice holistic medicine. I'm interested in using the physical, psychological and nutritional things that are needed for a person to achieve a state of health. I check every person's nutritional and biochemical status, always. I'm always interested in what's going on in their head, what's happening on the job, what's happening at home.

If I have someone come in with high blood pressure, I'm not happy with just giving him a high blood pressure pill. I want to find out what's happening with his boss, with his workers, with his colleagues, with his wife, what he's worried about, what he's doing.

If you have a man who's working two jobs that he hates, coming home after driving an hour through bad traffic, smelling exhaust every day, plopping down in front of a TV set with a six-pack, smoking two packs of cigarettes a day, eating a greasy hamburger for lunch, and then he gets high blood pressure—I think it's the height of idiocy to treat him with an antihypertensive alone.

Q: Could you mention some cases that illustrate this holistic approach?

Dr. Fried: I recently had a little girl who was having seizures despite the fact that she was on very high doses of Dilantin, an antiseizure medication, and a good one. She couldn't talk, she was drooling, and she couldn't pay attention to anything. Her balance was so bad that her father had to carry her into the office.

Among other things, I did a complete neurological workup on her. I checked her for vitamin levels and also for mineral levels. I did a hair and a nail analysis on her.

Now, this little girl, even though she was on Dilantin, had never been given any folic acid (folate). She was extremely low in folic acid. She was very high in copper, very low in zinc, and had a lot of lead in her.

Just by removing the lead, increasing her zinc, decreasing the copper and giving her lots of folic acid, as well as other B-complex vitamins, I had this girl off Dilantin within two months' time. She's walking on her own now. It's very gratifying. In fact, when her parents got her off the Dilantin, they came in here with a big bottle of champagne to celebrate.

I'm not saying that Dilantin should never be used, and I'm certainly not saying take everyone off Dilantin and give them folic acid and zinc. If you take someone off Dilantin right away, you can cause tremendous seizures. The point is that everybody who is given Dilantin should be given extra folic acid, and doctors who prescribe Dilantin should have enough knowledge of nutrition and biochemistry to know that. Unfortunately, some of them don't.

This child was treated basically nutritionally and by keeping in mind the ecologic factors that are involved in medicine.

For example, what toxic substances did she have in her? She had too much copper. She got that from her copper pipes at home and from the fact that she wasn't taking enough zinc. She had a big magnesium shortage, too, incidentally, and we had to get her magnesium up. These are the kinds of things that physicians are going to be doing more and more. They're going to be looking for ecological causes of illnesses.

Q: Do you think the medical profession is prepared to make these changes?

Dr. Fried: I think there should be some very big changes in medical education. Together with medical educators and some other physicians who specialize in nutrition and metabolism, I'm working to set up an American Board of Nutritional Medicine and Metabolism. It's pretty close to being formed. The purpose is going to be to examine and certify people who want to practice as nutritional medical people. We want to certify them so that the public will know that the person has an expertise in what he claims to be doing.

We also want to stimulate the education of physicians along nutritional lines. We'd like to get nutrition into the medical schools as a separate clinical science, so that people can really learn how to take care of patients by using nutrition and clinical biochemistry.

I think medical education has not gotten better over the years. I think it has gotten worse. It has become very narrow. You get people today who are graduating who know a tremendous amount about practically nothing. They're like people with tunnel vision.

That's not an educated person; that is a technician who's ignorant of even the things that his own work accomplishes, except in terms of his own procedures. And that's the fault of the medical schools.

CHAPTER
104

WANTED: A SCIENCE OF OPTIMAL HEALTH

Milton Saunders, Jr., M.D., is a man with a mission. Just don't call him a zealot. What drives him is not his unshakable belief in a given set of principles, but the fact that he doesn't know what to believe. Ask Dr. Saunders a question about nutrition, and the three words you will most likely hear in reply are *I don't know*.

The Virginia Beach, Virginia, dermatologist wants to know, badly, and is in the process of setting up a nutritional research organization, the Optimum Health Foundation, to give us all an education. The first of the foundation's centers is to be established in the Virginia tidewater region, with the possibility of further expansion into California, Texas and Massachusetts.

The nonprofit foundation will be designed to help the patients of participating doctors maintain the best health possible through individualized programs of nutrition and exercise. Research at the foundation's center will attempt to nail down the specific effects of nutritional therapy and find new ways for people to achieve optimal health through nutrition and physical activity.

Question: How do you establish what will produce optimal health in a particular individual?

Dr. Saunders: I don't know the answer to that. That's something that will have to be figured out through the foundation's efforts. Our objective is to be totally scientific about this, and totally specific if we can.

Nutrient levels which may be normal for you and make your system function at its best may be too high or too low for me. The Recommended Dietary Allowances for various nutrients laid down by the government are only the most crude guidelines that can't really tell you much about yourself.

To be able to be totally specific, to be able to meet your needs exactly for each nutrient, is something that will take a lot of time and effort. But it can be achieved, if only we channel the kind of talent and brainpower that took us to the moon toward furthering our own health, preventing disease rather than waiting for it to occur.

Q: How did you get the idea for this kind of research effort?

Dr. Saunders: It started a long time ago, actually, when I was back in dermatology residency. I began to notice that certain diseases that we just couldn't treat with standard medicine seemed to be very amenable to nutritional approaches. I started to use vitamin E in a couple of dermatologic disorders that don't respond to conventional therapy at all. One is called necrobiosis lipoidica diabeticorum.

Q: What does it do?

Dr. Saunders: It causes ulcerative patches on the shins of patients, usually women in their 30s and 40s with a predisposition to diabetes. Standard therapy for this disease is very poor, and the results of allowing it to go forward without check are catastrophic for some of these people.

At one point, out of desperation, I put several patients with necrobiosis on a relatively high dosage of vitamin E. Lo and behold, all but one of the patients in the initial trial got better. I tried the same regimen on patients with rheumatoid nodules, a disorder that occurs when people have rheumatoid arthritis but which, as far as the tissue is concerned, is related to necrobiosis. Again, some of the patients, a smaller percentage, responded to the vitamin E.

My interest was stimulated, and I turned to other dermatologic problems such as hair loss. Some of these cases were obviously nutritional problems, such as women on crash diets who suddenly began to lose their hair three to six months later. Also problems caused by nutritional deprivation due to the fetus' development in the last trimester of pregnancy. Others were a little less obvious, such as the women who were losing hair as a result of birth control pills and subsequent vitamin and mineral deficiencies.

I just sat down and said to myself, "What is needed for hair growth?" Well, I'm not a biochemist, but I had a basic idea that we needed the essential amino acids, we needed some zinc and we needed some vitamin E. I tried this regimen on some of my patients, and blam! They started growing hair.

Q: It is pretty impressive.

Dr. Saunders: Well, for a long time I just went along being satisfied with the fact that I was doing something effective, even though I didn't really understand how or why.

Then an arthritis specialist referred two of his patients to me because they also were suffering from necrobiosis. I put them on my usual vitamin E therapy. Both these patients had been on all kinds of arthritis medications, most of which had significant amounts of potential toxicity and side effects, to say nothing of the expense.

When they came back in about a month, their necrobiosis was somewhat improved, maybe 20 percent or so, but they were ecstatic. I didn't understand why.

One patient said, "Dr. Saunders, can't you see, my hands were crippled before, and now I can move them! I'm off medication; all I'm taking is vitamin E!" Not only was her necrobiosis getting better, but she was essentially cured of the debilitating part of her arthritis.

I convinced these two women, both of whom had responded in the same way, to go off the vitamin E and see what would happen. Both of them called, one in about six days, the other in about ten, and said they were right back where they started. They had constant pain and asked that I allow them to go back to vitamin E. I did and, of course, everything cleared again.

Q: Have the things you've discovered about nutrition caused any changes in the way you live?

Dr. Saunders: Well, I'm still learning things about nutrition and how it affects me personally.

In March of 1978, I was in the hospital with a cardiac problem. I had ventricular arrhythmia, an abnormal beating of the ventricle of the heart. It was the kind of thing where I suddenly realized that nutritionally and physically I was in sad shape. I had been getting fat and sloppy. I'd been drinking a lot. I wasn't an alcoholic, but I was a pretty regular drinker.

I had already begun experimenting with the effects of vitamins on my own health. Now I limited my diet and quit drinking. I began to feel better but not outstandingly better. But when I started jogging, combining good physical activity with the nutritional approaches, I really began to feel like a million bucks.

If you pump nutrients into a person and don't accompany that with physical activity, it's like putting gasoline in a car and having it sit in the driveway. It isn't doing anything. It's when you get the metabolism of the body going that you are able to utilize nutrients to their maximum efficiency.

I now run 2½ miles a day. I have a pulse of 68, a slow, powerful, regular pulse. I'm literally running for my life, if you want to look at it that way.

Q: What nutritional supplements do you need to keep yourself in condition?

Dr. Saunders: The formula I've arrived at is without any real scientific basis. As a matter of fact, I think it's not unlikely that I'm presently way off base, so I'd rather not tout what I do. I will say that when I take multivitamins, minerals and amino acids, as I do regularly, I find that my ability to function, both physically and mentally, is considerably enhanced.

In the last couple of days, I stopped taking everything, for a reason. I wanted to see if there was any difference. I don't want to get into a rut thinking, "It's obvious that this is helping me." Well, this morning my usual 2½ miles felt like 20. I mean it really was tough. It's the first time I've had cramps in ages.

One thing I might mention is the effect of red meat. I've always been a big carnivore. It was nothing for me to sit down and eat a 2-pound steak in one sitting. Afterwards, though, I would always feel a kind of nonspecific malaise. So we've cut back the consumption of red meat in my family to once or twice a week. We eat fish and poultry at other times, and I feel like a different person. It's made a big difference.

Q: How has the medical community reacted to your plans for the foundation?

Dr. Saunders: I think we're beginning to get an awareness in the medical community of the importance of nutrition. There is a growing number of closet nutritionists out there, doctors who use nutrition but don't make a big noise about what they're doing. I talked to a fellow the other day who's an ophthalmologist. He was telling me how you can't find salt, sugar or sweets of any kind in his house. His wife makes their bread, and makes it with unrefined flour. They make sure they get their supplements.

So I said, "Gee, that's great. Have you been spreading the word?"

"Oh, no!" he said. "You're the only one I can talk to about this!"

Q: Why wouldn't these doctors want to talk about nutrition?

Dr. Saunders: They're afraid that they'll be laughed at, that they'll be maligned, that they'll be thought of as being weird.

I think the medical profession has failed to recognize that there's a great deal more potential in nutrition than is being tapped. We are suffering today from the effects of having too many wonder drugs, too many "magic bullets." We don't cure disease anymore, the pharmaceutical companies cure it.

As a result, the average physician has not been educated enough in nutrition. It's not any fault of his own but really the fault of the establishment through the years. The magic bullets were there. Why should you have to turn to the prevention of strep throat when all you have to do is shoot the patient up with penicillin?

But I think people are ready for a change. They're almost demanding it. They're just this side of pounding on the doors of the physicians and saying, "Get thee to a nutritional course!"

Q: Other people seem too busy breaking down the doors of their local fast-food outlet to start lobbying for nutrition.

Dr. Saunders: Yes, that's outrageous, really. That's very bad. Here we are, one of the most affluent nations on the face of the earth, and we're nutritionally deficient. We eat gluttonously of the wrong types of things. We eat 125 pounds of sugar a year per capita in the United States. One hundred twenty-five pounds a year—that's a lot of sugar.

It's ironic. We should be the greatest nation in the world in terms of our physical and emotional states, and yet we have high levels of mental and physical illness.

One thing I find disturbing is the possible connection between sugar and learning disabilities in children. When our daughter first started school, we thought she might have minimal brain dysfunction. She was hyperactive and had a very poor ability to concentrate. We put her on Ritalin, and she went through a very difficult period for a while. Her teacher asked us to take her off the medication because it just turned her into a zombi.

Then she suddenly came out of it. We didn't know what had happened. In retrospect, we realized that she had made considerable changes in her diet on her own. She stopped eating sweets and cut down on meats tremendously. We don't know why she made the changes. It was as if something inside her was telling her to do this. That's kind of strange, isn't it?

Q: It is, and fortunate.

Dr. Saunders: I think kids are an important aspect of this fight. Take the fifth and sixth graders in a New York City school who were given a nutritional course and got so turned on they petitioned the school administration to change the diet in their cafeteria. They succeeded, limited the serving of french fries, got more salads, fresh fruits and yogurt all by themselves. It was

Kid Power. If we can reach the kids at an early age like that, we can really make a dent.

Q: Do you think we're making any progress in nutrition?

Dr. Saunders: We're only scratching the surface right now. Just think of the increase in the human resources of our country that would result if we could prevent a significant percentage of the illnesses we suffer. If we could increase the effectiveness of the average person to a point where he is superproductive, where he enjoys life, where his emotional problems are no longer a drain on our society—it's very challenging.

CHAPTER

105

DEATH'S DOOR
OR LIFE'S DOOR?

If most medical schools are ivory towers, then the Johns Hopkins School of Medicine in Baltimore, Maryland, is an ivory fortress. Since its opening in 1893 when, according to the *Encyclopaedia Britannica*, "it set a higher standard for admission than any other medical school in the country," the name *Johns Hopkins* has come to stand not only for medical excellence, but for medical orthodoxy.

So it was with some surprise—and a little hesitation—that Barbara Solomon, M.D., an internist from the Baltimore area, whose approach to medicine is anything but orthodox, found herself speaking to doctors and students of the Johns Hopkins School of Medicine on a subject which the organizer of her lecture, a graduate student at the Johns Hopkins School of Hygiene and Public Health, aptly called "new to the Hopkins community"—nutritional therapy.

"I've been interested in nutrition since I was a child," the energetic Dr. Solomon told the group of over 300 who had gathered for her lecture. "My aunt was a so-called health food faddist. My father was a doctor. And they were in constant debate— my aunt for treating diseases with good diet and supplements, my father for the conventional methods." She paused and added with a smile, "Sometimes it seems as if my whole career has been nothing more than an attempt to find out which one of them was right—but I think my aunt is right about some things."

That career has included earning an M.D. from George Washington University in 1960 and a master's degree in biochemistry from the University of California in 1954. It was her knowledge of biochemistry—and the experience of curing her own migraine headaches through a change in diet—that first led Dr. Solomon to make nutrition the mainstay of her practice.

She Cured Her Own Migraines

"While I was doing my residence at George Washington, I had terrible migraine headaches," Dr. Solomon told her audience. "I would have them three or four times a week. They were really putting a dent in my effectiveness. At the time, I was working with terminal cancer patients, most of whom were nauseated, vomiting and rapidly losing weight. What a situation that was! They were vomiting, I was vomiting. Well, at that time, a friend of mine recommended I take a course in modeling for a change of pace. I took her advice and, after listening to a presentation on diet, thought it would be a good idea to improve mine, especially since it had consisted solely of hospital food for the previous four years. So I followed the same diet as my modeling teacher, who ate only fruits, vegetables, nuts, seeds and fish. I not only stopped eating beef, but gave up poultry, too—for good measure. Within a week, I stopped having migraines! Not only that, whenever I ate beef, they came back. Was I excited—and relieved! Then I had the thought, If eliminating these meats from my diet cured my headaches and nausea, perhaps doing the same to my cancer patients' diets might help rid them of the same symptoms."

Translating that thought into action, Dr. Solomon removed both beef and poultry from the diets of some of her cancer patients. "They stopped feeling nauseated, they stopped vomiting, they started to gain weight. Often they stopped having pain. I was, to say the least, very pleased."

An article by Dr. Solomon in an issue of the *Maryland State Medical Journal* reported similar experiences with three terminal cancer patients.

With two of these patients, however, she eliminated not only beef and poultry from their diets, but *all* solid food. Fed nothing but fresh fruit juices or vegetable juices, the patients quickly stopped vomiting. Dr. Solomon then put them on progressively heartier diets until they could eat—and tolerate—normal meals which offered eggs, cheese, nuts and seafood as main sources of protein.

"The improvement in these patients—and other cancer patients I have treated who are not mentioned in this study—was dramatic. In fact, sometimes their tumors actually regressed. Other doctors couldn't seem to get it into their heads that it was the patients' diet that was causing this to happen. They often insisted that the original diagnosis had been wrong!"

To this day, Dr. Solomon eats no other meat than fish. And at lunch after the lecture, we sat next to Dr. Solomon as she ate a tuna salad—or at least tried to. Between bites, a crowd of medical students, doctors, health professionals and health seekers besieged her with questions about nutrition.

"Is too much vitamin C toxic?"

"My uncle is constipated, should he take bran?"

"Dr. Solomon, is vitamin E good for varicose veins?"

In a rare lull, when the consultation room turned back into a cafeteria, we asked Dr. Solomon if she was always showered with questions about nutrition when she appeared in public.

"Always. Almost everyone knows that diet is important for health, but very few can get specific information about their own diet from a doctor, information they feel safe with. Nutrition is the basic dimension, and I can't see why doctors remain so ignorant about its importance. In fact, most doctors' knowledge of nutrition lags about 20 years behind their knowledge of biochemistry. But even though I treat patients mainly with nutritional therapy, there's nothing I can do for them unless they change their dietary habits—stop eating white sugar and white flour, start taking the nutritional supplements I suggest. The first thing I tell patients when they come into my office is: 'You are responsible for how you feel. If you eat unbalanced meals, you'll feel unbalanced.' "

"Dr. Solomon. . . ?" someone asked.

Luckily, we had a personal interview scheduled that evening.

The First Step to Health

And that evening, over a fish dinner, Dr. Solomon told us more about her use of nutritional therapy in private practice.

"The very first thing I ask every patient is to stop eating refined carbohydrates—white sugar and white flour. Now, most of the people who come to see me have already seen other doctors and have been treated with conventional methods. But they still feel lousy. When I explain to them that their problem— arthritis, diverticulosis, depression, whatever—probably has its basis in many years of wrong eating habits and that the first step in treating their disease is to change the most damaging of these habits—eating sugar—they're usually eager, or at least they *say* they are eager, to modify their diet.

"So they stop eating white flour and white sugar. This change alone makes a big difference in their health. White sugar and white flour burn up vitamins and minerals without replacing them, lower immunity, foul up the digestive tract and complicate diabetes, kidney stones, osteoporosis. Also, they cause fatigue.

"In a week or two, they often experience a decrease in pain and an increase in energy. Then, of course, they cheat. They binge on ice cream or cake or cookies. And the next day, they feel terrible. Headachy. Sluggish. Depressed. It's at this point that they begin to really understand, through their own experience, that they can actually control how they feel by what they eat. And for most of my patients, this is a real revelation, a startling discovery."

Not eating white sugar and white flour is a real boost for those with osteoporosis, a crippler of thousands of elderly women. In osteoporosis, bones lose their strength and mass, and break easily.

"Eating white sugar really steals calcium from the bones, and it's calcium that gives bones their strength," Dr. Solomon told me. "So in addition to getting the sugar out of the diet of those with osteoporosis, I give them a calcium supplement and a trace mineral supplement. Also a multiple vitamin."

Arthritics May Have an Allergy

Arthritis is another bone disease that cripples millions. Dr. Solomon has had striking success relieving the pain of arthritic sufferers by eliminating from their diets not only white sugar, but citrus fruits and eggs, as well.

"There's nothing unusual about this. Over and over again, arthritic patients would come to me and say, 'When I eat oranges, my joint pains are worse.' 'When I eat eggs, my arthritis flares up.' So I've experimented. I always eliminate these foods from the diets of those I see with arthritis. And by and large, they do better. Also, I've heard of quite a few other doctors who are doing the same. It seems obvious to me, on the basis of my experience, that for some reason arthritics are hypersensitive to—that is, they have an 'allergy' to—citrus fruits and eggs."

Along with eliminating fruits and eggs, Dr. Solomon gives arthritics mineral supplements. "Zinc, in particular, relieves bone pain," she said. She also gives a calcium supplement that contains vitamins C and D.

Psoriasis, a skin disease, is another disorder which often yields to dietary restriction. "I have found that my psoriasis patients do much better when I take them off dairy products and anything with gluten in it. That includes wheat, oats, barley and rye."

All doctors treat diabetes at least partly with diet, and Dr. Solomon is no exception. "I give diabetics the conventional diet: no sugar, no honey, no molasses, more protein. I also substitute whole grain bread for white bread. And I give them a supplement of brewer's yeast because it has been shown that diabetics are low in chromium, and brewer's yeast is the best source."

Nutrition and Outlook

Dr. Solomon recommends a daily dose of brewer's yeast as one of the best all-around nutritional supplements.

"It not only contains all the B vitamins but is a cheap source of the important trace minerals, as well, and an excellent source of protein. So you're getting all three things at once."

Dr. Solomon's treatment for patients with heart conditions focuses on lowering their cholesterol and triglyceride levels. "I always prescribe a low-carbohydrate diet for my patients with heart troubles. If they must eat bread, I only allow them to eat whole wheat bread. I also give my heart patients niacin, a B-complex vitamin, because it is a natural vasodilator—it improves circulation. If nutrition doesn't work, then I go to drugs, but only after I've tried nutrition first."

But Dr. Solomon puts another aspect even *before* nutrition.

"I must say that over and above the physical aspects of healing there is the mental aspect—both the attitude of the patient and my attitude. If the patient has a negative attitude toward the possibility of his being healed, or if he dwells on his disease, moping and pouting in self-pity, constantly complaining, then although nutrition will of course help, it will be very difficult for that person to get better.

"Of course," she added with a smile, "I don't have any controlled studies that actually *prove* this, But over and over again I have seen patients with positive attitudes quickly improve while patients with negative attitudes continue to be sick.

"It's really fulfilling to see my patients improve," she continued. "Not *all* of them do, of course. But many, many come back to me after three or six months of eating very little junk and taking supplements and they are, well, *new* people. They're alive again, not just merely living. They have purpose, energy, they are enjoying themselves instead of barely making it.

"So many doctors can do nothing more than keep their patients—if the disease is serious—from death's door and often worsen or simply mask a patient's illness with drugs. But in my practice, people actually become healthy. And that makes my work tremendously enjoyable."

CHAPTER
106

HOW VITAMINS REVOLUTIONIZED MY PRACTICE

by Harvey Walker, Jr., M.D., Ph.D.

During my first ten years in the practice of internal medicine (1957 to 1967), I was very frustrated to discover how many of my patients had health problems for which I had no solutions. Then in 1967, while convalescing after a hernia operation, I read Adelle Davis's book *Let's Get Well,* which was given to me by a friend. After reading the book, nonstop, I realized that, even though I had gone to one of the most prestigious medical schools in the country, the few hours my instructors had spent discussing nutrition were totally inadequate to meet the needs of my patients. From that point on, I vowed to learn everything I could about the rapidly expanding field of nutrition and health.

I began experimenting on myself with vitamins and minerals, particularly the B vitamins, vitamin E, lecithin and vitamin C. I discovered that large doses of the latter helped reduce serious allergy problems which I had been experiencing. As the results became evident and my health and confidence grew, I began recommending nutritional supplements for my patients.

I'd like to share with you some typical case histories that illustrate how vitamins have revolutionized my medical practice.

A number of years ago, my wife, Kay, complained about her hair becoming thinner and thinner. It became so bad that she had to wear a wig for two years. But after several weeks on large doses of every B-complex vitamin known, the hair fall stopped, and her hair became thicker and more manageable.

A 57-year-old chief engineer came to me complaining of severe fatigue. I started him on a B-complex formula containing 10 milligrams of vitamins B_1, B_2, B_6 and para-aminobenzoic acid (PABA); 20 milligrams of niacinamide (a form of niacin); 10 micrograms of biotin; 100 milligrams of calcium pantothenate; 50 micrograms of folic acid (folate); 5 micrograms of vitamin B_{12}; and 500 milligrams of vitamin C. He took two of these tablets four times a day. Within a few days, he called me to complain that he now had so much energy, he was unable to sleep at night! After eliminating his bedtime dose of B complex, this man was able to work hard in the daytime without tiring and still sleep at night.

Vitamin C and Viruses

Since I started emphasizing nutrition in my practice, requests for flu vaccine by my patients have declined markedly. In former days, they would come in and ask for flu shots every fall. More recently, however, they say that, as long as they take 500 to 1,000 milligrams of vitamin C four times a day, they are able to avoid colds, flu and respiratory infections. And they would much rather take the vitamin C than have a flu shot.

I'm convinced that vitamin C is nature's virucide (an agent that kills viruses). When my oldest son was a junior in high school, he had a severe case of infectious mononucleosis which caused him to miss about four weeks of school. Unfortunately, I knew little about nutrition at the time. Later, when his younger sister developed mononucleosis, it was after I had become familiar with the great power for good of megavitamin therapy. I placed her on 1,000 milligrams of vitamin C every two hours, and within one week she was back in school and feeling fine.

A boy of 18 developed infectious hepatitis. Once again, I turned to my newfound ally, vitamin C, prescribing 1,000 milligrams every two hours. Within one week, his liver function tests had returned to normal and he was back on the job. I have not seen remarkable results like this reported in the standard drug-oriented medical literature.

A 58-year-old laborer came to me for help. His job required him to walk at least 3 or 4 miles a day through the factory where he was employed as a maintenance man. He said he was going to have to take a disability retirement because pains in his legs were preventing him from doing his work. I started him on vitamin E, 400 international units four times a day. He was also given lecithin capsules, 1,200 milligrams each, four capsules four times a day. After about a month, he reported his legs had improved so much that he had canceled his application for retirement.

I feel that vitamin E and lecithin make a good pair to be used together. Vitamin E helps to improve blood circulation, while the lecithin seems to solubilize fats in the blood that would otherwise precipitate and form deposits. I have many diabetic patients taking both vitamin E and lecithin who report much better circulation in their lower extremities. If they stop taking those nutrients, their feet get colder and feel less comfortable.

Using Vitamin E to Protect the Heart

Another man in his mid 50s reported terrifying anginal pain in his left chest when he walked uphill into the wind on his way to the local hockey arena. Although he was popping nitroglycerin tablets under his tongue, he still had anginal symptoms severe enough to force him to cancel his season tickets for the hockey games. After a few months on vitamin E, lecithin and other supplements, his chest pain subsided. He no longer needed nitroglycerin and was able to make it to the hockey games without pain. He achieved this result even though he was overweight and smoked heavily.

Incidentally, the use of nitroglycerin among my heart patients has practically ceased. But those who have stopped taking their vitamin E—or reduced the dose—have had a severe recurrence of their problems.

A young mother who consulted me had an enlarged heart and an abnormal electrocardiogram. I sent for the records of her previous health care in various hospitals, and she and I were amazed to discover that her heart problems had been known by doctors for three years, but no one had ever told her about it. Her heart problem was now causing her so much pain and disability that she was admitted to one of our local university teaching hospitals where cardiac catheterization was performed. It was determined that she was suffering from cor pulmonale, which is heart disease caused by lung disease, and that she had less than five years to live. This put her young husband into shock as he contemplated life without his wife and with two preschool children to raise.

It was theorized that, during the four years that this woman had been on the Pill, showers of pulmonary emboli traveled as tiny clots from her legs and pelvis into the arteries of her lungs, clogging many of them and greatly raising the circulatory pressure in her lungs. I placed her on large doses of vitamin E, along with B complex and the other usual supplements, and am very pleased to report that, five years later, her heart and lung function have improved. Yet, the university experts predicted she would be dead by now.

I believe that if all women on the Pill would take 1,200 international units of vitamin E daily, the incidence of complications like heart attack, stroke and thrombophlebitis would be greatly reduced.

Once, when my wife had been sitting at a desk for a long time typing, she got a blood clot in her leg. I sent her home with a bottle of vitamin E, and she was back to work in a couple of days. My experience before with thrombophlebitis was that people were in the hospital for three weeks getting over it.

One of our most tragic cases was a young diabetic girl who was almost blind and came to St. Louis for an eye operation. It was successful, but the doctors at the hospital where she went completely ignored my pleadings to put her on the nutritional regime which she had been on before she went in the hospital, and they sent her home without it. They did not tell me when she was discharged, and her nurse-sister did not realize how vitally important we felt these supplements were. And a week after she was discharged from the hospital—she'd been off her vitamin E then for about three weeks—she had a stroke and has never recovered from it. I think that was preventable, and it's just a tragedy. I think the world is full of tragedies like that.

Of course, vitamin E isn't the whole story in my practice. I've already mentioned the value of the B complex. And for those who have special skin and mucous membrane problems, I've found that vitamin A may be helpful. For those who have difficulty assimilating calcium, extra vitamin D may also be indicated.

The vitamin C dosages I recommend vary from 250 milligrams twice a day for a young child to as much as 1,000 milligrams every one or two hours for an adult battling a severe virus infection or the stress of surgery, burns, fractures or other major trauma. I recommend a routine adult dose of 1,000 milligrams four times a day and believe that, at this level, very few if any virus infections will occur.

I start most adults on 400 international units of vitamin E three times a day. (There is one precaution, however, regarding vitamin E. Those with rheumatic heart disease or high blood pressure should start with 100 units and gradually increase the dosage while watching their heart function and blood pressure levels closely.)

You will probably need more vitamin E if you are taking birth control pills, have had a heart attack, are very sedentary or have severe arteriosclerosis.

During the first ten years, I had some patients die from heart attacks, strokes and postoperative pulmonary emboli. Since all my medical colleagues had similar experiences, I was resigned to accepting those deaths. However, looking back over the last ten years, when most of my patients have been on an adequate nutritional regimen, I have had very few patients die from heart attacks or strokes. I have read that the noted surgeon Alton Ochsner, M.D., used vitamin E in his practice for several decades and reported excellent results with no postoperative blood clots in his patients. I have told my local surgeon friends of Dr. Ochsner's good results, but I cannot get them to try vitamin E. My patients, of course, receive vitamin E before, during and after surgery, and they have had no postoperative blood clots.

I build up all my patients prior to surgery. I give them extra zinc before and after the operation, along with vitamins A and E for better scar healing. Almost every surgeon consultant I have comments to me on how rapidly my patients get well and get out of the hospital and how few complications they have compared with other patients.

A Thorough Exam

In dealing with new patients, I believe that there's no substitute for a very careful, thorough examination and personal-history taking. Each new patient who comes to our St. Louis office first fills in a comprehensive health questionnaire with 1,566 questions. This is then processed by computer. He or she may also complete a computer-processed nutrition and activity questionnaire, which gives the patient a thorough analysis of previous diet with suggestions for improvement. This second questionnaire also analyzes the patient's exercise habits and prescribes additional exercises as needed.

After the questionnaire printouts are back, the patients are examined in the office by me or my associate. We review the quesionnaires with each patient and do a complete physical exam at that time.

Since food allergy is proving much more common than earlier believed, many of our new patients receive a food intolerance test. Many patients also have a hair analysis test, which gives us good guidance in prescribing mineral supplements. It is our goal to have all our patients knowledgeable enough about their own conditions and their own health so that they can take good care of themselves and avoid the need for extra office visits or hospitalization.

But they have to realize that, unlike drugs, natural treatment methods take time—sometimes several months—to produce important results. Since beginning to prescribe vitamins and minerals for my patients, I have observed a lot of remarkable things that I can't explain. I have a lot left to learn, and I probably always will. But practicing medicine has become much more pleasant since I now know that there are simple dietary measures and nutritional supplements that can benefit so many of my patients.

Because the nutritionally oriented practice of medicine is increasingly popular with the public, requests for such services are multiplying. I urge any physician who is interested in joining such a practice to contact me.

CHAPTER
107

MUNG BEANS AND COTTON SWABS

From the cross-legged patient paging through *Good House-keeping* to the proud diplomas displayed next to the nurses' niche, it looks like any other doctor's office.

But this one belongs to Victor L. Pellicano, M.D.—the soft-spoken, Lewiston, New York, internist who carries a bottle of vitamin C instead of a prescription pad in his coat pocket. And it may well be the only M.D.'s office you'll step into where you'll find a jar of mung beans sprouting next to a canister of cotton swabs.

"I'd been preaching the nutritional value of sprouts so often that a couple of my nurses decided to take up sprouting," the slim doctor chuckled warmly during our visit. "Now, when I get hungry for a snack, they whip me up a sort of sprout sandwich on Triscuits, and I have that with a cup of Red Zinger tea. It's just delicious. And, more than that, it's a highly nutritious snack!"

Actually, Dr. Pellicano is the last person you might expect to be expounding on the benefits of sprouts or good nutrition. A long-standing member of the American Medical Association, Dr. Pellicano has also served as president of both the Western New York Heart Association and the Society of Internal Medicine.

"It's true," says the kindly doctor, "I haven't always been geared toward nutrition. Medical school didn't train us in it the way it should have. And, let's face it, most doctors are pretty closed minded when it comes to vitamins and minerals.

"It took my youngest daughter—who was just entering college at the time—to introduce me to nutritional therapy. She asked me what I knew about organic food. I really didn't know too much about it. So she bought me Adelle Davis's book *Let's Eat Right to Keep Fit*. Reading that book set me off on sort of a nutrition hobby. I read more books and attended meetings on nutrition. Gradually, I changed my own dietary habits and began to incorporate nutritional therapy into my medical practice."

Of course, Dr. Pellicano continues to practice conventional medicine. He'll prescribe conventional treatment when it's indicated but, he told us, that's often after he has given nutritional therapy a chance.

"There are many times when conventional therapy is absolutely indicated and when nothing else will do. But there are other times when vitamin therapy works just as well—and better because it doesn't subject the patient to the risk of conventional drugs."

Vitamin C Stops Shingles

"A few years ago, I was visiting my daughter in Albuquerque, New Mexico, and I developed shingles. So I took between 10 and 12 grams [10,000 and 12,000 milligrams] of vitamin C a day. It stopped them almost dead in their tracks. Which really isn't so surprising, since shingles are caused by a type of virus, and vitamin C has already demonstrated itself in a number of viral diseases—including the common cold.

"All my patients who come into the office with symptoms of a cold are told to take 1 gram (1,000 milligrams) of vitamin C every hour for the first day and every other hour for the next few days thereafter. I've found that in most cases the vitamin C reduces the severity of the cold, and most of my patients can get through the course of a cold without the extra boost of an antibiotic.

"I also prescribe vitamin C for my patients with back trouble. They heal faster and their problem doesn't usually come back, as it does in patients who get the same treatment but who do not take vitamin C.

"You see, vitamin C is essential for maintaining collagen, the fibrous connective tissue between the bones. So if you've got disk trouble, it makes sense that vitamin C would help by strengthening the connective tissue in these joints."

You can probably tell by now that Dr. Pellicano is a real believer in the power of vitamin C. How much does he take each day to maintain his good health? Dr. Pellicano smiles as he pulls a bottle of Cs from his coat pocket and pops a jelly-bean-size vitamin C tablet into his mouth. "Each of these tablets contains 1 gram of C, and I take three to five of them every day." That's a far cry from the RDA (Recommended Dietary Allowance).

Preventing Scurvy Isn't Enough

"The trouble with the RDA is that it keeps changing. I think right now it's about 60 milligrams of vitamin C. That much will prevent scurvy, but it won't keep you in good health. When you compare the human body, pound for pound, with the body of an animal capable of synthesizing its own vitamin C, you realize that man would have to take between 5 and 12 grams of vitamin C each day to be on the same level."

And our basic requirement is one thing. What about the need created by outside influences like smoking, drugs and stress? "One cigarette neutralizes 25 milligrams of vitamin C in the body," Dr. Pellicano warns. "So if you're a pack-a-day smoker, you have to take 500 milligrams of C just to break even."

Don't believe those reassurances that if you eat a well-balanced meal you don't need the supplements. "In the first place, 90 percent of the people—especially the doctors—don't know what a well-balanced diet is," charges the Lewiston internist. "It's unfortunate that much of the nutritional information we have comes to us from industry. So, naturally, it's slanted in their direction.

"The reason we don't hear more about the benefits of vitamin C from the medical world is that there's no money in it. Look at the trouble Linus Pauling has run into with his work on vitamin C and cancer. No one is willing to give him financial backing. Yet, his work definitely seems to be leading to something. After all, we know that vitamin C has a beneficial effect on the white blood cells, which are involved in the body's immune mechanism. Apparently, the vitamin helps the white blood cells engulf harmful organisms more readily and render them harmless. And if this is the case, well then, why not help cancer victims? That is, if we accept the theory that cancer is caused by viruses and that persons who are cancer prone have flaws in their immune mechanism."

Good Health Starts with Cutting Out Junk Food

"I know what's right for me and my patients. For one thing, I've cut out all junk food—that includes everything that contains refined flour and sugar. I don't eat much meat anymore, either. Or poultry, for that matter. When I dine out, I try to order vegetarian platters, and if that is impossible, I order fish. And when it comes to fresh produce, I think organic is better. Here in New York State, we have a Natural Food Association which certifies organic produce—that way you can be pretty sure that, when you pay for organic, that's what you're getting.

"In the summer, however, I don't have to rely on those producers. I've got my own little garden in the back yard. It isn't much. But it's amazing how much you can get out of even a small plot such as mine. Tomatoes, peppers, cucumbers, squash. I've even got some Jerusalem artichokes—a patient gave them to me."

And what about vitamin supplements? "I take almost everything. Actually, it varies from day to day. Usually, I try to include brewer's yeast and lecithin in my morning grapefruit juice and crystalline vitamin C in my Tiger's Milk. I also take 3 to 5 grams (3,000 to 5,000 milligrams) of vitamin C each day as well as a multivitamin and mineral tablet, 400 to 800 international units of vitamin E and 25,000 to 50,000 international units of vitamin A."

Is that how he manages to stay so slim and healthy, we asked. "Yes, that and exercise. I do 15 minutes of calisthenics each morning, and then I make it a point to get as much walking into my day as possible. I don't take any elevators. If I have a patient in the cardiac intensive care unit, I run up the seven flights of stairs to see him.

"I know it all pays off," Dr. Pellicano smiles. "I weigh the same now as I did in college."

CHAPTER

108

THE "HEALTHY HOUSEBOAT" IS MAKING WAVES IN NUTRITION

"All aboard!"

Johanna Hall's voice is as clear as the cool waters of the Chesapeake Bay, her tone as warm as the sunshine that bounces off the water's surface and lights up her blond curls. Like a vision out of Mark Twain, she stands on the deck of a white wooden houseboat, beckoning to the 30 or so visitors who are approaching from shore.

Cast her as Huckleberry Finn's mother; the fictional waif would adore her. One thing she would do is feed him well. That's because Mrs. Hall is no ordinary skipper, and this is no ordinary houseboat. She's a teacher, dietetic assistant and nutritional counselor; the houseboat is her office and lecture hall. Twice a month, people crowd the two-story ship's cabin to hear her tell how making a small change in their diets can make a big change in their lives.

She makes it easy for her listeners: The advice is sensible and her step-by-step method is sound; her houseboat is moored in a cove that's an easy 10 minutes from downtown Norfolk, Virginia.

But Mrs. Hall, herself, walked the plank to get where she is now.

Seven years ago, she was a typical Virginia Beach housewife with two kids, a husband and a home to look after. She had never planned on getting a job. But then, her husband Don had never planned on getting hemorrhoids, either.

"What hit us as a misfortune turned out to be a blessing in disguise," she recalls. It was bran—and Mrs. Hall's hobby of reading every new book that comes to her local library—that saved Mr. Hall from the surgeon's knife.

"He came home from the doctor in despair. My husband Don is a big man, but he crumbled like a little boy at the thought of an operation. His hemorrhoids were prolapsed and the doctor scheduled the surgery for three weeks from then.

"It just so happened that I was reading a book called *The Save Your Life Diet* by David Reuben, M.D. (Random House, 1975). The gist of the book is that you can protect yourself from many degenerative diseases by eating a lot of high-fiber foods, especially bran. Normally, I would have thought, 'That's interesting,' and then forgotten all about it a week after I finished the book and took it back to the library. But the book mentioned conditions such as Donny's, and so I figured, 'What have we got to lose by giving it a try?' "

For the next two weeks, Mrs. Hall put bran in nearly everything her family ate: breakfast eggs and cereal, baked goods, casseroles and meat loaf, soup and salad, even juice. Three times each day, she had her husband drink 2 tablespoons of bran in a glass of orange juice: at breakfast, at bedtime "and after work, when I would meet him at the door with a glass of orange juice laced with bran instead of a cocktail!

"I did it partly to humor him," she confides, "to lift his spirits and get him to laugh about his condition. I really never expected it to help.

"A week before he was to undergo surgery, my husband started saying he felt so much better, he thought his hemorrhoids were gone. I didn't believe him; I figured it was just wishful thinking on his part. But he went back to the doctor, and the doctor agreed with him. The doctor called off the surgery and said, 'I don't know what your wife is doing, but tell her to keep doing it.'

"When Don came home and told me that, I was elated. And then I was scared. It was as if I had been handed a marvelous trust, a secret weapon, and I had no idea how to handle it."

So she went back to the library and read every book on diet and health. Then, she came home and purged all her kitchen cabinets of things like white flour and sugar, salt, convenience mixes, hydrogenated fats and oils, cookies and candies, coffee and soda. She replaced them with whole grains, wheat germ and bran, honey and molasses, herbs and spices, brewer's yeast and lecithin granules, fresh and dried fruits and nuts, herb teas and spring water.

Her husband supported her. Her kids did not.

"Danny was five and Michael eight and I had raised them on chocolate chip cookies and soda pop. They craved those things as if they were addicted. In America, we are consuming about 75 pounds of sugar (sucrose) per person per year, and they haven't declared that dangerous. Well, if that isn't dangerous, I don't know what is!"

Mrs. Hall knows what she's talking about when she inveighs against sugar. After getting her own kitchen in order, she enrolled in a degree program in dietetics at Tidewater Community College.

Her studies included a coordinated practice in the kitchen of a local hospital. After graduation, she started teaching nutrition to elementary-grade children at the Virginia Beach Friends School. Meanwhile, a manager at her favorite health foods store told her that the owner was looking for someone to edit a nutrition newsletter and conduct a few seminars in healthy eating. She made quite an impression on the owner, Bill Colonna, and her knowledge made quite an impression on Virginia Beach audiences. When her following grew, he asked her to set up shop on his old family houseboat.

Gaining Energy

During her lectures, she talks openly about her past: "I was the biggest junk-food junky in Virginia Beach. Now, my husband is strong and healthy, my kids don't get cavities anymore and they're better behaved.'' And she herself has lost a sinus condition and several pounds, gaining worlds of energy and the kind of figure that women envy and men admire. She freely admits her age: It's 39. She smiles when people say she doesn't look it.

"Often, they're the same people who say life is too short to deprive yourself, and I say, 'Sure, but don't you want to stay healthy and good looking well into your old age?'

"And besides, who says the foods I eat don't taste good?''

Mrs. Hall lugs pans of delicious, wholesome bread and cookies to her lectures so the audience can sample wholesome treats made from wheat germ and carob, molasses and peanut butter. There's always more than enough, and while her listeners feast, she fills them with helpful tips.

She tells them how to "make your own peanut butter in a blender, using fresh peanuts and a tiny amount of unsaturated vegetable oil, just enough to keep it smooth.''

She also tells them how to shop at the supermarket: "in a U. Go up the dairy and produce aisles that form the perimeter of the store. That way, you'll avoid most of the convenience foods and all their temptations. That way, it's also 'out of sight, out of mind' for the kids,'' she adds. "Did you ever notice how all the cookies, sugary breakfast cereals and soda pop are shelved low? The processed-food industry is wise. But you be wise, too. Learn how to say no.''

She also shows people how to read labels, locating hidden sugar in everything from catsup to canned beans. She uses charts to show how much salt you can easily consume without ever once lifting a shaker, while explaining what salt can do: "Sodium can raise your blood pressure and lead to coronary artery disease. I lost my mother at age 58 from a stroke. I have no doubts that she would be alive today if I knew then what I know now.''

By the time Mrs. Hall is finished talking, her audience is convinced, willing to jump right in and do anything she says. She says, "Take it easy. Don't expect to change years of habits and acquired tastes overnight. I did, but that way is drastic and I don't advise anyone to do it that way.''

Start off by getting rid of white sugar and all store-bought sweets, she tells them. "Introduce whole grains gradually. Start off by substituting half whole wheat in any recipe calling for flour." Going off salt should also be done slowly, by replacing it with herbs and spices. "Be creative. Experiment with new flavors," she tells them. She also suggests they buy a copy of *Confessions of a Sneaky Organic Cook* by Jane Kinderlehrer (Rodale Press, 1971). "The book offers good hints and recipes and is fun to read."

To ease people through the transition, she and other Virginia Beach mothers have formed SNAK. The acronym stands for Sharing Nutrition and Knowledge, and the group is basically a recipe exchange club. Members also discuss common problems and give each other support. Mrs. Hall thinks mothers should consider forming similar groups in their own communities.

Not all SNAK members are quite as fastidious as Mrs. Hall. "It takes time. It's the awareness that counts." She is trying to help people increase their awareness, but sometimes her mission takes a strange turn. Recently, a television news crew came to the houseboat to tape a feature that called for her to be shown throwing out a bag each of white sugar and white flour.

"I hadn't used those items in seven years, so I had to go out and buy them as props for the show," she recalls. "But I saved the receipts and, when the taping was over, I took them right back to the store and got my money back.

"I told the clerk that buying them had been a mistake."

CHAPTER
109

A THOROUGHLY MODERN NUTRITIONIST

She calls herself the Billy Graham of the Parkersburg, West Virginia, nutrition scene. But intelligent and charismatic Rebecca Riales (rhymes with *dials*) is more. She's a thoroughly modern nutritionist. And it didn't take us long to find out why.

No sooner have we settled down to chat in her comfortable professional quarters when confrontation strikes. A registered nurse from the local hospital rushes into her office bemoaning some flap among the hospital dietitians over a peculiar diet ordered for a teenage diabetic. The diet was ordered by Dr. Kenton Harris, Rebecca's physician-husband. But there is no mistaking the architect behind its design. It is Rebecca Riales' work, all right!

A far cry from the long-accepted American Diabetic Association diet, this diet is unusually high in carbohydrates. And, as everyone "knows," diabetics can't tolerate starch.

Or can they?

Rebecca Riales listens calmly. Then—as the nurse's recounting of dietitian opposition winds down—she sighs almost disbelievingly, "Don't they know that every medical study which puts a diabetic on a high-carbohydrate diet finds that the diabetic improves?''

By *carbohydrate,* she explains to us later, she doesn't mean a carte blanche to sugary desserts. On the contrary, she bids her patients to make do on less of that powdery white stuff. What she'd like to see more of on everyone's plate is complex carbohydrates. Beans and potatoes and whole grains. Starch with fiber as opposed to sugar without. To her, the difference is like day and night.

And Rebecca Riales has the know-how to know why. With a master's degree in biological science and a Ph.D. in human nutrition, she boasts a background which neither the American Medical Association nor health food enthusiasts can find fault with.

But as that enthusiastic sparkle in her eye tells you, Rebecca Riales doesn't lean much on laurels of past degrees. Instead, she prides herself on her open-mindedness and on her unquenchable thirst for new scientific information on nutrition. Moreover, with these solid scientific facts and a little friendly persuasion, she's hoping to integrate nutritional biochemistry into the heads of practicing physicians.

One wedge she has in the medical establishment is her husband, Kenton Harris, M.D., a practicing internist with whom she shares an office and clinical practice. Another is her position as an assistant professor at Ohio University where, one morning a week, she teaches nutrition to sophomore medical students.

In fact, the day we visited, Dr. Riales fortified herself with a morning meal of melon, raisin bran muffins and skim milk before embarking on the 45-minute drive across the state line to Ohio University. School had just let out for the summer. But two students who missed the final exam made an appointment to discuss the make-up final.

Interestingly enough, what began with questions like "Did we cover this or that?" and "How much text material are we responsible for?" ended up with probing inquiries on nutritional therapy for actual patients the students were managing in other courses.

One woman brought up the case of a physically active young man with a lactose (milk) intolerance who repeatedly broke bones in his ankles and wrists. The other student inquired about supplements for pregnancy.

Dr. Riales was, of course, eager to discuss nutritional alternatives. But she was careful to point out that her role has certain innate limitations. "Total care is in the hands of the physician. And technically you—not I—are the ones with the authority," she told the two students. "I just want you to be aware of the fact that total medical care is a big, multifaceted endeavor and that nutrition is one of those facets."

From the intent expressions on the students' faces and their interested remarks on nutrition, it was obvious that Dr. Riales had raised the consciousness of these two doctors-to-be.

Heading back to Parkersburg, Dr. Riales talked about the clinical practice which keeps her busy the remaining 4½ days a week. She accepts patients on referral from her husband and other open-minded M.D.s. She then talks to these persons (mostly diabetics and cardiac patients) about how they might alter their diets and perhaps take some vitamin and mineral supplements to improve specific conditions.

"It's more analogous to marriage counseling than a physician's appointment," says Dr. Riales. "I don't just sit behind a desk and say, 'Take this and this and this.' First we must chat. I want to know what the patient is already eating. What he likes and dislikes. Then I try to tailor a more optimal diet around his."

That's a major difference between a typical hospital dietitian and this unusual nutritionist, we found out.

A dietitian merely instructs the patient in standard diets taken from the hospital diet manual or the American Diabetic Association manual, Dr. Riales explained. And by "merely instructs," she means just that. A hospital dietitian has no say in the selection of the diet. It is predetermined by a written order from a physician who, of course, has no academic background in nutrition, in most cases.

But because Rebecca Riales is not affiliated with a hospital, she writes her own diet orders. She gets the lab work and medical histories of a patient and chats with the patient's doctor. Then, utilizing the latest nutritional information, she personalizes a healthful diet to fit the individual's lifestyle.

"I'm very cognizant of the fact that you can't change people very much," she admits. "So I start with the patient's own diet and modify it to its best advantage. I look at it this way: If a person doesn't like milk, what good would it do to write four glasses of milk on his menu? I'd just as soon have him take a calcium supplement—which, incidentally, is another difference between a dietitian and me. A dietitian never prescribes supplements."

But Dr. Riales does—and quite liberally if the need is there. That afternoon, while we played dormouse and listened in on a counseling session with a 61-year-old gent, Dr. Riales recommended dolomite for his nighttime leg cramps, vitamin E for intermittent claudication (leg pain after exertion), vitamin A for poor night vision and vitamin B$_6$ for numbness and tingling sensations in his hands.

"The leg cramps will probably vanish overnight with dolomite, but the intermittent claudication will take longer to remedy," she told him. "Don't get discouraged. Just keep taking the vitamin E. And remember, because vitamin E is an oil-soluble vitamin, it cannot be absorbed by the body unless it's taken with a fatty food—like salad oil, cheese or whole milk. Never on an empty stomach."

She also proposed that he take a good multivitamin and mineral supplement with folate, an extra dose of vitamin C and a course of brewer's yeast every day to offset nutrients missing in his low-calorie diet.

"Vitamins and minerals piggy-back on calories," she advises her patient with motherly concern. "Based on what you filled in on the diet questionnaire I gave you, I think you've gotten yourself into quite a few nutritional deficiencies as a result of your extremely low-calorie diet. Only 800 calories! You can understand why I'm asking you to take these supplements."

The elderly man nods his head and smiles approvingly. Rebecca Riales has won over another patient—not so much because she has taken the time to explain why she is prescribing all those pills, nor because she has given equal time to his minor complaints, but because, by the end of the session, she has tailored a diet around his favorite foods: bread and potatoes.

A little background on the patient we'll call Mr. Samuels: First and foremost, he is a diabetic—has been for more than four years, ever since his third heart attack. He's 5 feet 11 inches tall and weighs 191 pounds. A little on the heavy side.

Mr. Samuels says his biggest problem is weight. "The only time I can lose weight is if I have the flu and don't eat at all," he tells Dr. Riales. "Otherwise, every doggone time I eat something, it goes to weight."

She leans over the desk as if she's about to let him in on a secret. "Are you aware that the high levels of insulin you're taking to control your diabetes are working against you on your weight problem?" she asks. "Insulin's role is to get sugar out of the blood and into the cells that need it for fuel. But if you have more blood sugar than the cells need for fuel after lunch, insulin also helps to convert the extra blood sugar into fat, which is stored for future fuel. So if we can reduce the amount of insulin you take each day by virtue of improving your diet, then it may be possible to help you lose some weight."

And how does Dr. Riales propose that Mr. Samuels improve his diet? By stepping up his carbohydrate intake, of course. Mr. Samuels looks puzzled. "You mean I can lose weight on bread and potatoes?"

Losing Weight on Bread and Potatoes

"People make the unfortunate assumption that a carbohydrate is a carbohydrate when, in fact, there are four very different types of carbohydrates," says Dr. Riales. "There is sugar with and without fiber and there is starch, again, with or without the fiber.

"The rationale used to be that if starch turned to sugar then the diabetic can't have either one," says Dr. Riales. "But the rate at which the complex carbohydrate or starch turns to sugar is very slow—so slow, in fact, that the benefit derived from eating starch is as great as the harm derived from sugar.

"So everything you've ever been told about staying away from sugar still holds. But the diet that I'd like to see you go on has a very high proportion of calories in starch—especially starch with fiber."

With that, Dr. Riales sets off on her favorite spiel—on fiber. "I have this bias that, aside from indolence and inactivity, the biggest single contributor to obesity is eating foods without fiber," she says. "The reason is simple: Fiber fills you up on fewer calories. If you eat a lot of fiber, you won't have room in your diet for fat (which pound for pound or gram for gram is 2¼ times as fattening as carbohydrates), for animal protein (which is innately bound up with fat) or for simple carbohydrates without fiber.

"Besides, medical studies have shown that, all else being equal, the diabetic (whether on insulin or not) has lower blood sugar on a high-fiber diet than he does on a low-fiber diet.

"Unfortunately, between the grain in the field and the white dinner roll you eat is the mill which throws away the fiber. And between the apple on the tree and the juice you drink is the juice-making factory which throws away the fiber. What I'm saying is that you're better off eating whole food—whole grain products (like whole wheat and rye bread) versus refined; whole baked potatoes with their jackets, in place of instant potato flakes; whole fruit instead of fruit juice."

Mr. Samuels cheerfully agrees to the diet—"I should have come to you a long time ago!"

Just as Mr. Samuels leaves, Dr. Harris approaches and entreats his nutritionist-wife to see a patient in his office. Then he turns to me. "Eighty percent of the patients I see have self-inflicted problems," he shakes his head. "If they took care of themselves and ate right, they wouldn't need my help in the first place. Rebecca's gotten me into a lot of good habits. For one thing, we practically never eat meat. She makes delicious vegetarian casseroles. And although I still eat meat occasionally, I don't enjoy it anymore."

With Dr. Riales returned from her impromptu counseling session, we head for home. And home for Rebecca Riales and Kenton Harris is an ultramodern house of natural cedar and glass, situated in the shady midst of an old oak forest—just one more extension of their wholesome life style.

The Little Yeast Study with Big Results

We sink down into a modern sectional next to the baby grand (our clinical nutritionist admits to being a not-bad classical pianist). Her eyes light up. "June 19th was the biggest day of my life, and I've been 6 feet off the ground with excitement ever since," she exclaims. "That's the day I received a letter from Walter Mertz about the results of my little study on brewer's yeast and HDL [high-density lipoprotein] cholesterol."

She plops a large box of clippings from medical journals in my lap. On top is the letter from Dr. Mertz, the prominent chromium researcher and chairman of the USDA's Nutrition Institute.

"Dear Dr. Riales: . . . Thank you so much for your letter and the outstanding results that you reported," Dr. Mertz writes. "To my knowledge you are the first person who has shown a clear-cut dietary effect on HDL. My sincere congratulations."

Before we could read further, Dr. Riales interrupts with a backtracking to the details. For some time, she explained, she had been fascinated by research done on the glucose tolerance factor, or GTF, a chromium-containing compound found in large amounts in brewer's yeast. Convinced of its importance in improving the efficiency of insulin, she prescribed a trial course of brewer's yeast (2 teaspoons or 12 tablets a day) to the majority of her diabetic patients. While some of her patients did not seem to benefit, many did. Their too-high blood sugars came down to normal.

Meanwhile, she had been reading everything she could get her hands on about HDL cholesterol. Total blood cholesterol is made up of three types of globules: low-density lipoprotein (LDL), very-low-density lipoprotein (VLDL) and high-density lipoprotein (HDL). The HDL fraction appears to actually protect against heart disease, so the higher your HDL cholesterol level, the slimmer your risk of heart disease.

Gradually, all this GTF and HDL information began to congeal. Dr. Riales reasoned that, since insulin has important roles in connection with fat metabolism (in addition to sugar metabolism), perhaps something which improves the efficiency of insulin might have beneficial effects on blood fats, too—especially on the most important blood fat fraction, HDL.

"Last January, I persuaded Kent to take a daily dose of brewer's yeast so that I could measure any changes in HDL cholesterol," Rebecca smiles as she glances over toward her hubby on the other side of the room. "His HDL cholesterol levels were high-normal to begin with. But after six weeks on brewer's yeast, they jumped from 50 to 66—higher than any jump anyone else had ever reported. You can imagine my excitement!

"So I enlisted the cooperation of eight physician friends. Believe me, I couldn't have found a more skeptical group, but with a little persuasion they agreed to take yeast for me for six weeks. All but one were healthy, physically active, nonsmoking men between the ages of 35 and 45. The exception was a man of 50 recuperating from a heart attack."

Dr. Riales methodically measured 2 teaspoons of yeast per vial and placed a six-week supply of vials in a shoe box to give to each participant. To boost the morale and motivation of the troops, she added a touch of Rebecca Riales humor on the lid— a cartoon picturing a store front with a sign in the window reading Health Food Store Closed: Due to death of family member at age 106.

All went well. All but one participant completed the study. And all but one of the seven subjects completing the study showed increased HDL levels after six weeks of brewer's yeast supplementation. In fact, HDL cholesterol levels rose an average of 17.6 percent. In one person, the level increased by almost 38 percent!

"Another significant finding from my little yeast study was that, as HDL cholesterol levels rose, total fat in the blood decreased by 10 percent," Rebecca explains. "This just happens to be in perfect harmony with the studies in the literature which suggest that HDL removes fats from the body."

Of course, research aimed at HDL cholesterol-raising treatments is still in its infant stage. Quitting smoking and losing weight seem to be of some benefit. And we know that vigorous exercise can have a very positive effect on this cholesterol fraction. But not everyone is willing to go the route of a marathon runner. We also have some evidence that vitamin C and lecithin may help boost HDL cholesterol. But so far, Rebecca Riales' glowing results boast the most potentially astounding effects.

"Right now, there isn't really a whole lot Kent can tell a patient with low HDL cholesterol," Dr. Riales notes but then adds with a disclosing smile, "except that he's married to me and I tell him this crazy thing about taking brewer's yeast!"

OPHTHALMOLOGIST

CHAPTER

110

YOUR EYES
ARE WINDOWS
TO HEALTH

We're sitting in a modern medical conference room, not far from Peachtree Street in downtown Atlanta. Morgan B. Raiford, M.D., founder and one of the leaders of the Atlanta Eye Clinic and Atlanta Hospital and Medical Center, is explaining—with the help of a globelike plastic model of a human eyeball—some of his findings about nutrition and disease. An independent thinker and dedicated healer, Dr. Raiford has reached some basic fundamentals about the foods we eat that go far beyond the traditional domain of an eye doctor.

Dr. Raiford likes to paraphrase the words of the eminent 19th century British scientist Thomas Henry Huxley: "If everybody thinks alike, nobody's thinking very much."

Question: As an ophthalmologist, your primary interest is the eyes. Yet, your findings have broad implications for all doctors. Why is that?

Dr. Raiford: It's been said, "The eye's a mirror of our soul." Now we can also say, "The eye's a mirror of our physiology." Modern ophthalmology gives us a window through which we can observe the body's inner workings.

For example, the greatest killer, the greatest crippler, and the greatest cause of blindness in this country is atherogenesis—

the clogging up of our blood vessels that causes heart disease. And it's increased tremendously in the last 50 years.

Now, the eye is the only source where we can view the blood vessels directly. Under magnification, we can see these harmful changes taking place in the vessels of the eye long before the classical signs of high blood pressure and coronary heart disease appear.

We can also see inflammations and other problems that may be emulating other organs mirrored in the eye's blood vessels, nerve fibers and connective tissue. You could say that the eye is like our bodies' Yellow Pages, an index of activities elsewhere in the system.

Q: But how do you read those Yellow Pages?

Dr. Raiford: Here at the clinic we've pioneered a technique for taking color photographs of the eye and magnifying them many thousand times. We've taken nearly 100,000 such photos over 14 years. We've also made color video tapes.

Using this technology, about 3,000 different disease entities could be evaluated. This is a whole new era, a whole new ball game in understanding what's going on in the circulatory system.

Q: Where does nutrition enter the picture?

Dr. Raiford: The eye is an extension of the central nervous system, which makes up a total of only 2 percent of our body weight but demands 25 percent of our total nutrition. So the visual pathway requires more fuel input than any other organ system. The photoelectric cells in the eye, for example, do not wear out. They are programmed to last as long as the proper fuel mix is provided.

We have to have the right food ingredients. Those of us who grew up in rural areas know that. We know full well that, if farm crops and livestock are to develop, they must have the right ingredients. Well, human beings are no different.

Q: What happens if they don't?

Dr. Raiford: To understand what can go wrong, let's take a look at the tiny vessels called capillaries that make up 99.99 percent of the body's 60,000 miles of blood vessels. These capillaries are very delicate structures, and they all carry a very tiny negative electric charge. Now, the red blood cells that pass through the capillaries also carry a negative charge—it's a very small electric current, but it's there. So it's just like two little magnets. If we put two negatives together, they'll repel each other. That repulsion helps push the red cells through the capillaries. It makes it easier for the heart to pump blood.

But when we eat junk foods such as refined sugar (which I consider to be the greatest culprit in America today), we throw ourselves out of chemical and electrical balance. The little capillaries gradually lose their negative charge and become neutral or positive. Then the red cells, calcium molecules and other material floating in the bloodstream are attracted to the vessel wall. They adhere to it just like soap on a windowpane.

Gradually, they clog up and block the capillaries. Multiply that process many times over, gradually and quietly through the years, and you'll eventually see atherogenesis throughout the body.

The heart starts pumping harder to overcome all that resistance, and finally it goes into a spasm that we call a heart attack. There's no great mystery to it.

But the important thing is we can detect these changes in the eye in the very early stages. We've seen this literally thousands of times in the human eye, and we have photographs to prove it.

Q: So what we eat can be a critical factor?

Dr. Raiford: Absolutely. And not just in terms of heart disease. People who are excessive sugar eaters during the first 40 years of life are much more prone to develop diabetes. They wear out the pancreas trying to produce enough insulin. It's just like whipping a tired horse.

The human body is just not geared to eat the amounts of sugar that we are eating today. And when we upset our body chemistry, we are going to have to pay the price. It's like trying to drive an automobile 80 miles an hour in a residential area instead of on a raceway. You're going to damage something before you get through.

Nutrition spills over into other areas, as well. Without the proper fuel, for example, our visual reception, interpretation and storage—the whole learning and educational process, in other words—is impaired. So you could say that the total social structure of our nation suffers from inadequate fuel nutrition to the visual pathway.

We must learn how to provide a high-quality fuel mix to our cells if we wish to maintain our tissues and our immunity over the course of a lifetime. To disregard such basics is inviting bankruptcy.

Q: What turned your own efforts in this direction?

Dr. Raiford: In 1955, I heard a lecture by Dr. J. R. Maxfield, a pioneer in nuclear medicine, which really opened my eyes. I realized how limited I had been in my perspective on the health sciences, and I knew that I would have to restructure my entire education. From that day on, I have endeavored to find out why certain things happen at the cellular level.

In some health circles, asking the reason why may make some people uncomfortable. But a sense of inquiry has to be established in life to get anywhere.

Q: So it all comes back to the cell?

Dr. Raiford: All of our 100 trillion body cells have basic similarities, whether they be brain, bone, eye or liver. To function properly, they all need good nutrition.

Q: Can you be more specific?

Dr. Raiford: We're just beginning to realize that collagen, or connective fiber, is a common denominator for practically everything in the body. It's like the steel scaffolding in a large office building that holds everything up. Collagen supports the retina, ligaments, capillaries, everything. It holds the cells together.

Each collagen molecule is made of four different amino acids or building blocks. Let's compare them with four freight cars on a track that are not coupled together yet. In order to link them, we need certain essential cofactors that are not found in the body itself. We have to get these cofactors from our food—nutrition, if you please. These essential cofactors are the couplings that lock those four freight cars together. They're the binding units. Without these cofactors, we fall apart.

Q: Have these cofactors been identified?

Dr. Raiford: Yes. These factors—which are absolutely essential to life—include ascorbate (vitamin C), zinc, magnesium, manganese, copper, iron and vitamin E.

The interesting thing is that, when we get many of our patients off junk foods and increase their intake of cofactors, we see reversals of disease—reversals we can measure in the eye.

Q: Can you give us some examples?

Dr. Raiford: One patient was a schoolteacher who enjoyed her alcohol a little in excess. Her mind had become so dulled, she couldn't carry on her teaching duties. When she came to us, we saw clogged-up blood vessels in the retina. We got her off the alcohol and junk food and started her on high doses of ascorbate and other cofactors. Her blood vessels cleared up. Her memory is all right. She's intellectually alert. And she's gone back to teaching.

Another patient was a pilot, entrusted with testing a new military aircraft that represented billions of dollars of investment. He was under so much stress that his blood pressure went up and he had a blood leak in the eye. That's when he came to us.

We discovered that the stress of his work schedule had undermined his eating habits. He was way out of chemical balance. We got him back in balance, and he's perfect again. His vision is 20/20. He's all right. No problems. Last time I saw him he was a brigadier general.

There are other benefits. We find in our eye surgery that, if we put people on a good nutritional program, they will require fewer sedatives and they will heal faster—especially the elderly.

Q: What specific dietary advice do you give?

Dr. Raiford: You have to treat each person as an individual. But basically, I recommend four things.

First, they have to get rid of junk foods, especially sugar. When my great grandfather practiced medicine in the 1850s, the average American consumed between 15 and 18 pounds of sugar a year. Today, it's more than 100. If we can cut out sugar alone, we've eliminated a tremendous cause of ill health.

Second, I tell people to minimize alcohol consumption. Alcohol is also a sugar, an incomplete sugar.

Third, never use a cooking fat that is solid at room temperature. Vegetable oils are good, but if the same oil is reheated over and over again, it forms little globules of fat, called wax. When the melting point of this wax is higher than body temperature, the globules can make the circulation sluggish and clog up capillaries.

The retina of the eye can also be affected, particularly the macular region where the circulation is rather unique. We get many patients coming to see us with macular degeneration. The tragic thing is that we can't turn back the clock 30 or 40 years; we can only teach them about the proper foods and cooking oils.

The fourth recommendation we make is to increase the intake of nutritional cofactors.

Q: How can we do that?

Dr. Raiford: First of all, you have to eat more fresh fruits and vegetables and whole grains. One of the greatest criminal acts we have in America today is refining flour. Why take out 23 nutrients, put back 2 or 3, and call it enriched? Meanwhile, the food processors sell the nutrient-rich by-products to the cattle and poultry industry to double their profits. That's stupid! We need the whole grains.

We can also learn a lot from our Asian friends and not cook foods to death. The Japanese and Chinese do a beautiful job in food preparation.

Q: Do you ever recommend food supplements?

Dr. Raiford: Many times we have to. When we see people with acute swelling of the retina, for instance, we can suspect a chemical imbalance. And as the old saying goes, you can't drive a railroad spike with a tack hammer. You've got to start giving them nutrients in large amounts to make up for the deficit.

At times like that, you don't have time to play around with diet alone. When the barn's on fire, you don't go around wondering who did it. You put the fire out and you save the barn.

Q: Speaking of fire, what about smoking?

Dr. Raiford: We've taken a moving picture of a person's eye with a television camera and asked him to smoke a cigarette. We can see the blood vessels contract! I tried to get a major tobacco company to finance a research project on this, but I got turned down real fast.

Victory over Allergies

Q: Has nutrition helped you personally?

Dr. Raiford: I happen to have many allergies. My oldest brother died of a milk allergy, in Virginia, before we understood it. When I was a little kid, I always liked to climb the magnolia trees at my uncle's farm. But when I got to a magnolia blossom, I would have an acute headache and become nauseated. That was my first recognition of personal allergies.

I also found out, as I got older, that I would eat chocolate and break out in a rash. And then my ligaments would get stiff. But I can eat carob and it doesn't bother me.

I'm allergic to ragweed, too. I found out that, in order to build up my resistance to ragweed, I also have to avoid the other things. I had a flare-up of my right eye in 1955 due to ragweed. The retina was swollen. That really scared the daylights out of me. I was under a great deal of stress in my work and not eating the right foods.

So I got to work on it and reversed the swelling.

Each day during ragweed season, I take ascorbate in powder form—anywhere from 4 to 6 grams. I even take it at bedtime. I also take some zinc and magnesium for support. I haven't taken an antihistamine for my allergy in over 11 years.

Q: If enough people did that, the health care system as we know it would be turned upside down.

Dr. Raiford: Traditionally, the health sciences have been treating the tip of the iceberg and having no idea what keeps the iceberg afloat.

We now have many of the tools to create a whole new approach to keep us well, rather than to go from crisis to crisis, as present health care is structured. Nutrition is the answer. This is the medicine of the remainder of the 20th century.

When a patient can understand what's happening to his blood vessels, he's going to start rectifying his life style and his health maintenance—which is basically nutrition. That's when prevention will reach its zenith.

Of course, getting each patient to take some responsibility requires time. It slows you down because you've got to take a lot more time with each patient. When I was doing graduate work in New York, the hallmark of a successful ophthalmologist was how many patients he could see in a day. My philosophy is: How much can I see in a patient?

So we have a challenge here that is absolutely fascinating—what can we do to help our fellow man? And that's what life is all about.

CHAPTER
111

SEEING BETTER, FEELING BETTER

"It's so trite because it's been said so many times," Robert Azar, M.D., said to us, "that the eyes are the mirrors of the soul, but they're also reflectors of the physical condition of the whole body. When the eyes start to go, you almost invariably find that there are other degenerative disorders present in the body."

Dr. Azar, his young nutritionist colleague, Mackie Shilstone, Ph.D., and the other doctors at the Azar Eye Clinic in New Orleans have found that treating the deterioration of the whole body may be the best way to respond to the degeneration of the eye. A change in diet and scientific use of vitamin and mineral supplements have led to postponement and even cancellation of costly eye surgery.

A good many of the patients Drs. Azar and Shilstone see suffer from a disorder called macular degeneration. The condition, which commonly occurs in the aging process, is a deterioration of the central part of the retina of the eye. The retina is the screen at the back of the eyeball that registers the images we receive through the lens of the eye. The central part of the retina, called the macula, receives the central part of our vision—what we see when we look directly at something.

Macular degeneration cannot be corrected with glasses or surgery. "But," Dr. Azar told us, "with the nutritional approach, we've even seen that we can stop the progression of the disease, and we've seen some regression of the process. I think that's an exciting thing."

Even more exciting are the side effects of that nutritional therapy. Lester Villa, 72, came to the Azar Eye Clinic complaining not only about his eyesight, but of a general sense of fatigue, as well. "I felt very tired. I wanted to lie down all the time," he says. Dr. Azar examined Mr. Villa's eyes and then sent him to Dr. Shilstone for a complex series of tests to determine his nutritional status.

"There are a whole host of different things we're looking for to try to pinpoint the problem," Dr. Shilstone told us. "We recommend specific doses, micrograms and milligrams, of different vitamin and mineral supplements, depending on what we see." Dr. Shilstone routinely takes a dietary history and requests tests of his patients' blood, urine and hair. He describes it as a "detective program," a sifting through of all the available clues to arrive at a solid determination of the patient's nutritional needs.

In Mr. Villa's case, Dr. Shilstone found that his intake of refined sugar and starches was five times what it should have been. Mr. Villa's diet history showed a low intake of a number of vitamins and minerals, and the biochemical tests indicated that he was deficient in chromium. Dr. Shilstone and Dr. Azar prescribed a number of dietary supplements, including chromium, bioflavonoids, and vitamins B_1, B_2 and C. They also put Mr. Villa on a low-fat, low-sugar diet. In two months, Mr. Villa's fatigue vanished, and he was able to return to his job.

Mr. Villa's eyesight has not yet improved, but Dr. Shilstone has not given up on the case. "It doesn't happen overnight," he says. "Dr. Azar deals with a lot of elderly patients whose nutritional support system is below par. We see over and over what a lifetime of misuse of the body can do. You're asking patients to try to stop some of their bad habits, and they're asking for a miracle. It appears they're asking you to reverse their life. You can stop the macular degeneration process or slow it down. You can help the body catch up, but you'll seldom reverse the process."

Drs. Shilstone and Azar were able to turn things around in another patient, whose body responded very well because she was younger. That patient, a vigorous woman in her 60s, came to the clinic suffering from cataracts, cloudings of the lens of the eye that can result in blindness.

Dr. Azar regularly performs cataract operations at a local hospital in which he removes the clouded lens and installs a clear plastic replacement. The procedure is called an intraocular implant. This particular patient also showed degeneration of the macula, and Drs. Azar and Shilstone wanted to see if nutritional therapy might improve that condition before they resorted to surgery.

"We decided to really go the full route," Dr. Shilstone told us. "We put her on a complete supplementation program, vitamins and minerals in the right balance, and I started her on a walking program, four times a week for 20 minutes, because she had a circulation problem. She came back later, Dr. Azar examined her eyes and said, 'We've lost a surgery patient.' " The circulation to the macula at the back of her eyes had improved so much that surgery could be postponed.

To Dr. Azar, the loss of a surgery patient is no great tragedy. "The ideal here is to cancel the surgery cases," he told us. "This morning, I performed nine cataract operations with nine intraocular implants, a very sophisticated type of treatment. We have finer equipment and finer surgical instruments today than ever before, so in a sense we're performing surgical miracles on a daily basis.

"But for every one of those patients that I operate on, there are at least several that I can't help. I can take out the cataract and give them a plastic lens, but the retina and the inner lining of the eye have been so affected by the degenerative process that the operation is simply not going to help them. I got into the nutritional approach out of frustration at my inability to help the majority of the people that were coming in for help.

"We're realizing that, if a patient comes in and he doesn't have advanced disease, we can schedule our surgery a couple of months ahead of time. We have a chance for eight weeks to build him up with the appropriate vitamin and mineral supplements. I think more and more we're going to find an increasing number of these people who are going to be able to avoid surgery." Even now, Dr. Azar estimates, less than a quarter of the patients who come to him requesting surgery eventually get it.

For people suffering severe macular degeneration as well as cataracts, nutritional therapy might improve their condition to the point that corrective surgery can really benefit them. With his cataract patients, Dr. Azar estimates a value called the *target acuity,* which represents the best vision that might be achieved through replacing a patient's clouded lens.

Diseases like hardening of the arteries, high blood pressure and diabetes can lower target acuity by disrupting circulation to the retina of the eye. "If someone comes in with diabetic bleeding, high blood pressure, advanced arteriosclerosis, any of these degenerative conditions, then the retina of the eye is generally completely shredded," Dr. Azar says. "The target acuity on people with the degenerative diseases is very low, and they won't benefit from surgery. But if we treat them nutritionally and the condition of their retina improves, we may reach a point where they would get some benefit from putting in a new lens."

Both Drs. Azar and Shilstone say the partnership has been especially rewarding. "We're a funny team," Dr. Shilstone says. "You will rarely see nutritionist and M.D. work so closely, so close sometimes that you don't know which of us is pushing nutrition harder. It's a nice meshing of two fields that have been fighting each other for years. The partnership gives credence to what I do, and it gives Dr. Azar a way to treat problems he couldn't do anything about until now."

Dr. Azar has benefited personally from the relationship. He first got in touch with Dr. Shilstone after seeing him on a local TV station, where Dr. Shilstone served as the news department's health editor.

"I had gotten up to about 196 pounds," Dr. Azar recalls. "One evening, I was watching television, and they had Mackie and one of the other announcers running the marathon. It just embarrassed me that two healthy people were out there doing that while I was getting fat."

Dr. Azar called Dr. Shilstone and asked for his help in getting back in shape. Dr. Azar says his weight has now dropped to 170, and "Mackie and I ran two miles in 13 minutes the other morning. Of course, he walks backwards while we do this, but for someone my age that's a remarkable feat."

Dr. Azar says his diet has changed radically since he has known Dr. Shilstone. "In the beginning, it was a little difficult," he says. "It's a form of addiction, really. You almost get withdrawal symptoms when getting off junk food, but after a period of time the sight and smell of it is sickening rather than enticing."

Dr. Shilstone does his best to stress the importance of staying active at the same time that he counsels patients on nutrition. "They generally can't go out and run," he told us, "but if they can walk, fine. Any type of activity can help." Walking to the market is better than driving; taking stairs is better than taking the elevator. "We try to show them that you don't always have to take the easy way, that maybe the easy way isn't as good for you as the hard. It's just a matter of getting used to something."

It's not always an easy message to get across. Patients have a hard time understanding how changes in activity and diet can improve their eyesight, and many are perplexed by an approach that may take months to yield positive results.

"That's part of the American mentality," Dr. Azar says. "It's always been that, if we feel tired, we go down to the drugstore and get a quick fix. The younger generation is accused of being the 'now' generation, but older people are the same way. It's the whole society. Those are the attitudes we're trying to change, and it's not going to be easy.

"Mackie isn't coming in here with some sort of miracle cure for everything. He's sitting people down and saying, 'Look, you've got to be part of the team now. You're going to have to get down and work.' It's understandable that a man would be perplexed by that. It's a totally different approach.

"In an operating room, we take a diseased part and replace it, but we can't replace all the parts. We can only do so much mechanically. The rest of healing is all regenerative. You have to, in some way or another, assist the body in repairing itself, and that's where nutrition comes into play. It's an embryonic science, to say the least, but I think we're on the verge of a tremendous explosion in nutritional medicine."

CHAPTER
112

BETTER VISION
NATURALLY

Honey and vinegar, cod liver oil, vitamins and bed rest. In an age of expensive and sophisticated therapies like laser beams and corticosteroids, most physicians ignore these cheap and simple remedies. But in a small town in New York State lives one old-fashioned doctor who still uses natural cures—and seems to use them effectively—in the treatment of serious eye diseases such as cataract, glaucoma and corneal ulcers.

He's an ophthalmologist, Henry O. Little, M.D., and, at 83, he's virtually a legend in Hudson, New York, a village on the Hudson River north of Manhattan, where he's practiced since 1943. A salty old Yankee who wears lumberjack shirts and bow ties, Harry Little keeps office hours four days a week and gets around town in an old black Lincoln. He's still vigorous in spite of two hip operations, and his hair is remarkably brown. Only the sideburns are white. He's descended, he says, from a long line of Scotch-Irish "bone setters" as durable as he is.

"I believe in him," says a 73-year-old patient whom Dr. Little treated for an eye-related neurological problem. "A lot of people say, 'Oh, Little and his vitamins,' but I respect him. He takes time to sit and talk to you." Another patient, who went to Dr. Little with corneal ulcers, says, "Some people say he's just a country quack, but I have a lot of faith in him. He's quite a remarkable guy."

In a time when a lot of ophthalmologists spend only a few minutes with you, Dr. Little might talk for a half hour or as long as it takes to explain his prognosis. And where few ophthalmologists ask about personal habits, Dr. Little wants to know whether you smoke, whether you eat oatmeal for breakfast, whether you eat white or whole wheat bread, if you "burn your candle at both ends" or if you can stand the taste of cod liver oil. He also advises everyone to start taking a vitamin tablet of B complex with C daily.

"Everyone who comes in here gets put on vitamins," Dr. Little declares. "Unless they're stubborn."

Less Cataract Surgery

In the standard treatment of cataracts, a surgeon removes the clouded lens from the eye and replaces it with an implanted lens, a contact lens or special eyeglasses.

But any artificial lens is a poor substitute for the one we were born with, and surgery sometimes fails.

Surgery is also expensive. About 400,000 cataracts are removed annually in the United States at an estimated cost of $1 billion, or an average of $2,500 per operation. Preventing or arresting the growth of cataracts, many people agree, would be a much cheaper and safer route to take.

Dr. Little believes that he can arrest cataract growth with vitamins and cod liver oil. Fifteen years ago, he says, he performed cataract operations at the rate of one a week, but in the past five years, using nutritional therapy, he's seen only four cases that he felt called for surgery. "Since I've been in practice," he says, "I've gradually come to discover that cataracts are not entirely a surgical condition.

"Cataract is a sign that you're slipping. Your tissues are giving way, and you're getting closer to dying.

"So I arrest the dying. I've arrested thousands of cataracts in the last 35 years with vitamins, and for the last 5 years I've also used cod liver oil. Ninety percent of the cataracts respond to this treatment, and I can almost guarantee that, if I can catch them when their vision is still 20/40, they'll never need a cataract operation.

"But they've got to stop smoking, too. Tobacco causes more blindness than anything else," Dr. Little told us.

He calls for surgery only when a patient's vision is already seriously diminished in both eyes. His policy is to detect the cataract early and arrest its growth with vitamins and cod liver oil. "In my opinion," he says, "cataract is almost an entirely preventable disease."

Two of his cataract patients, a woman in her 90s and a man who is 79, both told us that they were satisfied with Dr. Little's nonsurgical approach. The man, Harold Pepoon, who retired to Hudson after having been in the plumbing business in Yonkers, came to Dr. Little with cataracts in his left eye and with very limited vision in his right eye.

But the growth of the cataract in his left eye was arrested, he says, when Dr. Little put him on vitamins B and C and cod liver oil three years ago.

He can still drive a car. "If anything, it's slightly better," Pepoon said.

A Lucky Discovery That Saved Lives

Vitamin D is what attracted Dr. Little to cod liver oil. Forty-five years ago, while practicing general medicine in what was then the wilds of Saskatchewan, Canada, he said, he used it to save the lives of twin brothers dying of rickets, the vitam D-deficiency disease.

In 1939, when he returned to New York after studying ophthalmology in London, he used cod liver oil—not having anything better to use—to treat a phlyctena, or blister, on the eye of a 15-year-old girl.

His discovery of the value of B vitamins was equally lucky. Again, not knowing what else would help, he gave a sample jar of B-complex tablets, left behind by a salesman, to a man suffering from iritis. Iritis is an extremely painful inflammation of the iris. "He took them," Dr. Little tells the story, "and in ten days, by golly, it was cured! And that's how I got into B vitamins and eyes."

A concoction he calls "Dr. Little's cocktail" is another plank of his eye health platform.

The cocktail consists of an ounce of hot water, 2 or 3 teaspoons of apple cider vinegar and a "gob" of honey. "I can't prove it," he says, "but I believe the vinegar enhances the effectiveness of the vitamins B and C you take by mouth. It's also a wonderful cure for rheumatism, and it cured the arthritis in my fingers."

He feels just as strongly about whole grains. "For breakfast," he declares, "you should eat oatmeal every day, and white bread should be eliminated." He also favors yogurt, raw milk, vitamin E and a reduced amount of coffee.

A few more case histories demonstrate the range of Dr. Little's vitamin therapy:

Eleanor Whitbeck, a 45-year-old nurse who lives in Hudson, came to Dr. Little about two years ago suffering from severe iritis.

She'd already seen another ophthalmologist, who prescribed prednisone, a cortisonelike anti-inflammatory drug. But the prednisone's side effects forced her to stop taking it.

Dr. Little gave her a series of daily injections of megadoses of vitamins B and C. He also prescribed B complex and cod liver oil orally, and he told her not to shop or clean house or do anything very stressful.

The condition got worse. Her eye filled frighteningly with pus, but then it got better. By the third week, the pain in her eye began to subside and gradually her eye healed. Her friends say the eye would have healed by itself, but she doesn't think so. Two years later, she's still taking vitamins and cod liver oil.

Austin "Pete" Hull is a former school bus driver from Durham, New York, who first saw Dr. Little in 1964, when he was 52, for dendritic ulcers of the cornea. These ulcers are usually caused by a herpes virus infection. They often resist treatment and can lead to blindness.

Hull had 13 ulcer attacks in 16 years, and he says that Dr. Little cleared up 11 of them simply with a series of daily injections of B vitamins. Twice, the ulcers also had to be cauterized with carbolic acid. Hull says the ulcers left a little scar tissue, but not enough to prevent him from driving a school bus, which he did until his retirement. Since then, he said, he's been driving the town ambulance.

George A. Hutchings, who is in his 70s and lives in Valatie, New York, met Dr. Little at a free eye clinic set up by the local Lions Club.

Dr. Little diagnosed glaucoma and put Hutchings on vitamin C and B complex. He later performed surgery to reduce pressure within the eye.

"My sight had deteriorated to the danger point, and he arrested it," Hutchings says. "He's one of the great men to come down the pike, as far as I'm concerned. He instills faith and confidence in you."

Another patient, Frank Crocco, suffers from diabetic retinitis, or pinpoint hemorrhages on the retina. Laser beam therapy reputedly shrinks the hemorrhages, but Crocco told us that several laser treatments in Albany didn't help him. "It got so bad I couldn't see myself in the mirror," he said. "I could barely see to walk."

After the laser failures, Crocco went to Dr. Little and began receiving a weekly, then a biweekly, injection of B and C vitamins. He also takes E at night, vitamins B and C in the morning and a tablespoon of cod liver oil daily.

Crocco doesn't know how it works, he just knows that he can now read headlines and can mow his lawn, things he couldn't do before.

One more patient, Chester Groat, a 75-year-old resident of Hudson, came to Dr. Little with a paralyzed nerve in his left eye which doubled his vision and forced him to wear an eye patch. Like the others, Groat started taking B complex, C and cod liver oil.

He was also told to relax and stop smoking. The vitamins took as much as four months to work, but Groat told us, "I had faith in them.

"Now we usually go all winter without a chest cold," says Groat about himself and his wife. "I really believe in Dr. Little. Personally, I think he's a very smart man."

Dr. Little himself does not know exactly how the cod liver oil or the vitamins work or which of the two does what. And, perhaps for that reason, he's been unable to convince other doctors that they work. "Maybe future generations will know why it works," he says.

He admits that his remedies do not work for everyone all of the time and that, like many natural therapies, they may take several days, weeks or sometimes months to effect a cure. They don't offer what he called the "dramatic improvement" that people have come to expect from modern medicine.

While Dr. Little does not rule out surgery, he regards it as a last resort.

First, he'd rather see people relaxing, giving up cigarettes and eating rolled oats—or any whole grain of their choice.

"Altogether, from my 52 years in practice," he says, "I am beginning to believe that all diseases are associated with a lack of vitamins.

"And in the practice of ophthalmology, I have gradually come to realize that vitamins and good food are a large factor in the control and cure of many eye diseases."

ORTHOPEDIC SURGEON

CHAPTER

113

A NEW BREED
OF SURGEON

Everybody knows there are just two kinds of doctor. The "conventional" doctor is active in the county medical society; he plays golf on his afternoon off. Disease, to him, is something to be cut out with a knife or beaten down with drugs—the stronger the better. Nutrition? Mention it in his office and you'll be sorry.

Then there's the "holistic" doctor. He puts the American Medical Association in the same class as the American Nazi Party, and his colleagues put him in the same class as Oral Roberts. He runs a few miles every morning and does yoga in the afternoon. Drugs are evils that may occasionally be necessary, but nutrition, stress reduction and life style counseling are the heart of his practice—not just to help his patients get better, but to keep them well.

So much for fantasy. In reality, there are also doctors like Grant Lawton, M.D., who practices orthopedics in Salem, Oregon. He performs surgery and plays golf—but when he appears at lunch time in the surgery locker room, it's generally to change into his running gear. Dr. Lawton isn't just active in his county medical society, he's its president. His is a "relatively orthodox practice," he says. But he treats some common orthopedic problems with high doses of vitamins, and he hasn't written a prescription for Valium in three years.

Ringing the door bell at Dr. Lawton's suburban home, one recent evening, meant interrupting a passionate cascade of music—ragtime piano. The pianist was Dr. Lawton himself. Playing ragtime is one way he relaxes—something as important for doctors, he says, as for their patients.

Dr. Lawton seemed relaxed as we sat on the patio of his home, well into the night, and talked about health and medicine. Tall, slim and fit, earnest in conversation about his profession, he described growing out of his conventional medical school training into an approach that also embraces nutrition, stress reduction and exercise therapy. "I'm looking," he said, "for the best of both worlds."

How did he get from there to here? Even orthopedic surgeons, it seems, can learn something from their mothers. "Up until four years ago, I'd never thought much about nutrition," he recalled. "My mother was interested in it, though—she had bottles of supplements next to the refrigerator and copies of *Prevention* and other magazines lying on the table. She'd ask me questions about nutrition—she looked to me for answers, since I was the doctor, and my answer was 'I don't know.' "

Dr. Lawton started reading his mother's magazines, and one evening he found himself sitting down to write to *Prevention* columnist Jonathan Wright, M.D. "I said I was interested in nutritional approaches to orthopedic problems. If he knew of any specific conditions that responded well to this approach, I asked him, could he let me know?"

Three days later, Dr. Wright was on the phone to Dr. Lawton, and the orthopedist's nutritional education had begun. "I spent some two years just reading and digesting all the information I could, trying to make up for lost time. I wrote to William Kaufman, M.D., in Bridgeport, Connecticut, for a copy of his book on niacinamide [a form of niacin]. I got to know Jeffrey Bland, Ph.D., a nutritional biochemist. He supplied some solid information for me, which allowed me to build up a bibliography."

Learning this new approach to health problems was exciting, Dr. Lawton recalled. "Then you start trying these things and you get results and that makes it even more exciting.

"The initial successes really got me going," he said. He gave niacinamide to several patients with osteoarthritis (the most common form of arthritis, and one that afflicts many older people). "Over a period of months, it became clear that my patients could turn their symptoms on and off with niacinamide. It worked. It worked just the way Motrin or any other antiarthritic drug would work, but without the potential side effects that these drugs have."

In his practice now, Dr. Lawton gives osteoarthritis patients nutritional therapy that includes niacinamide, vitamin C, calcium and vitamin D. Patients with carpal tunnel syndrome—a painful inflammation of nerves at the wrist—receive large doses of vitamin B_6. For Dupuytren's contracture, an often disabling thickening of cords in the palm, he uses vitamin E. He has had encouraging results giving vitamin C to victims of degenerative disk disease: "When I put people on vitamin C, it seems that I see them much less than I used to—they don't have as many recurrent problems."

Among its other advantages, Dr. Lawton says, nutritional therapy makes it easier for him to avoid using drugs. For carpal tunnel syndrome, for example, the standard treatment would probably be Butazolidin, "the most effective, most potent and most hazardous of anti-inflammatory drugs. If you sat down and read the potential side effects, you would never take it. I would never take it. And I can't honestly expect my patients to take it either—when there are alternatives. So I say, 'First, let's try something that won't hurt.' I've managed, in the last three or four years, not to write a single prescription for Butazolidin."

When pain is involved—as it often is, in the injuries and conditions that he sees—Dr. Lawton will carefully explore alternatives to pain-killing drugs. For acute injuries, he'll try ice massage or transcutaneous nerve stimulation (a technique that uses electrical impulses to short-circuit pain) instead of automatically writing out a prescription for narcotics. Or he will use the simplest and most basic of healing techniques—compassion.

"Say a patient comes into the emergency room with a shoulder dislocation. It's typically a painful injury, and he's tense and uptight. The natural reaction is to say, 'Let's give this guy an IV dose of Valium, or a phenobarb.' I've found I get much better results simply by reassuring him, talking with him quietly, explaining that, if he can let his muscles relax, the bone will go right back into place. And it happens every time. The fact is that if a patient has control—if he's not drugged up with Valium or phenobarbital—this is much more effective."

Dealing with Stress

In general, Dr. Lawton says, helping patients deal with stress is an essential part of orthopedics. For one thing, the acute injuries and chronic illnesses that he treats create a lot of stress.

"You have a young man who's married and has two kids and is wiped out on his motorcycle. He has multiple fractures, and he's lying there in traction wondering, 'Will I work again? Can I pay the rent?' There's a tremendous amount of stress involved. For me just to focus all my energies on getting his bones straight and ignoring the rest—that's a good deal less than what can be done. You just can't take good care of an individual without considering him as a whole.

"It's a matter of awareness. Asking 'How's your wife doing? How are the kids?' Reassuring him. Just being sensitive to his problems, to the fears that are running through his mind."

Ignored and unmanaged, the stress of an injury may, in combination with a generally high stress level, trigger other illnesses, he speculates. "If an orthopedist is aware of his patient's problems, he may be able to prevent development of an ulcer."

Many orthopedic conditions are themselves caused or aggravated by stress, according to Dr. Lawton. "The most common is the upper back strain. This may start with a minor lifting episode, but it goes on for weeks and weeks of muscle tightness. Typically, this is a stress-related disorder—some people say it's symbolic of trying to carry the world on your shoulders. Rheumatoid arthritis, too, very possibly has its basis in stress.''

What Dr. Lawton does in such cases, he says, is "provide the patient with some degree of insight." He'll help him to understand what stress is, how to deal with it and prevent it from wreaking damage. "When someone gets some insight into stress, often he can look at his life, realize, 'Gosh, maybe I am trying to do too much,' and make appropriate adjustments in his schedule." Dr. Lawton may also suggest specific relaxation techniques to relax muscles. He'll make sure his patient has the support of a sound, nutritious diet, with special emphasis on the B vitamins. ("I concur with the general feeling that these are in greater demand in times of higher stress.")

Nutrients before Surgery

In orthopedics, holistic methods like stress reduction and nutrition aren't always enough, Dr. Lawton admits. Surgery is "something you avoid unless it's necessary." When it is necessary, he'll perform it—and make sure that the patient has the benefit of "the best of both worlds." At least two weeks before surgery is scheduled, when possible, he'll put his patient on sizable doses of vitamin A, vitamin C, vitamin E and zinc. "There's good evidence that zinc and vitamin C are important for tissue healing and wound healing. Vitamin A, again, helps wound healing and skin repair. I suggest vitamin E to reduce the danger of blood clots."

Far better than treating orthopedic problems, of course, is preventing them. And this, Dr. Lawton says, can be done, particularly in the older years—when osteoporosis (bone loss) and osteoarthritis are major dangers.

"You'll see one person, who has remained active and is eating well, fall out of his ladder and not break anything. He fell

6 feet, landed on his hip, and you think it's got to be broken! But it's not. His bones are strong and he was able to absorb the impact. The next fellow, who's inactive, whose diet is low in calcium, who doesn't get outside and doesn't get vitamin D from sunlight, is far more likely to sustain a fracture. As for osteoarthritis, there's some evidence that people who are active, who maintain a full range of motion in their joints, have a very low incidence of the disease.

"So the answer here, in terms of prevention, is for people with advancing age to get out, get some sun and some activity—perhaps do some stretching exercises or yoga—and eat a sound diet, one that is rich in calcium. And probably take calcium supplements in addition."

Preventing orthopedic disorders also means weight control, Dr. Lawton adds. "This is especially important with the weight-bearing joints of the lower extremities. When you walk, the force across your knee is some three to five times your body weight. When you run, it's seven times, perhaps ten. So if you lose 30 pounds, it's like taking a hundred pounds off that knee joint. That can make the difference in whether or not someone needs to have surgery for arthritis in his knee or hip."

A special source of Dr. Lawton's enthusiasm for holistic approaches quite possibly is firsthand experience. In recent years, his family's diet has come to reflect his knowledge of nutrition. "We've gotten away from sugar and refined foods; we eat less fatty meats and more fish, and we keep a lot more fresh fruit and vegetables around." Since he's taken to eating a heartier breakfast and snacking on an orange or apple at mid morning and mid afternoon, he's seen a definite improvement in his ability to function throughout the day. He gives himself a hefty dose of vitamins C and E each day, and a B complex. ("If I'm looking at a tough day, I'll take an extra one, without hesitation.")

His health, he says, is better than ever.

At lunch time, he'll walk the block from his office to the hospital, change into his running clothes in the surgery locker room, do 2 miles and be back for a light lunch. "I guard that time," he says. "I try to keep the lunch hour open so I can get my run in."

To reduce the stress in his life, Dr. Lawton does what he asks his patients to do: keeps aware of what's causing him tension and adjusts his attitudes when he can. "I ask myself: 'Why am I getting uptight? What unrealistic expectation or goal am I placing on myself?' " He also practices autogenics, a relaxation technique akin to self-hypnosis. "Once I get into a relaxed state, I imagine myself going through the day. I picture myself absorbed, concentrating with a clear mind while talking with a patient, or responding well to a problem in surgery. It works."

Whenever the opportunity arises, Dr. Lawton tries to share with his patients what he's learned about going beyond "normal" good health "and down the wellness road."

"When a patient's symptoms are gone, he's feeling better, he's looking good, then I'll suggest to him, 'Maybe you'll never have to come back and see me if you can develop a healthy life style.' "

The limitations of a busy practice, he laments, make it impossible to get deeply into such subjects as good nutrition, stress reduction and exercise, "so I keep to the basics. What I hope to do is build a little motivation, perhaps, strike up some interest, give references—'I suggest you read this and this'—and get the ball rolling so they can learn on their own."

The effort is often discouraging. Being a specialist, not a family doctor, his contact with most patients is fleeting. And people come to see him not because of his interest in nutrition, or their own, but because he's an orthopedist and they have orthopedic problems. "Most," he says, "do not want to assume responsibility for their health. They would rather smoke, they'd rather sit around and drink beer and eat chocolate sundaes and, when they get sick, come to me and have me fix them. A doctor has a lot of influence on people, but at times like these I wish I had more."

Making fundamental life style changes is a lengthy process, Dr. Lawton realizes, and motivation is not easy to stimulate.

"So I don't walk away depressed when they don't seem interested. I like to think that maybe down the road someone will remember what I said and think 'Hey, maybe that guy was right'—and it might help to get something going."

Educating Other Doctors

As important as educating his patients, Dr. Lawton believes, is opening the eyes of his colleagues to holistic medicine. "Doctors may not ask about it or talk about it, but I get the impression they're interested. Instead of the that's-a-lot-of-baloney attitude that many people ascribe to the standard physician, I think there's real interest in nutrition and how it relates to health."

Among his colleagues, for example, Dr. Lawton has found more curiosity than hostility toward his use of nutritional therapy. "When I'm off call, a patient may call up the doctor who's covering and ask, 'Should I continue taking my vitamin C?' And Monday morning, the doctor will ask me, 'What's he doing that for?' and I'll explain. And some have even begun asking me, 'How much B_6 did you say you prescribe for carpal tunnel syndrome?'"

Remaining "in the mainstream" of medicine, Dr. Lawton says, he can continue to share his holistic ideas with other doctors. At an executive committee meeting of his county medical society, he suggested bringing nutritional biochemist Jeffrey Bland down to speak on nutrition, "and I got a very positive response.

"Promoting interest in nutrition at our county medical society pleases me as much as helping an individual in my office," he says. "The potential for benefits, actually, is much greater."

The gradual change in his practice has been particularly satisfying—but also frustrating—Dr. Lawton says. He prefers the equal-to-equal relationship that holistic medicine fosters to the "dominant, sitting on a pedestal" role of the conventional physician. ("Five years ago, if a patient called me 'Grant,' it might have annoyed me. Now I like it.") And he's happier with the idea that he can "encourage wellness, and that my patients may not have to come back."

The frustration, he says, is in the fact that "I can only take a first step—I may want to talk about stress with a patient in detail, but there just isn't time, and he goes out the door. I'm frustrated because I can't take the second and third step, too.

"But at least," he says hopefully, "I am taking that first step forward."

CHAPTER

114

THREE HEART ATTACKS BY 29: A PHYSICIAN'S PERSONAL DRAMA

by John Cappello, D.O.

My grandfather had a heart attack when he was in his 60s. My father had one when he was in his 40s. I was only 29. It couldn't happen to me, I thought. But it did happen. On June 25, 1970, I was suddenly awakened about two in the morning with a crushing pain in my chest.

I was having some serious business problems at the time, and I was eating poorly—lots of fatty and fried foods—and drinking more alcohol than I should have. What's more, I was not getting the exercise and rest I needed. The total stress of this situation was apparently too much for my body's weakest link—the heart.

At first, when it hit, I didn't know what was happening. I thought that if I could just move my bowels the pain would go away. (I learned that this is a common symptom with heart attacks.) I was wrong. Even a bottle of citrate of magnesia did not help, and the pain lasted until four. With great relief, I went back to bed for a few hours and woke up at seven to go to the office.

There were no recurrences for the next few days. Then on

June 29, it started again. I was having an early morning snack in the company's coffee shop when I felt the pressure building on my chest; this time the pain radiated down both arms to my fingertips. I waited about a half hour, conversing with friends, not being able to sit still, before I decided to go to a physician. After all, I had never been sick, so I did not know what I was experiencing.

Another "great" experience awaited me as I got into my car to drive the 20 miles home. The power steering in my new Buick had failed. The car handled like a Mack truck and, as I look back on it, I sure wasn't doing myself much good. Mother Nature wasn't on my side either; the mercury hit 96°F that day and, with Philadelphia-area humidity, the perspiration was just pouring off my body.

After a torturous half-hour drive, I finally made it to the local hospital. Curiously, the pain started to relent as I walked into the emergency room. When I told the emergency room nurse what had happened to me, I was immediately seen by the physician, who set me up for an electrocardiogram. Five minutes later, I got the bad news.

"You have had a heart attack," the emergency room physician told me. "So we are going to have to keep you in the hospital for a couple of weeks." A few tears came to my eyes as I thought of my father and grandfather and how I had seen their activities greatly curtailed after their heart attacks. But just as quickly as these thoughts came to mind, I promised myself that this would not and could not happen to me.

I was taken right to the intensive care unit. There I had what was unquestionably the most frightening experience of my life. In the middle of the night, I was awakened with the most severe pain I had ever had; it was chest pain so excruciating that I cried out for help. I learned later that the damage to my heart muscle was extending, or in medical terms, additional heart tissue was undergoing *infarction*. The nurse was not permitted to give me anything for the pain until she reached my physician, who ordered a strong pain killer.

Heart Medicine—A Life Sentence

The rest of my hospital stay and initial recovery were laborious. But, somehow, I got to the point where I became an outpatient and was put on my daily dosages of "heart medicine":

- Coumadin—an anticoagulant also known (in error) as a "blood thinner,"
- sublingual nitroglycerin—thought to dilate coronary blood vessels,
- Nitro-Bid—a long-acting nitroglycerin,
- Valium—an antianxiety agent.

Still, I was never totally free from chest discomfort. Anxious thoughts or a hard day's effort would cause that old tingling feeling in my chest and arms.

My physician, who had done such a valiant job in helping me overcome the acute stage of my illness, was of little help in my efforts to rehabilitate myself. "John," he said, "even if you jump into the African jungle on a parachute and live with the natives, make sure you bring a good supply of the medications you are taking." He made no mention of diet or supplements, which were discussed in the lay press. Nor did he question my habits and life style, which I knew must be changed. But I did not know what or how to change and needed guidance. I realized then that perhaps his acute-care training was what I needed to get me over the initial hump, but now to further improve I must seek other avenues.

Discovering Medicine and Nutrition

It was during this four-year search (1970 to 1974) that I decided to make a career change. I had always wanted to be a physician, but I did not want to go through all of the red tape. Now, somehow the hassle of preadmission testing, letters of recommendation, interviews and waiting did not seem to matter. Fortunately, I had completed all of the necessary premed courses, so I was not confronted with that roadblock. And my reasoning that I should further pursue medicine as a career was further spurred, as I felt sure my background in laboratory research would be of great assistance in uncovering the answer to improving my own health as well as the health of others. Eventually, I was accepted at a well-known Philadelphia school of medicine for September, 1974—the class of 1978.

Luckily, the summer before I started school, I came across a book by Naura Hayden. In it, Adelle Davis was discussed and a couple of her books—including *Let's Get Well* and *Let's Eat Right to Keep Fit*—were mentioned. I eagerly read these books and a new world was opened up to me. What I found particularly interesting was the research on vitamin C, the different vitamins of the B complex and anti-stress studies. At last, I had some leads to work with.

While I studied the various aspects of medicine and the human body at school, I devoted practically all of my spare time to studying human nutrition. My body became a laboratory. And as I studied and experimented, I realized that I was overfed the wrong foods and essentially undernourished to cope with the demands I was placing on my body.

Gradually, over six months' time, I weaned myself from all of my heart medication by following much of the nutritional advice I uncovered during my research. Of course, this approach is not for everyone. I was pursuing a career in medicine and by this time was quite sure about what I was doing. I don't want to leave the impression that the average person who has a serious medical problem should try to go it 100 percent along.

But what a different some of these health-oriented changes made for me!

My typical day began at 5 A.M. and I was home at around 8 P.M. A few hours of studying usually took me to bed around midnight. If there was an exam the next day, I could easily be up to 2 or 3 A.M. Somehow, I did it without chest pain or discomfort. Before, if I tried to keep such hours, my body would cry "uncle." Now I was building endurance, and each month saw further improvement.

During the course of my journey to better health, I also discovered *Prevention*. I guess I kind of identified with this magazine, since its founder also had health problems and was looking for a better way. The inspiration of others with an active interest in preventive medicine helped to spur me along the way.

Many people have asked what the regimen I used consisted of. These were the main nutrients during the initial phase of my personal program:

- brewer's yeast with calcium and magnesium,
- lecithin,
- corn oil.

Also included as supplements were:

- pantothenate,
- vitamin C,
- vitamin E,
- B complex,
- magnesium oxide.

Here is the way I started and my reasoning at the time:

Brewer's yeast is a known source for balanced B vitamins. This balanced source is important because during illness the need for all B vitamins seems to increase. If you increase one and not the others, you may cause a B vitamin imbalance. I started with ½ teaspoon of brewer's yeast the first week, then built up slowly to 2 heaping teaspoons per day over a four-week period.

Lecithin I used to aid in the transportation of fat and cholesterol in my bloodstream. Many of the cases of hardening of the arteries that I researched were typified by increased ratios of cholesterol to fat in the bloodstream. While experimentally unconfirmed, the premise I worked with was that lecithin could conceivably help restore a proper fat-cholesterol balance.

Corn oil is a natural source of linoleic acid, an essential fatty acid. It is believed that this essential fatty acid helps reduce the amount of cholesterol circulating in the blood.

Depending upon what I had in stock, I would use 8 ounces of either skim milk or fresh orange juice as a base. Then using a blender, I'd add 2 teaspoons each of brewer's yeast, lecithin and corn oil and whip it up into a healthful froth.

After my one-two-three blend, I would then take the following supplements:

Pantothenate, 100 milligrams and **vitamin C,** 500 milligrams—my studies revealed that both are stored in the adrenal gland and are known requirements in stress-related diseases.

Vitamin E, 300 international units, appears to act as an antioxidant by reducing the need for oxygen in the heart muscle.

Multivitamin with B complex—one of these was taken as an added safety factor.

Magnesium oxide, 250 milligrams, was taken since magnesium is found in muscle tissue and is involved in many energy-producing reactions in the body.

In addition, my life style was drastically altered.

I sharply cut down on refined sugar and animal fat and, instead, switched to a diet high in whole grains, fresh vegetables and fruit in season.

Because of these and other life style changes, I no longer need to stick as closely to my crisis regimen. Under especially distressful conditions, though, I usually go back to some variation of my initial formula with rather good personal results.

CHAPTER

115

THE SUGAR GENERATION

When, 12 years ago, Hugh W. S. Powers, Jr., M.D., a general pediatrician in Dallas, Texas, started interviewing the parents of "problem" children, he heard many angry complaints about the generally accepted medical treatments for children with learning disabilities and behavior and hyperactive disorders.

"And they were dissatisfied for one very good reason: lack of results," Dr. Powers told us.

"The conventional treatment for these problems is the drug Ritalin. Now, the use of Ritalin has had considerable success with certain children. But the statistical breakdown is that only 50 percent partially benefit from it, while 25 percent don't get any benefits and another 25 percent get worse. And the only alternative to Ritalin that the conventional physician will usually consider is other tranquilizers or psychiatry.

"But what really galls these parents," he continued, "is the physician's attitude that there isn't some other solution when his methods fail. Here they are with a child who's doing poorly in school or running wild all over the place at home, and the physician is, in effect, telling them: 'My methods may not work, but I'm not going to try something else.' "

Dr. Powers is a physician who is willing to try something else. "You could say I've had a lifetime interest in nutrition. One of my aunts worked with E. V. McCombe of Johns Hopkins, one of the fathers of nutritional medicine in this country, and so I was getting vitamins even as a kid. Then, at medical school, I studied the physiology of nutrition. But it was about 12 years ago that I became interested in functional problems of the nervous system and learned that changes in levels of blood sugar affect behavior. So I got interested in how to manage blood sugar. I started educating myself further in nutrition, going around the country joining organizations, reading Adelle Davis, Carlton Fredericks and *Prevention* magazine."

From that beginning, Dr. Powers's background as a general pediatrician broadened naturally to a multifaceted nutritional approach. He now uses nutrition to treat not only problem children with learning or behavior difficulties, but also those with allergies or those who simply get sick a lot with minor illnesses.

The first thing Dr. Powers does when parents bring their children to him is to sit down with them for two hours and take a detailed case history, including family, pregnancy and past medical history, as well as a record of the family's daily diet. He does that for several reasons. "One is to rule out any serious hidden medical problem. Then, too, I want to know whether there's a hereditary pattern to the child's problem—whether his parents and siblings have had something similar.

"But most enlightening is to find out what sort of dietary examples the child is being given at home. Not only what his diet consists of, but also what kinds of foods he sees his parents eating. I need to know whether I'm going to have a hard time getting a child to cut down on sugar because his father sits at the dinner table eating tubs of ice cream."

Following indications in the case history, Dr. Powers may want to conduct a complete physical examination or laboratory studies such as blood count, urinalysis and a five-hour glucose tolerance test. These will help to narrow down the child's specific problem.

"In most cases," said Dr. Powers, "I begin treatment with

a general nutritional program. That consists of eliminating sugar, other simple carbohydrates and caffeine—including cola drinks—starting the day with a high-protein breakfast, and using appropriate vitamin supplements. I start with this because it's safe and effective with a wide variety of problems. Now, if the child's problems continue, I won't hesitate to try other treatments. But I seldom have to—the nutritional program usually takes care of the problem. In fact, I've had parents tell me that the results are often amazing."

Low Blood Sugar a Frequent Problem

"Take the case of learning and behavior difficulties," he continued, "kids who are either too tired or too restless to pay attention in school and those who are either mopey or running all over the place. In their extreme forms, such symptoms often indicate hyperactivity. Kids with these problems respond remarkably well to a diet that eliminates sugar and limits other simple carbohydrates—syrup, molasses, honey, corn sugar and so on. That's because the root problem here appears to be their blood sugar levels."

In a study that Dr. Powers conducted with 260 problem children, he found that blood sugar levels consistently correspond to behavior and performance in school. Sugar made them irritable or listless. "But after starting the general nutritional program," said Dr. Powers, "there was consistent improvement. One 15-year-old girl was a poor reader, doing badly in school, and had a history of headaches, fatigue and needing more sleep than normal. After a year on the program, she underwent a striking change. She gained three years in reading comprehension and became bright, cheerful and outgoing."

When you know these children's typical diet, it's not surprising that Dr. Powers's sugar control program helps their problems.

"These kids usually eat a terrible diet. Sugared cereal, jelly on cinnamon-sugar toast, cookies, cake and colas with almost every meal and lots of ice cream. Their consumption of whole grains, fresh vegetables and sources of protein such as legumes, fish and fowl is generally minimal. For a child to think and behave well, he needs to have the right food."

Caffeine is also a problem. "Kids are doing themselves a lot of harm by the way they down colas," says Dr. Powers. "There's about half a cup of coffee in a 10-ounce bottle of Coke— not to mention 6 tablespoons of sugar. Some kids drink the stuff by the quart. They're practically poisoning themselves. A quart of cola contains about 300 milligrams of caffeine; a toxic dose of caffeine is 500 milligrams."

Children who consume large amounts of caffeine as well as sugar may be plagued by chronic irritability, inattention, poor memory, psychosomatic complaints and hyperactivity, all culminating in severe academic or even psychological problems. "I've treated several psychotic teenagers who reported drinking 2 or 3 quarts of cola a day," said Dr. Powers. "But another of my patients, whom I call the 'queen of all cola addicts,' outdid even them. She used to consume a variety of soft drinks straight from the dispensing machine that her well-meaning father had placed in their home. That and a heavy load of sugary food were really fouling her up. She refused to do schoolwork, was sullen and fatigued, and would often break out into unprovoked crying. 'I just yelled out loud and broke my pencil in half,' she told me about one of these incidents. When she was brought to me, she'd already been seeing a psychiatrist. I put her on the general nutritional program, but she followed it very erratically. Still, the last word from her father was that she's definitely better without sugar and colas."

Foods That Build the Immune System

In addition to eliminating bad foods from the child's diet, Dr. Powers aims at increasing the good food. "Good dietary management should build up the child's resistance as well as limit harmful foods," Dr. Powers explained. "One of the most ignored problems in pediatrics is the chronically sick child who has no serious physical disease. Sometimes the condition is mistaken for an allergy. The child just gets a lot of minor illnesses—colds, sore throats, ear infections, bouts of diarrhea and vomiting.

"Now, sugar is often the culprit here, too. Research has shown that all sugars lower the phagocytic index, an important immune response in the body. Reducing dietary sugar helps, but it's only the first step. Real treatment must aim at producing a state of full health that will help prevent relapse. That means building up resistance."

How does Dr. Powers help children boost their resistance? "I prescribe a diet of fish and chicken, organ meats like liver, fresh vegetables, unsweetened yogurt and small servings of cheese. These are resistance foods. They provide the body with its raw materials and arm it against infection. And it's no accident that they also help to stabilize blood sugar, so the child will also feel better."

Resistance foods are especially important for the chronically sick child, but a good diet is obviously good for all children. Together with a group of his patients' mothers, Dr. Powers has compiled the guidelines shown in the accompanying table for a diet for children.

"I'll often supplement this diet with vitamins and minerals," the physician says. "Since most problem children aren't eating well, they need vitamin and mineral supplements to get proper nutrition. For instance, vitamins contribute to the physiological use of protein, in which these kids are frequently deficient. So I give a general supplement. But since these kids are under a lot of stress, I'll also give them a big dose of C and a B complex."

If you've ever tried sticking to a diet yourself, you might wonder whether it isn't especially hard for kids. Dr. Powers is the first to admit that it is.

Winning the child's cooperation is essential. "If you can't sell the child, he's not going to stick to his diet. And in the end, it's the child who has to do it. It's different from the conventional

[*continued on page 670*]

Dr. Powers's Diet
for Low-Blood-Sugar Control

Food Category	Foods to Use	Foods to Avoid
Meats	Beef, lamb, veal, pork, chicken, turkey, any fish.	Any processed or cured meat.
Vegetables	All kinds, at least two at a time.	None.
Vegetable Juices	All.	Processed with any additives.
Fruits	Fresh fruit in limited quantity (one-quarter piece per day for younger children).	Excessive amounts.
Fruit Juices	All natural. Dilute to 1 ounce of juice to 3 ounces of water one to three times a day for small children.	Added sweeteners.
Breads	Including rolls, muffins, crackers, biscuits all made from whole grains.	Breads with two or more sweeteners.
Cereals	Any made from natural, whole, unrefined grains.	Additives or preservatives.

Dr. Powers's Diet
for Low-Blood-Sugar Control—*Continued*

Food Category	Foods to Use	Foods to Avoid
Rice	Natural, whole grain.	Processed.
Pasta	Spaghetti, noodles, etc., all natural, whole grain, can be egg, spinach or Jerusalem artichoke enriched.	Those made from white flour.
Beverages	Emphasize water. Milk, herbal teas, diluted fresh fruit juices, vegetable juices acceptable. Sugarless, caffeine-free (light-colored) sodas infrequently.	Coffee, tea, all dark-colored sodas. Anything sweetened with sugar, sorbitol, mannitol, xylitol.
Sweeteners	Fructose, tupelo honey, molasses, carob syrup, rice syrup, corn syrup only in small amounts and *only* in low-sugar dessert recipes.	White refined sugar, brown sugar, honey, confectionary sugar in recipes. Any sugar or sugar straight out. Sorbitol, mannitol, xylitol.
Desserts	Ideally all no-sugar such as nuts or	All sugar-containing desserts.

**Dr. Powers's Diet
for Low-Blood-Sugar Control—*Continued***

Food Category	Foods to Use	Foods to Avoid
	popcorn. Low-sugar desserts (made with the allowable sweeteners listed above) in small portions and *only* on special occasions not to exceed twice a week.	
Chewing Gum	None.	All gums of any kind.
Condiments	All spices and herbs. Ketchup, mayonnaise, mustard in small quantities due to their high sugar content.	Excessive amounts. Remember that most ketchups, dressings, sauces contain 25 to 50 percent sugar.
Fats and Oils	Only lean unprocessed meats, lean fish, poultry without skin, low-fat and part-skim cheese.	Fried foods and snacks dipped in oil for crispening. All oily foods. Excessive use of butter and margarine.

treatment with drugs. I can't be in control all the time. The parents can't be in control all the time. We need the child's active cooperation. He has to want to take responsibility for getting better."

Dr. Powers has found that the whole tenor of nutritional medicine is different from the conventional medical practice. "It's cooperative medicine. I have to work differently with the parents, too. When I had a conventional pediatric practice, there were 40 kids in the office a day. But when you're using a nutritional approach, you have to sit down for a couple of hours and get to know a lot of things about your patients and their families."

But that's not the only reason Dr. Powers believes his nutritional practice has helped him, as well as his patients. "It's more fun," he says, "because the approach is more successful. And that's gratifying."

CHAPTER
116

GROWING UP HEALTHY— THE NATURAL WAY

Something was wrong with the baby. Seriously wrong.

The infant had come from the delivery room to the nursery 30 hours earlier and he wouldn't—couldn't—stop screaming. Not a normal baby's cry, but a high-pitched howl. He couldn't eat or sleep, only stare and scream.

The hospital's nurses and obstetrician were at a loss. The general physical exam didn't show them the problem. The newborn's head resisted rotation. His tiny thighs were drawn up to his chest and couldn't be made to relax. They couldn't guess at a remedy for the squalling infant's misery. The obstetrician called Dr. Dunn.

When Paul Dunn, M.D., arrived, he located the problem quickly. The child's cranial bones, compressed during the process of birth, were misaligned. Usually, a newborn's first deep breath expands the bones and they settle into place alongside one another. This time it hadn't worked. Dr. Dunn placed the struggling baby on a table and instructed two nurses to hold the infant carefully still. He stood at the child's head, turned it slowly to one side as far as he could, and held it in place, waiting.

Soon he felt a little movement building up under his hand, then quieting down. The movement stopped and he felt a little tremor of release. Moving the infant's head to the other side, he felt the process of movement and relaxation repeated. After five minutes of Dr. Dunn's manipulation, the baby stopped crying and fell into the first sleep of his young life. Dr. Dunn worked on for another ten minutes while the baby slept. He gently massaged the baby's head and neck until he could rotate the head easily from side to side and draw down the once-rigid legs. From that time on, the child slept normally, ate normally, and behaved like a normal newborn.

Dr. Dunn's osteopathic therapy was a double blessing for the youngster. It not only ended his suffering swiftly and effectively, it did so without recourse to drugs and their potential side effects. "I'm sure if the hospital had done the 'usual' things," Dr. Dunn said, "the kind of things I'd have done a few years ago—put him on phenobarbital and belladonna to calm him down and put him to sleep—he'd have gone home a colicky baby and at least have grown up to become a hyperactive child with a learning problem, if not something more serious."

Dr. Dunn is a pediatrician with a difference. He feels the medical profession has fallen short in fulfilling its responsibilities to its youngest patients. He chose pediatrics as his own specialty after his internship exposed him to the complaints of hundreds of adult patients who lived careless and unhealthful lives. After years of self-inflicted damage, they came to Dunn as they might bring a poorly maintained car to the repairman. "I didn't want to spend my life with these worn-out adults, listening to all their complaints," he says. Working with children, he decided, he could make an important difference early in their lives and help them grow into a robust adulthood.

Raising an unusually large family—he's a father of ten—Dr. Dunn became progressively more dissatisfied with the narrow approach to health offered by conventional medical training. He wanted to do better for his own children and the children in his practice, to incorporate as broad a field of knowledge as possible into his working methods. As Dr. Dunn's wife and partner, Kathryn, puts it, "We're just middle-of-the-road people who looked for better answers for our children than anyone else provided."

In his Oak Park, Illinois, office, Dr. Dunn employs, in addition to general pediatrics, a comprehensive program of testing and treating children with brain injury and learning disability. The program includes osteopathy, psychology, biochemistry, audiology, Montessori education, developmental optometry, physical education and nutritional guidance in an interdisciplinary effort designed for the needs of each patient. Dr. Dunn stresses the importance of such cross-disciplinary cooperation with these children. "Let's pool our knowledge and not be afraid that another disciple will steal our thunder."

The importance of proper nutrition in his overall treatment program is obvious even before visitors leave the reception room. One newspaper clipping on the bulletin board notes that undertakers find human bodies do not deteriorate as quickly as they used to. The reason, they believe, is that today's diet contains so many preservatives that the chemicals interfere with the natural process of decomposition. Beside it, another advises parents on a method to steer their youngsters away from heavily advertised snack foods, make them label conscious and improve their eating habits. The writer suggests taking the kids to the supermarket to read the labels, with the understanding that, if they can't pronounce the ingredients, they can't eat them.

Clearly, Dr. Dunn is interested in teaching parents new nutritional ideas so their children will stay healthy.

"Sometimes we assume everybody already knows the basics of sound nutrition," says Mrs. Dunn. "But there are a lot of people out there who think sugar is energy and our breakfast cereals are just great.

"When you consider how easy it is to shop when you don't care," she continues, "it only takes a minute to fill your cart with instant groceries for all week. But when I shop, there are whole aisles that I skip!"

Nutrition for the Whole Family

Many of the learning problems and other disorders Dr. Dunn is asked to treat can be traced back to parents who habitually push their shopping carts down the wrong aisles. According to

Dr. Dunn, the solution is "a nutritional program set up for the whole family, not just Johnny and Mary, so the entire family gets to feel better.

"From the newborn period on, I'm talking to the parents about the types of nutritional principles you read about in *Prevention* all the time," Dr. Dunn explains. "I advise sticking as much as possible to fresh fruits and vegetables, serving chicken and fish in place of beef and pork, serving some seeds and nuts— although, for the little ones, they should be ground up and mixed with something else, like applesauce. Serve eggs boiled rather than scrambled or fried. Avoid bleached-white-flour products and refined sugar products. Give kids additional vitamin C to prevent colds."

Mrs. Dunn acknowledges that this may mean asking a family to change their long-time marketing habits. They should also be prepared for some initial squawking at the table. "There's a lot of emotion wrapped up in the foods we're used to eating," Mrs. Dunn observes. But by changing the family's diet gradually, one daily meal at a time, the transition to healthier habits can be accomplished with a minimum of fuss.

How can children be weaned away from the junk foods their peers enjoy? Get them involved, urges Mrs. Dunn. Teach them what to look for, and let them help with the shopping. Encourage them to help prepare meals. Set a good example. Above all, don't try to impose good food on them, or there'll surely be resistance. Mrs. Dunn chuckled to recall one little boy who cleverly found a way to frustrate his insistent, health-minded parents. "He'd always trade his whole wheat sandwich full of everything good for his lunchroom friend's peanut butter and jelly."

"Once they find out the connection between what they eat and how they feel, they'll learn," says Dr. Dunn.

Early Stimulation

Dr. Dunn also reminds parents that children need more than good food to grow to their full potential. They have a tremendous appetite for stimulation, too. And in his opinion, it can't start too early.

"Playpens make great firewood," he declares. "The child's body, senses and capabilities develop through use, and without use they don't develop." It has been found in animals that 80 to 90 percent of the microneurons that deal with the thinking process develop after birth, mainly during infancy, and in proportion to the amount of stimulation the baby receives. "You can see how important it is to give the baby every opportunity to move through the environment from very early on," Dr. Dunn says. The more a baby is allowed to move, the more it can learn about its world.

"When I talk to mothers of newborn babies in the hospital, I tell them that even next week they can put the baby down on a blanket on the floor. Of course, he'll just stretch and look around, but he'll be getting accustomed to that level so that, when the time comes for crawling, he'll be able to do it as much as he needs to. The time may come at one or two months, or three or four. No one but the baby knows. So you can't say, 'I'll wait until he starts doing it'—you might miss the beginnings of it.

"From very early on, let him spend much of his time crawling on the floor, and more and more time as he gets older. Don't just let him spend hours sitting up immobilized in an infant seat, a playpen, a walker or a swing seat, because it restricts his early movements." Infant seats and the like are fine, he continues, so long as they don't become the place where the child passes most of his time. These early movements, incidentally, can also help prevent learning problems.

Dr. Dunn is a firm believer that youngsters from early infancy should spend time outdoors. "Try to get the child out every day except in severe weather," he recommends, "so he can see, hear, feel and experience as many things as possible. Walk him along the same route regularly, so he becomes used to orderly repetition. It's like listening to a favorite song over and over again. He knows what's coming next, and that's the beginning of attending."

And parents should not forget the importance of exposing their young ones to good speech. Read to the child, don't just cuddle and coo, even if he's only two months old, Dr. Dunn suggests. "He may not understand reading aloud, but it's still good language going in. And what goes in is what the mind stores and what later comes out."

For six years, Dr. Dunn was away from pediatric practice, working exclusively with children with special problems. After his return to the field, he remembers, he commented to Mrs. Dunn that the children looked different to him and acted differently. There seemed to be more irritable babies, more crying babies. "They don't seem to be at home with themselves. It probably has to do with prenatal nutrition and pollution. Alcohol consumption by the mother during pregnancy can have an effect. She doesn't have to be an alcoholic. There's evidence now that just a regular drink or two a day during pregnancy can make a difference.

"About 45 percent of the kids with learning problems that I see have increased lead levels from car and airplane exhausts in the atmosphere, hair sprays, newspaper print and about 100 other sources. We handle it with vitamin C and sulfur-containing amino acids. These pull lead out of the system and counteract other toxins in the environment. Vitamin E is another antioxidant that will counteract the effects of lead."

Overweight from Addictive Eating

Many of Dr. Dunn's preteen and teenage patients suffer from that almost universal American disease—overweight. Much of the time, he says, the problem is one of addictive eating caused by sensitivity to particular foods. Mrs. Dunn describes the therapy: "The doctor will oftentimes put adolescents on a complete detoxification program. This appeals to them because it's a very distinct change. We've used a juice-and-vegetable nine-day fast to get them away from the things they usually eat, get a thorough cleansing, break the old habits and get organized to start something new. It's amazing what this will do for kids.''

To a large degree, nutritional problems for adolescents begin early, when they're making their first independent decisions about diet, and end when independence matures them, the Dunns feel.

"Once kids get out in their own apartments—at least ours—they go in for the wok, the brown rice and vegetables, and making food becomes the center of their social life. They eat better because they're poorer,'' says Mrs. Dunn.

One of the greatest rewards of his work for Dr. Dunn is that he has very few in-all-the-time patients. "With the basic approaches I use, nutritionally and otherwise, I don't have nearly the number of sick kids that I used to have. I rarely get more than three or four phone calls over the weekend. I'll go weeks and weeks without having to put anybody in the hospital. They just don't get that sick.'' Today he's spending much of his time treating children with specialized learning problems, visual problems, and others suffering from hyperactivity. And despite his long-standing resolution to work only with kids, he has considered bringing his brand of preventive medicine to adults, but his present busy schedule prevents that.

"I feel sorry for them,'' he chuckles. "At the end of their children's exam, parents often sheepishly come forward and say, 'Er—um—I've got that problem, too!' ''

Fortunately, as the former president of the International Academy of Preventive Medicine, Dr. Dunn had the opportunity to encourage a growing number of other physicians to work with parents who are willing to take responsibility for their own health.

CHAPTER

117

A COMPLETE PRESCRIPTION FOR BETTER HEALTH

The woman walked into the prescription department of a Leavenworth, Kansas, department store, intending to buy a package of over-the-counter diet pills. She walked out with two bottles of vitamins and some sensible advice on weight control.

A local farmer received a crash course in vitamin therapy when he came in to pick up his wife's duodenal ulcer prescription. "A lot of research says vitamin C and zinc help the medicine work better," consultant pharmacist Tom Liederbach, R.Ph., told the farmer, who glared at him suspiciously. As Liederbach started to ring up the cash register, the farmer's glance shifted to a nearby vitamin display. He surreptitiously lifted a bottle from the rack, turned it over in his palm to read the back label, then returned it. He faltered, snatched the bottle again and plunked it on the counter.

"Exactly what does it do?" he demanded.

Liederbach told the farmer that zinc and vitamin C requirements are increased with mucosal wounds such as ulcers. Vitamin C, he explained, is needed for the collagen of connective tissue to cement the healing cells. The zinc also aids in wound healing and helps oxygenate the blood, which helps the healing process even more. "Until we see her progress, they are no substitute for your wife's medication," he warned. The farmer nodded, looked at the small plastic bottle with the typewritten label and child-proof top, then examined the larger, brown glass bottle with its fancy label and cellophane-sealed cap—and bought both.

As the day wore on, people dropped by to have prescriptions filled, buy vitamins or just chat with the pleasant young man in the white coat, name embroidered over one pocket. They found it easy talking to this pharmacist, who handed out affection and advice the way pediatricians do lollipops.

"People often feel they didn't get their money's worth if they walk out of a doctor's office without a prescription," Liederbach told us. "They may feel their complaints aren't being taken seriously. These people are often the victims of worries, stresses and depressions that no drug can help.

"What they often need is counseling. But most doctors honestly haven't the time for that, and when they do, usually it doesn't have the beneficial effect it could because patients aren't receptive.

"But here," he continued, indicating the expanse of store where his professional wares were housed in clinical array next to the tangled greenery of an adjacent plant department, "it costs them nothing. They are more relaxed when they come in here than when they walk into a doctor's office, and therefore they're more open. Too, they often are more responsive to the advice I give them about getting proper exercise, nutrition and rest than they are when the same advice comes from their doctor."

The physician's office, Liederbach contends, often presents an artificial environment substantially different from the patients' day-to-day lives outside. They endure it temporarily, in order to obtain symptomatic relief for what they hope is a temporary problem. Long-term solutions and radical changes are unwelcome; many patients are no happier accepting a diet or exercise program than a verdict of terminal illness.

A pharmacy, especially a pharmacy such as the one Liederbach manages, overlooking the toys and trinkets, tires and trowels that are displayed in the store, makes change seem more palatable than when it is demanded by the awesome patriarch they call "doctor."

People find it easy to relate to Liederbach, perhaps because his curls and boyish smile are so disarming, perhaps because his strong body is a testimonial to healthy food and regular exercise. He and his wife, Theresa, who rode her bicycle to the obstetrician's office through the ninth month of her last pregnancy, plan to open a preventive pharmacy center, incorporating a unique pharmacy practice with natural therapeutic alternatives including food, herbs and nutritional supplements.

Working with natural foods at a Kansas City health foods restaurant introduced Liederbach to herbs. His fascination grew. "I'm a voracious reader; I learned that a lot of medicines are naturally based. Penicillin, for example, comes from cultures of certain common molds. Digitalis is extracted from the foxglove plant.

"I sold my restaurant with the intention of becoming a physician," but he changed his mind when he saw how little emphasis the profession placed on disease prevention through nature and nutrition. In order to help people in that way, he decided to return to school and become a pharmacist—with a major emphasis on pharmacognosy (the study of medicinals made from herbs and other natural, biological sources).

Although his sounds like a new approach to pharmacy and medicine, "it's actually the oldest way," Liederbach explains. "Originally, pharmacists were herbalists—pharmacognosy is the word for what they practiced—and in addition to drugs with questionable efficacy, they employed the use of herbal extractives as effective remedies. Only in recent years, with the advent of chemical pharmaceutics, has the importance of pharmacognosy been sidestepped.

"There is a new approach coming to medicinals, however. A specialized consultant pharmacist in conjunction with the physician will prescribe the proper remedy, and a less highly trained retail pharmacist will dispense or compound the medicines.

"Physicians are not able to keep up with the enormous amount of pharmaceutical literature while maintaining their expertise with diagnoses," Liederbach thinks. "A lot of younger physicians realize this and are becoming increasingly concerned. A significant amount of what doctors know about drugs and medications has been told to them by drug salesmen. Perhaps that is one reason why three independent sources estimated that from 10 to 18 percent of all hospital inpatients studied were suffering from adverse medical reactions classified as iatrogenic [physician-induced] diseases."

A pharmacist, Liederbach believes, should make it his business to know about drug side effects.

"Did your physician tell you you need potassium with that?" Liederbach asked the woman who was buying over-the-counter diuretics on the recommendation of her physician. "Without additional potassium, there's a chance it could cause leg cramps." He told her bananas were a good source of potassium.

"So much potentially dangerous stuff is sold over the counter. A pharmacist should be aware of the danger they pose. For instance, a person who buys a dubious 'diet aid' containing phenylpropanolamine (PPA) could be in for serious trouble if he also is taking decongestants containing the same ingredient. And if he also drinks coffee. . . ." Liederbach shakes his head. On several occasions, he has intercepted such purchases and warned people of the possible consequences, including possible cardiac abnormalities.

Similar situations arise when people buy a prescribed medicine and also buy cold remedies or aspirin, which may interact with it. "Doctors realize I'm doing them a favor," he says, because most patients don't think to tell their physicians about over-the-counter preparations they consume regularly, because they are either embarrassed or ignorant of how dangerous these so-called safe drugs can be.

"That's one reason why you should always go to the same pharmacy and get to know your pharmacist. Usually, he knows a lot more about these things than either you or your doctor."

Concerned that the strength of his views may lead to misinterpretation, Liederbach stresses, "I am not out to undermine the medical profession or to disparage physicians." He just wants people to realize there are certain limits to what their doctors can do—in terms of time and training. There is nothing wrong with that. An architect is not a carpenter.

Patient, physician and pharmacist form a trinity that works to benefit them all, in Liederbach's view. Since he can get a glimpse of a person's life style that a doctor may never know, he can help the doctor's treatment reach its desired end. When he calls himself "a liaison between doctor and patient, medicine and nature," he means human nature, too.

CHAPTER

118

THE DOCTOR
WHO FOUND
WHAT HE WAS MISSING

"I thought I was living my life to the fullest. I had no nutritional orientation at all. I believed that to restore health you had to take drugs. If my friends would ask me about the need for vitamins, I would tell them not to bother, since they would urinate them all away." These are the words of Kenneth Hodge, M.D., of Sacramento, California. Dr. Hodge is now a nutrition-oriented physician. The following interview with Dr. Hodge tells the story of his conversion, the story of how a potentially fatal stroke brought him face to face with death or lifelong paralysis—and the power of nutrition to bring back health.

Question: Before your stroke, what was your attitude toward nutrition?

Dr. Hodge: My concept of nutrition was eating the four basic food groups and that was it. I told my patients they got plenty of vitamins from their foods. I preferred white flour, and I really enjoyed coffee and alcohol.

Q: Was there any warning that you might suffer a stroke?

Dr. Hodge: Yes. My father died of the same kind of stroke in 1951, while I was serving in Korea as a battalion surgeon. I had some symptoms, too. About three years before my stroke,

I began experiencing jagged lines of light around my field of vision. This is called scintillating peripheral optic scotoma. The zigzagging lights would move inward until my whole field of vision was pulsating.

Another symptom that started about that time was something called dyslexia. I was reading a medical text one day when I realized that I was unable to tell the meaning of the words. It was as though a portion of the word was missing. That was rather disquieting, especially when I saw that some of the words were simple ones, like *the*. I was also suffering from frequent left-sided headaches.

Q: Did you consult a doctor?

Dr. Hodge: Oh yes, a neurologist. He took a brain scan, but back then the scan was not very accurate as a diagnostic tool. The test came back normal. So I asked for an arteriogram, but the neurologist didn't want to do that test. It's very dangerous: Strokes or heart attacks sometimes follow it. I knew that, so I didn't insist. But I wanted to have something. I knew something was wrong with my brain. But I was able to function more or less normally for the next two years.

Q: Then what happened?

Dr. Hodge: About a year before the stroke, I went out into the kitchen one night to talk to my wife. I talked for about a half hour, and during that time she didn't understand a word I said. Words like *doo* and *dah* were coming out of my mouth.

Finally, my wife asked me if I had any idea what was wrong with me. I said the first English word she could understand: *aphasia*. She asked me what that meant. So I said the second English word that night: *Stedman*, which was the name of the medical dictionary I had in the house. She looked up *aphasia* in *Stedman's* and found that it means the inability to speak. That's all the book said, though, so she didn't find out the connotations of what was going on. But as the night passed, my speech slowly returned, but never quite to normal.

We never discussed that night very much, since I lost the word power for an in-depth conversation. My memory would lapse, too, now and then. I couldn't remember the punch lines of jokes.

Q: What did your doctor do this time?

Dr. Hodge: More tests. But all the results were normal.

Q: What did you do? Did you think there was anything you could do to prevent a stroke?

Dr. Hodge: No. There was nothing I thought I could do. Hearing from two competent medical doctors that the blood flow to my brain appeared normal, I began to think maybe there was something else wrong with my brain. Besides, I had always thought there was nothing that could be done about a stroke.

Q: What finally happened?

Dr. Hodge: Finally, about a year later, I was watching TV one night. I got up to change the channel, squatted in front of the set and fell over to my right side. As I fell, I put out my right hand to break my fall. But my right limb didn't have any strength. I could move it, but I couldn't support anything. So I lay there stupidly on the floor, looked at my wife with a sick grin on my face and said, "Honey, something's wrong here." I wasn't having any trouble talking then. I said, "It's too late to call the neurologist now, let's hold on and see how I am in the morning." Right after I fell, I was able to get right up.

At 7 A.M., I woke up and went out to get the paper. As I squatted to pick it up, I fell again. Same as the night before. I got up and walked through the bedroom and told my wife it was back again. I went into the bathroom and just as I went in, I fell again.

The neurologist came over and gave me a quick examination. He said I was probably cooking a stroke if not having one, so I'd better get into the hospital.

Q: What happened there?

Dr. Hodge: I had an arteriogram. A thin plastic tube was inserted in a leg artery and threaded through to the base of the neck, and a dye was injected. X rays then show any blockage of the blood vessels.

Q: What were the results of the test?

Dr. Hodge: I wasn't getting too much blood to my brain. My left cerebral artery was 90 percent blocked—so only 10 percent of the blood flow was getting through to the speech center and the motor center for the right side of my body. Both my common carotid arteries were 50 percent blocked, and both my vertebral arteries were 50 percent blocked. And two of my three coronary arteries were massively blocked. If coronary bypasses had been in vogue at that time, I would have been on the operating table as soon as my paralysis went away.

After the arteriogram, I found myself in this terrible predicament. I couldn't talk, couldn't move my right side and couldn't think very well, either. The only thought that came into my head for a long time was that I wished I would die. And actually, according to the tests, that could very well have happened.

Two hours after the test, the stroke got worse. The blood vessels apparently spasmed in response to the dye. It felt like somebody had put a red-hot poker in my brain. The doctors considered performing a bypass operation on my cerebral artery. When they mentioned the possibility to my wife, she asked one of my good friends, who is a neurosurgeon. He said, "The best thing that could happen to Kenneth is death."

Q: That was the very bottom, wasn't it?

Dr. Hodge: That's right. But my introduction to nutrition was to come soon. My daughter came in to visit me soon after my stroke and saw the hospital food, which at that meal happened to be pancakes and syrup. She asked me if I would take something nutritious if she made it and brought it in. I said yes, because I didn't want to start an argument. Then she asked the doctor and he said she couldn't do it, and he gave three reasons: It was against hospital policy; there was a dietitian who could look after my nutritional needs quite adequately; and he had no belief in it at all. Neither did I.

But my daughter did. So she went underground. She smuggled the pep-up drink—a brewer's yeast milk shake—into the hospital a quart at a time.

Q: How did you like that?

Dr. Hodge: It was a new taste thrill for me. I could hardly stomach it. But I drank it dutifully, in small sips. Of course, a quart of that stuff has enough nutrition to last you for a day, so pretty soon I was eating hardly any of the hospital chow at all. I stopped drinking coffee; I stopped drinking wine. I stopped pasta, pastries and syrups. I started physiotherapy. And a couple of weeks later I went home, I was able to walk. I walked to my 50th birthday party.

Q: Is that unusual?

Dr. Hodge: Pretty much, yes. Beyond that, though, it gets into the fantastic. Two months after my stroke, you could have looked at me from across the street and not have noticed anything that would give away that I had suffered a stroke—unless you stopped and talked to me. I was still very depressed, so much so that I was trying to think of cute ways to kill myself so my wife could still collect my life insurance. At that point, I was crying at the drop of a hat. If somebody would say something to me that was nice or not nice, I would cry. My emotions were extremely labile, which is typical of a stroke victim.

My wife thought a change of scenery might do me good. She knew I liked the seashore, so we went to stay at her parents' beach house.

Q: And there you found something that changed your life?

Dr. Hodge: On the bookshelf in the beach house was a book called *Food Is Your Best Medicine* by Henry Bieler, M.D. My wife said I should take a look at it, which I did—simply to avoid being pestered about it any further. I thought the author was nuts. No way in the world can he be right about foods causing disease, I thought.

Q: Apparently, something happened to change your mind.

Dr. Hodge: On the way home from the beach house, we had to pay a visit to my sister-in-law. I didn't want to go because she was the kind of woman who was always complaining about her health. But—to my surprise—she was a different woman! She didn't have any of her neurotic complaints. Her skin color was good and she was in good spirits. An entirely changed woman.

It seems she had despaired on conventional medicine, which had yet to do her any good, and had started going to chiropractors, faith healers—anyone who would hold out a shred of hope for her. Finally, she went to a biochemist-nutritionist. And that's when her problems started clearing up.

Q: Did your sister-in-law suggest that you see the nutritionist, too?

Dr.Hodge: Did she! It was my sister-in-law who had planted *Food Is Your Best Medicine* at the beach house!

Q: How did you feel about that?

Dr. Hodge: Well, I suggested—with my limited word power—that my wife ought to see if this nutritionist could do anything for her rheumatoid arthritis and her peptic ulcer. But while she was on the phone making the appointment, I told her I would go, too. I figured I had nothing to lose and probably nothing to gain.

Q: So you went to the nutritionist.

Dr. Hodge: We both went and spent an hour apiece talking about our health and dietary histories. Then we were each given individual diets to follow, including supplements.

Q: And the results?

Dr. Hodge: Two days later, Joyce, my wife, had no ulcer pain. Within a month, she had no joint pain. But what happened to me was even more fantastic. The first thing I noticed that was different was that mosquitoes were ignoring me—because I was taking a lot of B vitamins. The second thing I noticed was that two different types of backache I'd had since I was a teenager were gone. The perennial sneezing that I'd suffered since I was even younger was gone. My sinusitis disappeared. My intermittent hives also disappeared. Both the zigzagging lights in my field of vision and the left-sided headaches that had come before and after my stroke also disappeared. The prostatitis that I'd had for five years disappeared.

But the most beautiful thing of all was that my depression started to lift. As soon as we got home, I started to assemble a couple of bicycles we had bought. It took me a week to get them together, and I struggled for several days just to get mine to move forward. I was riding on a gravel yard, and when I lost my balance and fell—well, the front yard was a bloody mess because I was taking a blood-thinning medication at the time. But within a week, I was making the half-mile trip to the speech therapy class. And a month later, I was cycling 27 miles a day.

Four months later, I was getting into arguments with my speech therapist, so she decided I didn't need therapy anymore. I had totally lost my depression. And my memory was returning.

Q: And that's when you decided to return to your practice?

Dr. Hodge: Well, I decided I would take another whack at anesthesiology, which was my specialty before the stroke. But I was looking at things with new eyes. I started to see things about medicine that I had never noticed before. Physicians think of levels of disease; they don't think of nondisease. I was thinking about health.

I was thinking that if I'd been eating as I was eating now, I would never have had the stroke in the first place. That was a brand-new concept for me, thinking about health instead of disease. And I saw that many people who came into the hospital were turned out in worse shape than when they came in.

So slowly, but surely, that started to get to me. I would look at these physicians in their youth, with their pedantic authoritarian tones, telling patients how to do things, what to do, and not brooking any nonsense from them at all. And I thought, "Is that the kind of guy I was? If so, I don't want to be one anymore." So after nine months, I decided to quit.

Q: And you began your nutritionally oriented practice?

Dr. Hodge: Cautiously at first. I read every book I could lay my hands on that dealt with nutrition. Little by little, though, I accepted more patients.

Q: Do you remember your first patient?

Dr. Hodge: Yes, the nutritionist who gave us our diets referred a man to me. He had joint pain and angina. He was taking seven or more nitroglycerin tablets a day for relief of the heart pain. But within a week on the diet I gave him, he cut down on the nitroglycerin, and during the following month he took only two. His joint pain also improved.

Q: Now your practice is full time?

Dr. Hodge: I usually run from nine in the morning until five-thirty. But I don't see too many patients in a day. On a busy day, maybe 24 people. But if I have 2 or 3 new patients, I don't see more than 6 or 8 people that day.

Q: Do you ever prescribe exercise?

Dr. Hodge: Oh, yes. I think that exercise is also very important. And when I say exercise, I don't mean you have to be an athlete. Just exercise to your capacity. Extend your capacity as much as you can, little by little. Strength is not essential, just a good, pumping, functioning heart is essential to carry oxygen and nutrients to various parts of your body. A good wide-open cardiovascular system is essential, too, for clear thinking and proper functioning of the other organs.

Q: I suppose your experience has taught you a lot about the medical profession and health?

Dr. Hodge: Well, like the average physician, I was well educated, self-assured and felt I had the answer to everything. Today I realize that I did not have the answer to everything; as a matter of fact, I had the answer to almost nothing. My attitude toward life has changed drastically since the stroke, and I consider the stroke a beneficial event. I think that optimism is essential. Pessimism creates illness. Negative thinking of any kind— whether it's anger or pessimism or depression—ruins people. Any disease is made worse by negative thinking, whether it's cancer or arthritis or an ulcer or angina.

Q: Do you ever help motivate your patients to adopt a healthier life style by telling your own story?

Dr. Hodge: Sometimes I do. I kind of go at it briefly. I usually just tell them they don't have to suffer from depression, that they could lead their lives with much more enjoyment. I simply describe to them what they're missing in life.

119

MAKE YOUR BODY
A SAFER PLACE
TO LIVE

When Harry T. had his car accident a few years ago, he considered himself pretty lucky to get out with only a minor case of whiplash. But after several weeks, he wasn't so sure about his luck anymore. By that time, his neck had completely stiffened up. So had his shoulders and hands.

Instead of getting better, he was getting progressively worse. After visiting rheumatologists and other specialists at several prestigious California medical centers, he was told he had developed osteoarthritis of the spine. His doctors prescribed the usual anti-inflammatory drugs, pain-killers and physical-therapy treatments, but nothing seemed to help. He just got stiffer and stiffer while living with constant chronic pain in his neck, shoulders and hands.

For two years his suffering continued, and he adapted to it as well as possible. But Harry didn't give up. He had been a successful business executive for years and wasn't about to let this illness do him in. Besides, he was only 60 years old—much too young to sacrifice the rest of his life to pain and misery.

Lucky for him he found out about the Commonweal Clinic in Bolinas, California. "We first saw Harry about 20 to 24 months after the car accident,'' says Charles Thompson, M.D., former medical director of the clinic. "His range of motion was severely limited. He had a very hard time turning his head. In fact, he couldn't even move his chin a quarter of the way down to his chest.

"When I found out that Harry's arthritis had come on very quickly after his car accident, I couldn't help but wonder if there wasn't some physical and psychological connection between the two. Harry suspected the same thing, but he couldn't figure out exactly what it all meant. So we worked both tracks with him—the biophysical track and the psychosocial track,'' explains Dr. Thompson.

"From counseling, Harry discovered that he still had not dealt with the aftermath of his divorce. His guilt had immobilized him emotionally just as the shoulder and neck pain did physically. Clearing up the psychological problems produced some pain relief.

"As for the biophysical track, first we tested him for food, chemical and inhalant sensitivities in the laboratory. A number of the things he was tested for, particularly certain foods, produced a significant increase in the arthritis symptoms in his neck and hands. We immediately took him off the offending foods and then put him on vitamins C, A and D, as well as B complex and calcium.

"It took about six weeks until Harry noticed improvement, but then he knew he was on the right track.

"After about three or four months, he was incredibly improved—completely free of pain. And his emotional well-being was the best it had been in years,'' Dr. Thompson told us.

An Alternative to Despair

Even if Harry were an isolated case, the results would be worth pondering. But the practitioners at the Commonweal Clinic say that they've almost come to expect significant improvement in otherwise hopeless situations.

"We see lots of patients who have reached Harry's level of despair," says Susan Rutherford, clinic administrator, "and two-thirds of those people complain of three or more chronic illnesses. By the time they come to us, they have usually been through the million-dollar workups and been everywhere trying to find help. Often their doctors have just told them there's nothing that can be done for them and sent them on their way."

"We go about things differently here at the clinic," says Dr. Thompson. "Sure, we'll run the routine blood tests (if they haven't been done within the past six months) plus a thorough, overall examination. But where most traditional doctors leave off is where we really begin."

"An initial visit to the clinic takes about two hours," says Ms. Rutherford. "And subsequent visits usually take at least an hour each."

"That's because we do so much more than just a physical exam," continues Dr. Thompson. "We want our patients to become active participants in their own healing process, not the passive people that other physicians have come to expect. It is our aim to empower people, as much as possible, to understand more clearly whatever disease process they're dealing with, both physiologically and psychologically."

To do that, Dr. Thompson and Ms. Rutherford work as a team with each patient. They actually started the teamwork idea about five years ago in their preventive medicine practice in Seattle. Now, it's a routine procedure here in the Bolinas clinic, too.

Dr. Thompson brings his training in internal medicine into play, while Ms. Rutherford acts as a counselor and health educator with training in drug and alcohol abuse, nutrition and stress management. Eight other colleagues, including a child health care specialist and a clinical ecologist, round out a staff that includes both medical and lay practitioners.

"There's a certain amount of overlap in our expertise, but together we cover a lot of bases," Ms. Rutherford told us. "Besides, we find the patients appreciate having both the male and female perspectives on a given situation. And patients can relate to a lay professional; they're relieved to know there is someone here who speaks their language. Of course, Dr. Thompson does, too, but they may not realize that at first.''

Their innovative ideas in treating the chronically ill have led them into the classroom as well as the examining room. Medical students, nurses and doctors have been learning from Dr. Thompson and Ms. Rutherford.

''We've taught classes at the University of California medical center and, before that, in the Seattle area,'' says Ms. Rutherford. ''We've also taught our ideas in the local school districts, at colleges in this area and at a drug and alcohol rehabilitation center,'' adds Dr. Thompson.

''Through all of that contact I have come to sense that most of the people we see live in their bodies as if they were dangerous places to be—that their bodies are essentially a scary, unknown collection of organ systems and chemicals that could just go haywire at any moment. They believe that, without the skill and knowledge of a sort of 'factory-trained mechanic' (an M.D.) to manage it, their life is in peril.

''Actually, it's more likely the other way around. That is, recognizing what's good for you and what isn't, what makes your symptoms feel worse and what makes them feel better, can be used as an opportunity to learn and grow in terms of medical self-care,'' Dr. Thompson told us.

Trust Your Hunches

''Therefore, a lot of our work has to do with reawakening body awareness so that people can learn to trust their own hunches and intuitions about the physical and psychosocial causes and effects of their problems.''

And most do have hunches. ''The majority of our patients have had an intuitive sense (sometimes for years) that what's going on in their bodies physically has something to do with how they think and feel emotionally about themselves, their lives and their world. Unfortunately, not one of the physicians they've seen has ever felt it was important to pursue that line of reasoning.''

Yet, that's exactly where Dr. Thompson begins when a patient first comes to the Commonweal Clinic. "To make it easier to bring out all the information needed, we have a detailed questionnaire that every patient is required to fill out," he explains. "It asks patients about their basic life style choices and medical, nutritional and exercise history. Then, at the end of each section, we include open-ended questions such as: Do you have any suspicion that your symptoms are related to certain foods, or to your menstrual period, or to life style changes such as divorce, or even a promotion?

"You'd be surprised how many people have these strong, nagging intuitive hunches about their illnesses. Not long ago, we treated a young woman who was a classic example of that. She had been under psychiatric care for about ten years, and her family had a strong history of all kinds of physical and emotional problems. Yet she 'knew' there was a physical cause. She had spent thousands of dollars on various treatments by the time she came to see us. But she still suffered from periodic psychotic depressions that lasted at least five days at a stretch. During an episode, she would experience hallucinations and very strong out-of-body experiences. She was quite immobilized in the midst of an otherwise normal, active life.

"These attacks would occur every 30 to 40 days. What's more, whenever something like final exams or a date would come up (which added stress), she could almost count on having one of these psychotic breaks. After we completed a detailed medical history, it turned out that the attacks were most strongly correlated with her menstrual cycle and obviously correlated with other psychosocial stresses. She also had a long history of dysmenorrhea [painful periods], premenstrual tension, water retention and breast soreness."

Helped by B Vitamins

"I immediately started her on daily B_6, niacinamide [a form of niacin] and tryptophan supplements," Dr. Thompson continues, "and it completely broke the psychotic pattern. Vitamin B_6

is thought to be the cofactor necessary to convert tryptophan [an amino acid] to serotonin [a brain neurotransmitter], and a lack of any of these can cause severe depression.

"It bothers me that, during all those years, no one ever took a decent enough history to uncover what her real problems were— not the psychiatrists she saw and not the neurologists or endocrinologists, either.

"That's why we emphasize the importance of a good, thorough history. For example, as a part of all initial workups, we also evaluate the patients' total stress load by having them fill in a life-adjustment rating scale. This test assigns a certain number of points for major life changes such as marriage, divorce, death of a spouse, moving or promotion. The higher your total score, the more stress you are under and the greater your risk of illness or accident.

"If we see that someone scores high, we may suggest an adjustment in nutritional intake," says Dr. Thompson. "The tendency is for most people to have little or no breakfast, a light lunch and then pack in two-thirds of their daily nutrients and calories at dinner. But by then, roughly two-thirds of their total output of physical, emotional and mental energy has already occurred, so that they are running on a deficit. That can be critical for someone whose recent history contains 250 or 300 of those life-adjustment rating points. Statistically, that person is much more likely to experience a major illness or accident."

"We attempt to match input of nutrients with output of energy by having our patients spread out their calories more evenly over the day," continues Ms. Rutherford. "We suggest that they eliminate foods that contain a lot of preservatives, artificial colorings and other chemicals, as well as overprocessed foods like sugar and white flour. Those foods are stressors in themselves and don't always provide the kinds of nutrients (especially the B vitamins and minerals) that might be depleted during times of stress."

"Of course, complaints about stress are usually not what brings people in," Dr. Thompson points out. "But stress is often related to the other chronic ailments they may be suffering.

Whether it's asthma, gastritis, colitis, high blood pressure, psoriasis or whatever, we approach each patient as an individual. Even people with the same disease will probably be treated differently. That's why it's so hard to generalize. We don't have a special diet for this ailment or a special nutrient for that disorder."

Listening to the Body

"Each of our patients learns to use his or her uniqueness to help uncover the underlying answers to a particular problem. In other words, the body becomes its own biofeedback system," Dr. Thompson explains. "This is especially evident when we check for food sensitivities. From the history taken, we determine which foods are suspect. Then we do allergy testing for those specific items. During the testing, the subjective symptoms are noted—mental fogginess, agitation, anger, dizziness. We also note whether the symptoms they originally came in with are increased by the food in question. From all of that, we are able to determine what level of allergy response or hypersensitivity the person shows.

"Food sensitivities really matter," Dr. Thompson emphasizes. "Two or three years ago, I would have said, 'That's a lot of hokum.' But not anymore. I'm completely convinced. Our own laboratory experiments have confirmed the effects that foods can have on susceptible people. I have seen the elimination of allergic foods reduce the symptoms of migraine, depression, psoriasis, recurrent ear infection, colitis, arthritis, even high blood pressure.

"That last one was a real surprise to me. We've had four patients in the last year with moderately high blood pressure who did very well with food allergy elimination. Two, who were on antihypertensive medication, were able to cut their dosage in half."

In fact, Dr. Thompson is still amazed by the number of people who have been significantly helped at the clinic. "In the chronic disease population, the expectation is that you may be able to help 10 to 15 percent. If you can get that percentage up to 20 or 25, you are doing extremely well. Yet, in our experience with the chronically ill, we have better than 50 percent with significant improvement. And that includes a decrease in symptoms, a decrease in dependence on medication and an increased sense that the body is a decent place to live.''

CHAPTER
120

THE MEDICAL SCHOOL WHERE NUTRITION ISN'T A DIRTY WORD

"The graduates of today's medical schools know more about heart transplants than they do about basic nutrition. I would guess 90 percent of them couldn't describe an adequate, nutritious diet that was appropriate for people at various stages of life."

That was the reply of Philip R. Lee, M.D., director of the institute for health policy studies at the University of California medical school at San Francisco, when asked by Senator George McGovern whether today's new doctors were properly trained in the importance of nutrition.

This bad news about America's medical schools was also aired in another important forum, the official voice of the American medical establishment, the *Journal of the American Medical Association*. Esther S.Nelson, M.D., commented in the editorial column on the sad fact that, while every single veterinarian in the country had been thoroughly trained in nutrition, nine out of ten of the country's medical schools didn't adequately cover the subject.

That's the bad news. But there's good news, too. There is a doctor who's making sure every medical student that passes through one of the East Coast's most prestigious medical schools appreciates the importance of nutrition in maintaining good health.

Dr. Willard Krehl, although he is carrying on something of a revolution in the medical school curriculum, does not personally carry on like a revolutionary. The noise from the construction ten stories below, as the medical college at Thomas Jefferson University expands to fill up yet another two blocks in the center of Philadelphia, reaches up into his office but does not disturb his concentration. Dr. Krehl is a scientist, not an angry revolutionary. He has both a medical degree and a doctor of philosophy degree. His writings have appeared in nutrition and medical journals and in nutrition textbooks. He has the facts.

"I doubt there are ten hospitals in the country that can give a comprehensive nutritional evaluation of a patient. The idea that we're really all so well fed isn't true. Many of us are overfed. But many don't measure up to even a conservative estimate of what we need. As doctors, we should find out who these people are and educate them," Dr. Krehl said, commenting on "the skeleton in the hospital closet."

"But we often don't spend time with patients to see them through their troubles. Instead, we prescribe drugs."

Dr. Krehl doesn't want his students to make the mistake of ignoring nutrition. "All too often, one finds the nutritional status dismissed with the statement that the patient is 'well nourished' and 'well developed' or that the patient 'seems to be getting a balanced diet.' Nutritional deficiencies exist but not necessarily in the obvious form of traditionally recognized deficiency diseases.

"One may have malnutrition without obvious evidence of nutritional disease. The deficits may begin early in life and continue for long periods of time. It's just as important to diagnose these problems of malnutrition before these diseases develop in full-blown proportions as it is to diagnose appendicitis before the appendix ruptures. You know, preventive medicine is not new. Hippocrates said that the physician 'must look after the patient's regimen while he is yet in health.' "

Dr. Krehl admits to his students that "the concept of treating healthy—symptomless—patients is rather foreign to traditional concepts of medical practice," Hippocrates notwithstanding. But he also tells them, "It can be done. Illness can be prevented."

How? Well, the students are not left hanging on that question too long. "Frequently, the practice of preventive medicine involves efforts to change the behavior or life style of the individual. He may be advised to exercise more, eat less, relax more, discontinue smoking or the use of alcohol, or to change some behavioral pattern which may lead to future illness. The patient may also be encouraged to learn to swim or reduce weight."

The important act on the part of the physician, Dr. Krehl points out, is to communicate with the patient. "A huge communications gap exists between the doctor and his patient because the role of teacher is unfamiliar to most physicians. But to get the patient to take greater personal responsibility for health may require much greater skill, more time and understanding than knowing how to prescribe drugs."

Actually, Dr. Krehl believes, all medical care is preventive, even crisis-oriented care. The difference, he points out to his students, is in the moment when the physician intervenes in the patient's life to prevent further illness. Obviously, Dr. Krehl wants his students to learn to intervene before the patient needs crisis-oriented care.

To this end, Dr. Krehl instructs his students in how to investigate a patient's record and identify health problems that might develop in the future. For instance, students are taught to find out what patients eat, whether they use drugs, alcohol or tobacco, what occupational hazards or environmental pollutants they're exposed to, what they like to do with their leisure time and what psychological adjustments they make. The students also learn to look at a patient's record and identify what health problems might have been prevented by earlier attention.

Naturally, they are also taught to look for the signs of nutritional deficiencies. Dr. Krehl tells them, "Nutritional disease due solely to inadequate intake is rare, but it does occur if faulty dietary habits persist. Marginal nutritional deficits may occur commonly because of improper diet, poor absorption, decreased utilization, increased excretion and increased nutritional requirements. Moderate illness or injury does not necessarily cause nutritional catastrophe unless these stresses are prolonged or unless the nutrient reserves are too depleted. For temporary demands, reserves may meet the need. When stress becomes sufficiently great, the reserves no longer suffice and illness can result."

Dr. Krehl believes that "there is a great deal of variability in the nutritional needs of individual people. Some people may need many times the Recommended Dietary Allowance."

As his students learn to assess the nutritional status of their patients, they learn not only how to perform standard laboratory tests for nutrient levels, but also what to look for in a patient's appearance that might give a clue to a nutritional problem. "A number of complaints are often, but not always, associated with what we might call 'undernutrition'—fatigue, apathy, loss of appetite, burning or tingling sensations, palpitation, nervousness, headache, irritability, upset stomach, depression, muscle weakness, apprehension, lassitude, abnormal changes in weight, and, in a child, failure to grow."

Quickly, Dr. Krehl ran through some of the classical symptoms of vitamin deficiencies which he teaches his students to look for: "The skin very frequently gives the first signs of malnutrition. Not all skin changes are nutritional in origin, however. Certainly, dry, scaly skin should bring to mind the possibility of inadequate vitamin A. Seborrheic dermatitis in the area of the lips and nose could be a sign of inadequate pyridoxine [vitamin B_6] and riboflavin. Dryness and opacity in a patient's eyes could be caused by vitamin A deficiency.

"Anemias will commonly show up as a generalized pallor of the tongue and mouth. In fact, abnormal appearance or inflammation of the tongue or around the mouth should lead one to at least suspect nutritional deficiencies.

"A doctor should also be alert to the mental and emotional abnormalities associated with deficiencies of B vitamins, particularly thiamine and niacin.

"Muscular weakness, particularly if generalized, could be a result of nutritional deficit. The simplest test for muscular weakness is to have the patient squat and then attempt to stand. In thiamine deficiency, muscular weakness is severe enough that the patient cannot rise from the squatting position. Absence of the reflexes, particularly the ankle jerk, may also be present."

On the subject of meganutrient therapy, Dr. Krehl says he believes some beneficial effects may occur when high doses of vitamins are taken. "But," he adds, "I don't believe it's necessarily a nutritional effect. Using high doses of vitamins is really more like using a pharmaceutical. You create a 'mass action' effect on a particular biochemical process in the body, one which normally uses a vitamin in the first place. Of course, not too much is known about the biochemistry involved. But some of the effects are well documented. For example, the treatment of intermittent claudication, a condition in which walking becomes extremely painful, is possible with 400 to 600 international units of vitamin E per day. There's little doubt that it works. I've used it myself on patients with intermittent claudication. Another good example is that the Canadian epidemiologist Terence Anderson has proved that vitamin C—while not actually preventing colds—significantly reduces the number of days lost to cold symptoms."

Of course, not all physicians accept the importance of nutrition in health or that using large doses of vitamins might help a patient. As a matter of fact, on the day we visited Dr. Krehl, he was scheduled to debate another doctor on the merits of meganutrient therapy. The debate was part of a series of nutrition seminars set up by Dr. Krehl and Robert Karp, M.D., a pediatrician who was a member of Dr. Krehl's department, to expose the hospital staff to important issues in nutrition.

The outcome of the debate was best expressed by a young medical student who raised his hand during the question-and-answer period and told Dr. Krehl's opponent, "For someone who is supposed to represent the scientific position of honest skepticism, you have really failed to bring to the argument any real scientific information thatmight discredit anything Dr. Krehl says. All you've done is generalize from newspaper clippings, while Dr. Krehl has offered scientific evidence backed up by a stack of medical journal articles."

Apparently, the strength of Dr. Krehl's careful, scientific concern about nutrition promises to carry the day not only with his students, but also with the hospital's dietary staff, formerly under the direction of Gwendolyn Acker, R.D. Together with Mrs. Acker's department, Dr. Krehl's staff revised the diet manual for the hospital. Although it wasn't in print the last time we spoke to Dr. Krehl, according to him it takes into consideration a great deal more than the usual "four food groups" idea of nutrition. And in the community health aspect of his work, Dr. Krehl is trying to teach people how to avoid serious illness by taking care of themselves, rather than waiting for a crisis to arise.

Dr. Krehl reports that the response from other medical schools has been favorable. At a recent symposium held at Jefferson medical college, many administrators from other medical schools expressed interest in Dr. Krehl's program.

The vision of a new generation of doctors who pay attention to the nutritional needs of their patients can no longer be dismissed as an impossible dream. Dr. Krehl and his staff are making it come true in Philadelphia. And when you think about it, you realize that it's really not too much to ask, since, as Dr. Krehl says, "Food, aside from the air we breathe and the water we drink, is the most important environmental factor influencing our health. When a doctor is evaluating the health of a patient, the most important thing he can do regarding nutrition is to think of it."

CHAPTER
121

THE DOCTOR WHO TAKES HIS OWN MEDICINE

"I was just another medical doctor who followed the text-books and did what he learned in medical school," admits August Daro, M.D., of Wilmette, Illinois. "Then, about ten years ago, I became interested in applying nutrition to medical problems. I bought myself books on nutrition and books on biochemistry. I read all I could on the subject. I taught myself.

"Now, around that time, a very high executive of a baking company called me in. I was doing general practice at the time. He had suffered from osteomyelitis of the leg for about 18 years. That is a bacterial infection which can often result in the actual destruction of parts of the bone. I told this man that I didn't know why he called me, since I'm not a bone specialist. He said, 'I know that. I've been to the bone specialists. I want you to tell me what you would do if you had this leg.' Without any hesitation, I told him I would try to heal it from within. So I put him on a good diet. Raw vegetables, and some cooked just a little. Vitamin D and multivitamins. Liver two or three times a week. In a year's time, that leg healed up and the problem has never returned."

Though Dr. Daro hasn't always been what you might call a nutrition-oriented physician, he has always seemed to notice nutritional deficits causing problems in his patients.

"I once had a very large prenatal clinic, visited by 150 pregnant women in an afternoon. I observed two things. One: Some of the women had beautiful teeth and some had really rotten teeth, full of cavities, and swollen gums. Two: Those who had good teeth ate their vegetables. I questioned all the women about this. And those that did not eat vegetables or drink milk—their teeth were bad. But there was a *third* group. They ate a lot of vegetables and their teeth were still bad. So I asked them how long they cooked the vegetables. They said they cooked them until they were done. So I had to find out what that meant. It meant they cooked the vegetables anywhere from a half hour to an hour and a half! No wonder their teeth weren't helped by the vegetables."

Needless to say, Dr. Daro's present patients are no strangers to fresh, natural foods and vitamin-mineral supplements.

"I had a housewife of about 30 years of age come in complaining of nervousness and headaches. She'd had these problems for several years. I could find nothing wrong with her in the physical exam. I put her on a supplement containing magnesium, calcium and vitamin D, which controlled the headaches and nervousness.

"One of my patients was a 38-year-old woman who had been plagued all her adult life with premenstrual tension and severe cramps during her period. She was completely relieved with a supplement of magnesium, calcium and vitamin D. She was so happy when she came in after taking the supplements. She said it was the first time in her life she was without symptoms."

Treating Infections, Cysts

"I had a 40-year-old woman who was always bothered by sore throats and bronchitis. Now, I don't use antibiotics for that sort of thing. I treat them with vitamin C and vitamin A. I had her take 3,000 milligrams of vitamin C and 20,000 [international] units of vitamin A daily. She has remained free of both problems since.

"You know," the doctor continued, "breast tumors are of great concern to both doctors and the women that come into the office. The most common tumors we see are called chronic cystic mastitis. They're not malignant, but they may lead to malignancy. A number of women with these tumors are deficient in thyroid. These women were helped by thyroid supplements. But not all the women were helped. I began to use vitamin A for sebaceous cysts of the skin. And I thought that, since the breast tissues derive from the skin, maybe the breast tumors will respond to vitamin A, too. I noticed that these women had dry skin. So I gave them vitamin A, and it worked. I've seen cysts of the breast 2 to 3 centimeters in diameter disappear with vitamin A. I've had enough cases to be absolutely sure, too. And in some cases, I've taken a mammogram before and after the treatment to demonstrate the disappearance of the tumor."

Vitamin A and the Skin

"I use vitamin A for any cyst that appears on the skin. A 50-year-old woman came in for a gynecological exam and asked me to recommend an ophthalmologist that would remove a cyst from the upper right lid of her eye. I asked her if she was in a hurry to have it out. She said no. I asked her if she would like to try vitamin A to see if that would make it disappear. She said she'd like to try it. So I had her take 40 to 50,000 units per day and I also gave her an injection of vitamin A once a week. In about eight months, the cyst disappeared.

"There were never any adverse reactions to the vitamin A. As a matter of fact, I was in a confrontation once with a 'doctor of science' who was the chairman of the nutrition department of a large medical organization. The newspaper got us together and questioned us. They asked him about vitamin A first. He said it was dangerous because it can be toxic. Then they asked me. Now, I knew this man was not an M.D., so he had no clinical experience. So I said, 'I've been in practice for a long, long time and I have never seen a case of vitamin A toxicity. However, I have seen thousands of people who had a deficiency of vitamin A.' That took care of him. Some people are sensitive to vitamin A, of course. But you can be sensitive to anything—strawberries, eggs, milk. If someone is sensitive to it, you don't give it, that's all.''

Some of the people Dr. Daro helps with the healing wonders of nutrition happen to be other doctors. "One day I noticed another surgeon getting ready for surgery and his back was covered with acne. I told him to try some zinc. He knows me, has confidence in me, so he tried it. About three months later I saw him, again getting ready for surgery. His back was completely clear! It was as though he had never had any acne.

"Soon after that I played golf with the head of the dermatology department at one of the medical schools in Chicago. It made for some interesting conversation, believe me. I convinced him, and now we're doing some work together on the use of zinc in dermatology. I use zinc and vitamin A on acne—not only on older people, but on young women, as well. Women come in from age 14 to 30 with acne. The zinc and vitamin A are very helpful for most of them.''

Helping Other Doctors

"I took a trip to Florida a little while ago. A great surgeon, who is no longer practicing, came along. He didn't seem as active as I am, though. So while I had him in my apartment, I made sure he saw me taking my supplements every day. So pretty soon he started to cup his hand and hold it out and say, 'You can give me some of those to take, too.' Now, here was a man who had never prescribed vitamins and minerals. All of a sudden, he became interested. On the way down, we had talked a little about it—the value of vitamin A and zinc. He's very sharp. He wanted the names of the supplements I take. When we came back, he immediately went to the drugstore and got some for himself. And you know, I talked to him yesterday and his voice sounds stronger and he admitted that he feels much better since he's been on the supplements.''

These men weren't the only doctors helped by Dr. Daro's nutritional counseling. Dr. Daro takes his *own* medicine. ''The medical profession says: 'Cut cholesterol out of the diet to lower blood cholesterol.' They usually include eggs which I think are a most wonderful food. I eat two eggs a day. But I also reduce saturated fats, meats and creams. I eat lots of low-fat meat, lots of fish. I eat fish six times a week. And I use lecithin, 2 table-spoons of granular lecithin in the morning. I use safflower oil on salads. About two years ago, I took my cholesterol count for the first time. It was 280, which is high-normal. But with this diet, I've gotten it down to 180. And as a matter of fact, I went into the hospital about two months ago for a cataract operation, and they took my cholesterol level as part of the routine ex-amination. It was down to 150!''

Did Dr. Daro prepare for his own surgery in any special way? ''I increased my intake of zinc. With zinc, tissues heal better, faster. My regular supplements are magnesium, B_6, vi-tamin A, vitamin C. I amazed the doctors, you know. Just two weeks after surgery, I was back out on the golf course. Some people can't get back to their regular routine for months after cataract surgery.

''And you know the funny thing about this, the surgeon who operated on me is a good friend of mine. He never believed in supplements before. But when I was in there for a follow-up exam, his wife also happened to be there and I noticed she had a bit of a skin condition. So I mentioned to him that she should take some zinc and some vitamin A. And he took notes on this himself, what she should take. This amazed me. I think he saw the effect of the supplements on my healing. I kept telling him that the supplements and the good eating had something to do with my recovery. I said, 'I'm not trying to take away from your fine operating technique, but you've got to have tissues that will heal.' I saw his wife just yesterday, and she's taking the vitamins and minerals and improving.''

Dr. Daro's healthful diet works its wonder outside the hospital, too. "I graduated from medical school in 1925. I started practice in 1928. And I have a lot of energy. Yesterday, I was in the office here and I saw about 28 patients. I do that three days a week. I owe it to nutrition. I eat properly. I don't smoke or drink. And I try to get my sleep.''

Other things are important, too, Dr. Daro says. "I have a theory that it's just as important to exercise as it is to sleep. So I tell my patients to jog, even at home. Start slowly. Or use a bicycle either outside or in the home if they have a stationary cycle. I tell the older people to do some walking.''

Nutrition, Humor and Kindness

"I think a good sense of humor helps, too. If you're serious all the time, you get too much tension. What people don't know about stress is that, if you don't have any stress at all, you collapse. You need a certain amount of it.

"Not enough medical schools teach nutrition. But something else that interns and nurses should be taught is that the patients are human beings. You need to have a human hospital. One of my earliest experiences was at Chicago Lying-In Hospital. One morning, as I was just getting off my rounds, a husband who had both arms full of presents came up to me. He said, 'My wife said you were so wonderful to her that she made me go out and get you these presents.' I didn't know who it was, so I had to go out on the floor to find out. It turned out to be a young woman who had been crying the night before. I had said, 'Now you don't have to cry; you're in a good hospital, one of the best in the country. Your doctor is one of the best. And I'm on duty tonight and I'll watch you close to make sure nothing happens to you.' All I did was what any kind person would have done.''

CHAPTER

122

Dr. "Live-Right"

What do you find in your doctor's waiting room? Chairs and tables? Stacks of old magazines? Perhaps a radio playing soft music?

Well, how about lunch? Not just any old lunch, but a nutritious whole-foods meal prepared by your doctor's staff and served without charge. If you were a patient of Ray Wunderlich, M.D., of St. Petersburg, Florida, who specializes in preventive medicine, that's exactly what you'd be likely to find.

"We serve lunch every other week, and sometimes every week if the demand is great," Dr. Wunderlich told us on a recent visit to his office. Slender, bearded and, at age 53, obviously in great shape, Dr. Wunderlich is a runner, and several of his trophies are displayed in the office. (He had just run 15 miles before we met him!)

"We serve anywhere from 7 to 30 people right here in the waiting room," he continues, "and they share. They share experiences. My wife, Elinor, who's a registered nurse, or I give a short talk about the foods we're presenting. We'll explain why we're having vegetable quiche or buckwheat sprouts or whatever it might be.

"And the patients love it because it's very tasty stuff, and they're interested in getting the recipes. It's just a great way to convince people that nutritious food not only tastes good but is easy to prepare."

But that's not all. Just about everywhere you turn in Dr. Wunderlich's office you find useful and important health information—on bulletin boards in the waiting room and treatment rooms, in pamphlets that Dr. Wunderlich has prepared and in tape recordings that you can play at home. "Actually, right now we're in a period of transition," he says. "We hope to have an even better way of giving nutrition education soon with a slide-and-tape machine for the patients.

"Yes, we do an awful lot of passing out of material. First, there's a folder we give to every new patient. It contains basic information, such as practical suggestions about which foods to eat and which to avoid, how to gradually adjust your diet to get out of the typical American processed-food rut, what to pack in your lunch box, plus an important note about dietary supplements.

"Then we have more specific materials: signs of visual problems, biosocial factors in learning disabilities, suggestions for the food-allergic patient and much more."

Dr. Wunderlich graduated from the Columbia University college of physicians and surgeons. How much training in nutrition did he receive? "Not much," he says. "I don't remember any course on nourishment.

"Even today you won't find many articles about general nutrition in the journals that physicians read. You might find something on a highly specialized topic—for example, a fatty-muscle chemical and how it relates to a certain disease of infants. And that's called 'nutrition.' But those articles are for super-specialists. How it all relates to beans and peas and squash and milk and soils and fertilizers is seldom addressed.

"There's a sign up on one of my bulletin boards," says Dr. Wunderlich, grinning. "It says, 'The specialist is someone who learns more and more about less and less, until pretty soon he knows everything about nothing.' It's a beautiful saying. It's the old blinders business. We certainly need specialists and their skills, but not to the exclusion of generalists."

Emphasis on Prevention

In order to practice full-time preventive medicine for both adults and children, Dr. Wunderlich gave up a large pediatric practice about six years ago. "I found that patients who ate properly and took appropriate nutritional supplements were healthier than the rest.

"I could treat disease very well, indeed. However, I decided to turn my efforts toward the development of bright eyes, gleaming bodies and alert minds. I learned that wrong living habits discourage health and that right living habits generally lead to well-being.

"Of course, I still do treat disease. I'd say two-thirds of the people who come to me have chronic diseases. They aren't satisfied with the way they're functioning and the way they feel.

"Their diabetes doesn't get better, their arthritis doesn't get better, their lupus doesn't get better, their depression doesn't get better, their schizophrenia doesn't get better, their periodontal disease doesn't clear up. They don't want to take a bunch of medications over a long time, but they can't get well. I offer them the nutritional option with attention to body chemistry, allergy, nutritional supplements and possible toxic substances.

"And I also treat kids with learning disorders and hyperactivity. So we see most everything except very acute illness. We're always trying to educate the patients. We try to get our licks in, you know, and get them reinforced, because when the patients get out there in the world, they're not going to get reinforced too often. These people need all the help they can get to give up old bad habits and replace them with healthier new ones."

Patients come from as far away as Oregon to see Dr. Wunderlich and, of course, from all over the state of Florida. "I had one fellow in here from the center of the state," he says, "and he was scheduled to have a triple coronary bypass in a few months. We began to work on him, changing his diet and giving him nutrients. And he came back about eight weeks later, and his hair, which was white, was turning black!"

What was Dr. Wunderlich doing to him? "If I could do it again, I would!" he says. "I'd grow my own hair. But everything isn't the same for each one of us. Different factors operate in different people. With him, we had just the right combination of diet and nutrients. This gentleman had a rather dramatic change. He stood up straight, grabbed a new lease on life—and his hair began to darken. You could see it within an eight-week period.

"So he went back to his cardiologist. And his cardiologist talked to him for a long time and looked over all the things he was doing, and this fellow said his cardiologist was going to start coming to see me!"

Did he ever have the coronary bypass? "No, he never had the operation," says Dr. Wunderlich, "and we don't think he's ever going to need it. We think his blood vessels are going to open up."

Treating the Individual

Dr. Wunderlich does a good deal of his nutritional testing for allergies and vitamin levels right in his own office. "We do a vitamin C test with urine, which is very important," he says. "We can find out if a patient is excreting a lot of vitamin C or whether he isn't. Some patients are taking up to 10 grams a day and not spilling any vitamin C. So they usually need more.

"What we're doing is individualizing supplements for each patient. You see, what you have to always remember is to treat the individual patient—and not the patient's nutrient test. Everyone's needs differ. We've been giving lip service to that for a long time. But the more you can do it, the better results you get.

"Take me, for example. I know how to stay in balance pretty well, but what I do for myself doesn't necessarily apply to my patients. If I gave them what I take myself, it might not work. You have to look, and then you have to share information between patient and doctor."

Dr. Wunderlich is quite excited about a new test for nutrient sufficiency. "It's done with the eyes," he says. "A friend of mine, Dr. Jack Pierce, a professor of optometry at the University of Alabama, told me about it.

"I put a stain in the patient's eyes with a little stick of paper. It's not harmful and not traumatic at all. Then I take an ultraviolet light, shine it in the eyes, and look at the illuminated tear film of the eyes with a magnifying glass.

"I watch that tear film, and that tear film should hold in front of the cornea for ten seconds without breaking up. If the tear film breaks up before ten seconds, it's an indicator of nutritional deficiency. The biggest component in it is vitamin C, but the B vitamins are also involved—the water-soluble vitamins.

"So just that little test is an index," says Dr. Wunderlich, "and that's so important. Because a patient might say, 'Oh, I'm taking my vitamins.' And you might say, 'Oh, that's good.' But the fact is, you don't know whether it's too much or too little. So we look at physical signs in the patient, we measure blood levels, we measure what we can in the urine, we do hair mineral tests and we do the eye test. Plus we talk to the individual about past history, family history, allergies, intolerances and progress with nutrient supplements.

"You look at the tongue, you look at the skin, you look at everything. Then you put all that information together and say, 'OK, the evidence says you're just about right in your nutrient levels.' Or, 'The evidence says you're low in these areas.' And that's what we try to correct."

Hands-On Therapy

But there's still more. In addition to all those things, Dr. Wunderlich is now becoming involved with manipulative medicine. "I'm involved in what we call counterstrain, which is a form of hands-on therapy," he says. "It's a technique in which you find tender spots in the body pressure points. Then you position the body and hold it in a certain position, and those tender points go away, and the patient feels better. You relieve pain with practically no discomfort on the part of the individual. We're also doing deep muscle therapy, as well as counterstrain, because it helps people.

"Manual therapy is a great help in muscle inflammation and muscle tension. Sometimes also in osteoarthritis. Osteoarthritis is usually considered a disease of wearing out and degeneration. But it doesn't appear to be that way at all to me. It appears to be a disease of wrong living.

"Why? Because sometimes I can stop the Heberden's nodes—the tender swellings in the finger joints—in their tracks when the patients eat correctly and when their vitamin-mineral needs are met. And sometimes I can help to break up the nodes by appropriate physical therapy.

"For example, if you're using a high dose of alfalfa, and if you're using appropriate manual therapy on those nodes, sometimes you can mobilize the deposits. But the patients must be eating perfectly. They must have much of their food as raw food, they must have no foods to which they are sensitive, and they must have their mineral and vitamin needs met.

"Furthermore, they must be sure they have proper circulation in the arms. That means rehabilitation of all the muscle groups from the shoulder to the hand. Altogether, it means nutritional therapy, and it means consideration of sensitivities. That's not easy to come by, but that's what it takes."

What about osteoporosis? "We don't see osteoporosis in physically active women," says Dr. Wunderlich. "Of course, you have to be pretty active. You have to be stressing the body daily. But you don't have to jog. Walking can do it.

"In the prevention and treatment of osteoporosis, what you're looking for is a pull or stress on the bone. That's what stimulates bone to function. As soon as you have it, then that bone is going to keep rebuilding itself. It's similar to what happens in the muscles—tearing down and building up. It's a continual turn-over. That's how we keep it fresh, live and young.''

Helping Problem Children

Although he no longer practices pediatrics as a specialty, Dr. Wunderlich still has an abiding interest in the health of children. He has authored several books on the subject, and he has delivered a paper to a meeting of the Association for Children with Learning Disabilities.

"I see problem kids all the time," he says. "Kids who don't learn, who can't sit still, who have attention deficit, who have behavioral problems, who have minimal brain dysfunction—whatever you want to call the specific syndrome that they have.

"Now, when I see a child with a learning disorder, he will usually also have a language disorder: He can't spell or write.

"People recognize the language disorder—they call the kids dyslexic. And they recognize the learning disorder because those kids are different from other kids. But what they don't recognize is the living disorder they have.

"When you go into their homes or look into their lunch boxes, you see that they're not eating correctly. Or if you do body chemistry probes, you find that they're not absorbing food or they have serious allergies or vitamin-mineral deficits.

"And," Dr. Wunderlich continues, "they frequently have toxicity. The toxicity is all kinds of things. It may be chemical food additives. It may be toxic minerals—cadmium, lead, aluminum, copper, mercury and so on. So those kids have nutrient deficits, and they have toxicities. Some may have nutrient deficits along with minimal toxicity. and some may have major toxicity, but all of them have nutrient deficits of major degree.

"So when I see a kid with a learning disability, I say, 'Let's not just look at the LD that is a language disorder or the LD that is a learning disorder. Let's look at the LD that is a living disorder.'

"That's what's been overlooked all these years. The educators are looking at the kids, but they don't really see that what they eat before they come to school affects what they do there or that what they did yesterday affects what they do today. You see, all American children are born deficient."

We thought that was a fairly provocative statement.

"I firmly believe it has more truth than fiction in it," Dr. Wunderlich says staunchly. "My thesis is that many of us are drifting along on adequate nutrition but not on optimal nutrition.

"And so I see more and more children with puny chests. I see more and more children with failure to thrive. I see more and more children with allergies or behavior problems. More, not fewer. And I think the rates are rising absolutely, not relatively."

What, you may ask, do the Wunderlichs themselves dine on? We found out when they invited us to their home for dinner.

This is a very busy family, so Elinor Wunderlich prepares many meals ahead of time. Her freezer is chock-full of such goodies as a concentrated seafood gumbo to which fresh okra and tomatoes can be added, a black bean and cheese casserole, carob brownies . . . you get the idea.

For dinner that night, we had the black bean and cheese casserole as a main dish, and it was wonderful. Also included were alfalfa and lentil sprouts, beet greens and a salad with fresh everything in it. For dessert there were baked apples and muffins.

It was the perfect end to an enlightening day with a doctor who practices what he preaches.

123

BRAIN FOOD—
IT REALLY WORKS

Sarah never left her home. She couldn't, because she spent 12 hours each day grooming and washing her body. Mostly she washed her hands. From the elbows down, the skin was raw, chapped and at times even ulcerated. She used incredible quantities of creams and ointments, but it didn't do much good.

Sarah underwent ten years of psychoanalysis. She took every antidepressant available, as well as every major and minor tranquilizer on the market, in an effort to break out of her destructive behavior. She even underwent six series of electroshock treatments and was hospitalized for three of them. And still the washing continued.

Yet, today Sarah is free of her obsessive-compulsive disorder and leads a normal, productive life.

What made the difference?

In Sarah's case, says Jose A. Yaryura-Tobias, M.D., it was doses of the amino acid tryptophan, niacinamide (a form of niacin) and vitamin B_6 (pyridoxine). Dr. Yaryura-Tobias, a native of Argentina and medical director of Bio-Behavioral Psychiatry in Great Neck, New York, says the therapy increases the blood level of serotonin, an agent responsible for promoting nerve impulses which, in the brain, dictate much of our behavior. Tryptophan is a precursor of serotonin and is also a source of niacin, a vitamin. When niacinamide is given with the tryptophan, less tryptophan will be converted into the vitamin, and more of it will be used to make serotonin. Vitamin B_6 is essential to that conversion.

"But there's more to it than that," says Dr. Yaryura-Tobias. And he should know. For over 20 years, he's been doing research while practicing medicine, first as an internist and then as a psychiatrist with a strong background in psychopharmacology (drug therapy). "I realized early in my practice," says Dr. Yaryura-Tobias, "that psychoanalysis and drugs were not enough.

"In medical school in Argentina, we had to take one year of nutrition. We could not practice medicine if we didn't study nutrition first. When we examined a patient, we not only had to make a diagnosis at the bedside, we also had to prescribe an appropriate diet. After all, if you have a gallbladder problem, you must follow a certain diet. If you have diarrhea, you need a certain diet. As a psychiatrist, I reasoned, Why not a diet for the brain? That's as much a part of the body as the gallbladder or intestines."

Still, psychological problems are as varied and complex as the people afflicted. Faulty nutrition may play an important role in the development of symptoms, but so do childhood trauma, genetics, society and environment. The solutions to those problems must therefore involve numerous therapies in order to gain the maximum chance of recovery. No one method covers it all. Rather, a mixing and blending of philosophies is the best bet.

"And that's what we practice here," says Dr. Yaryura-Tobias. "I call it an integrated approach to psychiatry. We have 15 people on our staff, including 2 psychiatrists, 6 psychologists, 1 neuropsychologist, a nutritionist, 2 research assistants, an art therapist, a psychiatric social worker and an EEG-EKG [electroencephalogram-electrocardiogram] technologist. We each contribute our special area of expertise to the diagnosis and treatment of our patients so they get the benefit of the various disciplines. By working together, we find the best approach for each particular case. Because people are different, what works best for one may not work for another.

"Take the case of Sarah, for example. For her, diet alone was enough. For others, a combination of diet and medication may be necessary. But even if a drug is used, adding the appropriate nutrients allows us to cut the dose of the drug by about half, eliminating annoying or damaging side effects."

For still others, a behavioral approach might be added to the nutrition and drug therapy. Fugen A. Neziroglu, Ph.D., specializes in behavioral therapy and is the clinical director of Bio-Behavioral Psychiatry. She explains that traditional behavioral therapy focuses on changing a person's habits without trying to form a diagnosis or explain the cause.

"My behavioral approach is somewhat different from that," she says. "We want to rule out physical illness, and in order to rule it out and to see what treatment is really appropriate, we have to have a diagnosis."

"To aid us in that area, each new patient is given a physical examination," adds Dr. Yaryura-Tobias. "Our psychiatric social worker, Audrey Harbur Bershen, takes a complete social history. Blood tests measure liver and kidney functioning, vitamin and amino acid levels and proteins. A five-hour glucose tolerance test is done to rule out hypoglycemia [low blood sugar] or diabetes. We do an electroencephalogram and an electrocardiogram and hair analysis for trace minerals and toxic chemicals. And, of course, we conduct a thorough neuropsychological evaluation.

"When a patient is diagnosed as an obsessive-compulsive, the nutrients that we use are tryptophan, niacinamide and vitamin B_6. Those elements appear to participate in the biochemistry of the illness. We don't say that obsessive-compulsive disorders are a unique disease of the tryptophan-serotonin metabolism, but our research has shown us that a good amount of people with that problem could be categorized in a biochemical classification."

Help for Depression

"A person suffering from depression may also do well with tryptophan," he continues. "I like higher doses of vitamins B_1

and B_6, though, because they help activate the energy transport system in the body. We also use phenylalanine. That is an amino acid which in the body is converted to phenylethylamine, an antidepressant. At times, drugs are a necessity, but they are never used without the nutrients.

"The point is we don't limit ourselves to one type of therapy. It wouldn't make sense to do that. Illness has many causes, so how can we expect to help all our patients with only one method of treatment?

"The patient must understand, too, that results will take longer with the natural therapies than with the drugs. When a drug is used, the results are very dramatic. But you can have bad side effects, too. With the tryptophan and vitamins, results will be gradual, taking maybe ten weeks to reduce symptoms completely. But the benefits here are obvious—no side effects to mess you up in other ways."

Still, those methods may not work completely, and other therapies will be called into service. Here's where behavior modification comes in.

"Behavior therapy is really down-to-earth," Dr. Yaryura-Tobias told us. "It's faster than psychotherapy. It goes into the problem and modifies the habits that have become imprinted over the years. After all, you can take away the chemical reasons for the illness, but the behavior has been learned for years and has to be unlearned."

When behavior therapy is called for, it is usually in conjunction with a proper diet and supplements, most often tryptophan, niacinamide and vitamin B_6. The behavior modification itself begins with an intensive two-week program, after which symptoms are reduced by about 60 to 70 percent.

"For example," says Dr. Neziroglu, "we had a patient who was afraid of glass. He feared that glass would get on his hands, then circulate through his body and contaminate everything he touched, including his wife. His fear of glass caused him to wash everything in sight. He had freshly washed dollar bills hanging on a clothes line in his house. His dry-cleaning bills were over $200 a month.

"We went to his house, and we put glass everywhere. He even had to carry a piece of glass in his pocket all the time, and he slept with fiber glass under his pillow. This process is called flooding. We flooded him with anxiety. His level of anxiety remained elevated for two hours or so. And then we saw, after that time, the anxiety just came down. He began to see for himself how ridiculous his fears had been all along. After about two weeks, there was a tremendous reduction in his symptoms. And after several months, all symptoms were gone.

"And what's so encouraging," Dr. Neziroglu told us, "is that relapses are infrequent, even though some of these people have been ill for many years."

The Bio-Behavioral Psychiatry group has done wonders also with people suffering from severe aggression associated with hypoglycemia. Of course, not all people with low blood sugar have a violent nature. But the ones who are violent often have an abnormal EEG (brain wave test), too. Just giving them an anticonvulsant to straighten out the EEG (which is what most doctors do) won't bring results.

"What we did," Dr. Neziroglu told us, "was to divide 45 patients with this disorder into four groups. One group was placed on a special diet to alleviate the hypoglycemia; another group got an anticonvulsant for their abnormal EEG; the third group got traditional tranquilizers; and the fourth got a combination of the diet, vitamin B_6 and an anticonvulsant. The only group that improved statistically was group 4, the one receiving the combination.

"We believe that about 33 percent of all aggressives can be helped by the combination of diet, B_6 and an anticonvulsant," she adds.

Brain Fatigue Is Common in Everyday Life

Fortunately, most of us never reach such a desperate stage. Still, we all go through our own daily cycles of highs and lows.

It's important, says Dr. Yaryura-Tobias, to recognize your own symptoms so they don't get out of hand. Specifically, he is referring to a condition we've probably all had at one time or another—brain fatigue.

"The brain tires like a muscle," explains Dr. Yaryura-Tobias. "When a muscle is fatigued, it gives you a signal—pain or cramps—which is due to the lack of oxygen in the muscle. You have to rest to recover.

"The brain will also give you signals when it is overtired—inability to concentrate, inability to put thoughts together, a sense of irritability to minor things. You feel jumpy, nervous. You may have difficulty in falling asleep or staying asleep. You go from lows to highs. The brain cannot control itself any longer. The brain works by excitation and inhibition. When there is fatigue, those things begin to be altered, and they do not coordinate. The incoordination of the brain will bring incoordination in the thought process, in the mood, in intellectual capacity—in all the functions that you have."

For most of us, brain fatigue is part of our normal daily cycle. But then we eat a good dinner, read a book, do some exercises. We have switched from doing one thing to doing another that is unrelated, and that rests the brain so we are ready for the next day's work load.

But for many others, brain fatigue becomes a chronic condition.

Fatigue builds upon fatigue with no recovery period in between. You can't catch up with just a night's sleep anymore. You find yourself unable to concentrate or put thoughts together. You have pushed yourself to an extreme and you can't return any longer.

"I think there is an amazing amount of brain fatigue that exists," Dr. Yaryura-Tobias told us. "People come here and I tell them they must stop working right now. It's reached that level.

"Unfortunately, because brain fatigue is not a visual thing, no one believes it exists, not even the patients who are describing the symptoms. They keep on trying to work, and to do that they take stimulants—coffee and amphetamines. They go out at night and have cocktails.

"A lot of them are on tranquilizers and sleeping pills. They do all that because without it they could not function."

Daily Exercise Is Important

"By the time they come in for a consultation," he continued, "they may have a drug problem to go along with the brain fatigue. That is when I feel the nutritional approach is best, along with resting the brain. We give supplements, especially the B-complex vitamins, and a program of exercises along with a good diet. Physical exercise is very important, too. It is one of the most perfect things to reduce anxiety and tension.

"When I recommend physical exercise and nutrition, it's not for one week—it's forever. It's a life style that one has to adopt permanently to remain in good mental health."

But, of course, good habits should be started before you reach the breaking point.

"I exercise every day," Dr. Yaryura-Tobias points out, "and I take supplements—about 1,000 milligrams of vitamin C, plus B complex and dolomite. And I give my brain a vacation by switching to nonpressure pastimes such as reading novels or poetry, listening to music or watching a good program on television. Then I am able to resume my schedule refreshed.

"That's important because most of the people we treat here are very sick. They've usually been all over trying to find help. When a patient brings us 30 years of illness, we must work out 30 years of illness. Sometimes it's almost impossible.

"But I can tell you this, something we are doing here is good, because even with the very sickest patients, we get about 50 percent to improve. And it's not the medication. As a psychopharmacologist, I am sure of that. It's the addition of the vitamins. I'm positive. We also see that behavior therapy is helpful and so, too, is working with the patient's family.

"That's our approach and it works. I think that an integrated practice is in medicine of the future."

Apparently others are starting to agree.

"Hofstra University in Hempstead, New York, sought us out when we started our group here," Dr. Neziroglu told us. "They sent a faculty member to observe our methods and asked us if they could send interns. Now we have four interns working with us toward their doctoral degrees."

"Setting up this type of practice is not easy," warns Dr. Yaryura-Tobias. "It's very difficult to have real teamwork. Your pride has to go down a little. You get embarrassed if you make a mistake. But don't tell me that there is no chance to do this type of work. The fact that it is not done doesn't mean it will not work. Because it will work if you try. We are living proof of that."

CHAPTER

124

PSYCHOLOGICAL HELP THROUGH BETTER DIET

If you suffer from a stress-related complaint such as depression or anxiety or even ordinary insomnia and you'd like to find a treatment more natural than antidepressants or tranquilizers, there's an herbalist-psychologist in the Philadelphia area whose ideas might interest you.

His name is Arthur Hochberg, Ph.D., and he tries to provide what he calls "an alternative to conventional psychology and medicine." For him, that means using herbs, food, vitamins and minerals instead of prescription drugs. It also means treating the whole person by combining psychology and nutrition.

"How people feel emotionally and how they feel physically are absolutely connected," Dr. Hochberg told us. "In every physical problem there's a psychological counterpart." The attitude of the therapist seems to matter, too: "People are happy to talk to a doctor who listens to them. Ultimately, what heals patients is compassion."

For one of Dr. Hochberg's patients, a 49-year-old woman who teaches at a high school in a depressed part of Philadelphia, his method provided an alternative to using estrogen for menopausal symptoms.

"I was skeptical. I frankly didn't think it would work," the teacher (she requested anonymity) told us. "I was planning just to 'wait out' menopause without medication. I don't normally go to a doctor. I'm a no-nonsense person."

She waited it out successfully for two and a half years, but finally stress in the classroom brought on overwhelming hot flashes. "A tremendous depression would sweep over me, and I'm not normally depressive at all. The heat would rise from my feet, go up through my body and hit my face with a shock. My face turned beet red. I felt incredible heat, nausea and dizziness that lasted two to three minutes. It happened 20 to 30 times a day."

Dr. Hochberg questioned her about her diet and medical history and suggested brewer's yeast, pantothenate and vitamins B_6, A and E, along with tea made from rue (in very small amounts), horsetail and black cohosh root. Although she discontinued the tea after the first day ("It was bitter"), within a week she felt an improvement, and after a month her symptoms subsided to four or five mild hot flashes a day.

"He was square with me," the teacher told us. "He said the herbs and vitamins wouldn't eliminate the symptoms, just reduce them. He said, 'See what happens and if it works, it works.' "

For Cathy Bath, a 30-year-old mother of two with one more on the way, Dr. Hochberg offered an alternative to cortisone and several years of postpartum fatigue.

Mrs. Bath had suffered from eczema on her hands since the age of nine and had controlled it with a standard prescription—cortisone cream. In early 1981, however, the skin condition spread to her face and she was catching colds every couple of months. She sought medical help.

Dr. Hochberg advised her to cut white flour and sugar out of her diet and recommended large amounts of brewer's yeast, vitamin C and water-soluble vitamin A. The regimen also included chamomile tea, kelp, spinach and beet greens, cod liver oil and the exclusive use of olive and safflower oils in cooking.

"Now my face is perfect," Mrs. Bath says. "It used to be awful. It was swollen, it itched, it was red and scaling. Now my only problem is protecting it from the sun.

"I also feel energetic for the first time since my first pregnancy. I don't need naps in the afternoon anymore." She has cut her use of cortisone. "It amazes me that I only have to use it once or twice a week, because I was one of those people who couldn't go anywhere without a tube of cortisone."

Battle with Depression

In one especially dramatic case, Dr. Hochberg helped a 37-year-old insurance executive overcome half a lifetime of depression and dependence on candy bars and caffeine.

The executive, Dave Richards, had suffered from mood swings and depression since high school. He could barely keep awake in class and relied on coffee to pep him up. He was a top student, but his self-image was very poor and life was "a daily battle." He saw several psychiatrists without success.

About three years ago, he went to Dr. Hochberg, who spotted a severe problem with sugar intolerance. He prescribed tea made from small amounts of licorice root or goldenseal or juniper berries and hops, or a mixture of valerian and other herbs. He also put Richards on a strict low-sugar diet of fresh vegetables and whole grains, fruits, seeds, garlic and spring water.

Now when he starts to feel moody or "unbalanced," Richards says, he sips herb tea. "It smooths me out, helps me to avoid mood swings. I like that."

About Dr. Hochberg's natural therapy, Richards says, "It really changed my life."

Dr. Hochberg's forte is herbs and he used a battery of them, along with a broad spectrum of nutrients, to help one woman recover from severe intestinal pain and anxiety.

He advised the woman, Zainab Bauman, a 33-year-old mother of one, to use a lot of garlic. It cleans the system, he said, to boil a bulb of garlic every day with parsley, then drink the broth and eat the bulb. The therapy also called for a relish of turmeric, spearmint, cayenne, tamarind and lemon. He suggested teas from slippery-elm bark, fenugreek and other herbs, as well. Mrs. Bauman says it worked.

"In about three weeks, my whole state of mind changed," she says. "Everything changed. I felt like a cloud had been lifted off of me. I realized that my depression was rooted in my mind, not in reality."

Another young woman, who also requested anonymity, told us that Dr. Hochberg helped her recover from anxiety and depression with tea from sage, raspberry and chamomile. Her therapy, which included vitamins, minerals, papaya enzymes and bran, also relieved a long-standing problem with water retention. "Whatever it was he did, I'm grateful," she said.

Herbal Formulas

Dr. Hochberg was willing to share some of his herbal formulas, which are used in conjunction with exercise and the elimination of white flour, sugar, caffeine, alcohol and nicotine.

For colds, nausea and headaches: Dr. Hochberg suggests preparing a tonic by mixing small pieces of ginger root, coriander seeds and garlic with water and honey to taste. Then boil off half the liquid. Throughout the day, periodically drink what's left.

For instant stimulation: Mix ⅛ teaspoon of cayenne, 2 tablespoons of apple cider vinegar, a cup of warm water and ¼ teaspoon of molasses.

For insomnia or tension: Steep half a teaspoon of valerian root in hot water for five minutes (do not boil the root). Sip it gradually through the day or take at bedtime. For taste, valerian should be mixed with honey, spearmint or clove. One precaution: Valerian is a strong herb and should be used moderately.

For cleansing the body: Garlic, dandelion root tea, chamomile tea or valerian root tea (in small amounts).

For low blood sugar: Licorice root tea (also to be used in moderation), juniper berry tea (again, in small amounts), spearmint tea or dandelion root tea.

For migraine headaches: Strong peppermint tea and niacin.

Dr. Hochberg says he often tries several combinations of herbs and nutrients before finding the blend that suits the patient best, and sometimes he uses hair analyses to pinpoint deficiencies. About 70 to 80 percent of his patients achieve good results in about two months if they stick to the program, he says.

People who can purge themselves of anger, Dr. Hochberg says, also stand a better chance of recovery. And it helps if they participate in their own cure by preparing teas and keeping busy with gardening, exercise and other activities.

Dr. Hochberg, who is 40, traveled a long and winding path to his present office on the second floor of a small building in Bala-Cynwyd, a suburb of Philadelphia. Born in Brooklyn, he earned a doctorate at the University of Utah and later learned how to live on herbs and berries in the wilds of California. He has taught at colleges in Indiana and New Jersey and has worked at several health clinics in eastern Pennsylvania.

He has visited Africa, Mexico, Israel, Switzerland and the Far East, looking, he says, for bits of wisdom about the human mind and body.

A good part of his zeal as a therapist, Dr. Hochberg notes, comes from dissatisfaction with conventional medicine. His patients often tell him horror stories about undergoing unnecessary and expensive tests and about meeting doctors who refuse to listen to their opinions.

"I feel strongly," he says, "about people being harassed and intimidated and manipulated by the medical profession. The more patients I see and the more stories I hear, the more I realize that part of their illness is fear.

"Doctors pretend that there's a great mystery about illness. And when they don't know what to do, they tell their patients that nothing can be done. The patients suffer from helplessness and abandonment. Distrust of doctors is one of the most rampant feelings I see in patients.

"What heals patients is compassion," he emphasizes. "The patient must trust the doctor, and the doctor must have confidence in the patient. It's distrust that makes people seek alternative treatment."

CHAPTER

125

A LIFE-EXTENSION PROGRAM FROM A DOCTOR WHO'S BEEN THERE

Forty years ago, future physicians learned even less about nutrition in medical school than they do today. "Until four years ago, I didn't know enough about nutrition to help myself, much less my patients," Robert I. Lowenberg, M.D., of Atlanta, Georgia, a vascular surgeon for 31 years, told us. "My diet consisted of beef two or three times a day, lots of margarine, lots of salt, and candy bars when I was in a hurry. The best nutritional advice I could give my patients was: Lose a little weight and stop smoking. Most physicians don't realize the importance of nutrition until they're slapped in the face by it."

Dr. Lowenberg was jolted into nutritional awareness four years ago by a heart attack. Though he recovered, a year later he started having chest pains and suffering from fatigue. Tests indicated that blood vessels to his heart were blocked and that he needed a coronary bypass. "I began to realize that I wasn't headed in the right direction, and I became interested in what nutrition could do to help me."

He started listening to things other people were saying about nutrition and degenerative diseases, and he started reading and researching. "I soon discovered that the nutritional factors in degenerative disease had been pretty well worked out. But each researcher had put his work into a a small pigeonhole and left it there to be forgotten. A better approach seemed to be putting it all together into a nutritional program people could live by."

As a former vascular surgeon, Dr. Lowenberg used to treat with the scalpel the diseases he now treats with nutrition. "I've been in there—I know how the blood vessels of someone with heart disease, angina, atherosclerosis and diabetes actually look. Vascular surgeons know that if one blood vessel is narrowed or blocked, chances are that others in other parts of the body are, too. Atherosclerosis, for example, affects not just one set of blood vessels—it affects many of them. It's only that one vessel occludes before the others. Symptoms don't appear until the blood vessel has narrowed 70 to 80 percent. But if someone has trouble in the left leg, he almost certainly also has trouble in the right. It may be two or three years behind, but arteriograms will usually show significant narrowing in both legs.

"Now, surgery can help only blood vessels in the certain area operated on. If I perform a bypass in someone's left leg—at great cost—I haven't done anything for the right leg or the aorta or the renal artery or the brain."

But the former surgeon sees no contradiction between surgery and nutrition. "It's a question of which comes first. In emergencies, of course, surgery is necessary. But many other cases could be treated nutritionally. Surgery can open a vessel to the point where it was when the patient was 25 years old. But that's not always necessary. Often, an increase in flow of 5 or 10 percent is enough to start improvement, and proper nutrition can often do that. If nutrition should fail, you can always go on to surgery."

Keeping Bypasses Open

Yet, even people who do undergo corrective surgery should, Dr. Lowenberg believes, change their diets afterwards to prevent recurrences. "Everybody who has a coronary bypass—and this year there will be about 100,000—should go on a nutritional program immediately after the operation to keep the new graft open. Risk of closure is high: A significant number of bypasses close each year, and a high percentage of patients die of stroke within 5 years. One reason is that bypass grafts harden five times faster than their parent vessels. After 1 year, they're equivalent to 5 years old—after 5 years, 25 years old. A proper nutritional program can undoubtedly delay closure of those grafts.

"A good case in point is a 44-year-old man I treated before I knew anything about the importance of nutrition in degenerative diseases. He was a heavy smoker and had hardly any blood flow in his left leg. The threat was gangrene. I had to operate, and fortunately the leg was saved. But I didn't run enough tests on his blood chemistry or even ask him about his diet to discover how those factors were affecting his condition. Nor did I alter his diet. Over the next 13 years, he suffered additional occlusions in the upper as well as the lower extremities. All in all, I had to perform 43 further operations on this patient, including diagnostic probes. And still, he continued to suffer complications—some of which involved those operations.

"If I knew then what I know now about nutrition, I feel confident that I could have spared the poor man many operations. That's because a nutritional approach, unlike surgery, affects every blood vessel in the body."

Fats are blood vessels' big enemies. "High levels of fat in the blood do two things," Dr. Lowenberg explains. "They leave deposits on the arterial wall, narrowing the blood vessel; and they neutralize the negative charge that separates red blood cells, making them stick together like a stack of wet dishes. In a healthy person, red blood cells float through blood vessels in single file, absorbing oxygen and discharging it to the tissues. When high fat levels make them stick together, a lot of surface is lost for picking up and delivering oxygen. Tissues begin to suffocate. To make matters worse, the clumped blood cells also get jammed at bends in the capillaries."

Unfortunately, most of us are up to our eyes in fat. "The typical American diet derives most of its calories from fat—45 percent. Another 15 percent comes from protein, with the balance being supplied by carbohydrates. The main goal of a life-extension diet is to cut fat calories down to 15 percent or less. Simultaneously, one should reduce cholesterol intake from 600 milligrams a day—the American average—to 100 milligrams a day, a very safe level. Another important step is the elimination of simple carbohydrates, such as sugar, and the substitution of complex carbohydrates. In addition, fiber intake of 25 grams a day is advisable. That's because fiber has been shown to control fat levels and to help prevent blood clotting and reduce the impact of diabetes, as well.

"Reducing the deposits on the arterial wall may take months or years, but with this diet the microcirculation improves within days. And that in turn helps everything."

Dr. Lowenberg has treated many patients using a life-extension diet and has seen impressive results. "A 61-year-old man who had already suffered several heart attacks and one stroke came to me for help. He was a nonsmoker but overweight and also had diabetes. He could barely walk—he used a cane and had to be helped into my office.

"The first thing I did was get him to cut down on fatty foods. No butter, margarine, eggs or salad oils. But the biggest reduction came from eliminating meats, which I do entirely in high-risk cases, at least at first. Meat has no fiber. And as for protein, legumes can supply, pound for pound, just as much protein as steak—but without the fat.

"Next, I increased his fiber intake: whole grain cereals—millet, brown rice, bran, whole wheat.

"Then I concentrated on getting him off less obvious troublemakers—sugar, salt, coffee and tea. Sugar is a nutritional no-no. For people with blood sugar problems, it's even worse. Salt makes the body retain water, putting a burden on the circulation. It also makes it hard to lose weight. Caffeine is a stimulant—it speeds up the heart rate, putting unnecessary stress on it. It's good to put a little stress on the heart by exercising. Exercise speeds up the heart for only a few hours and builds up endurance. But a big coffee or tea drinker stresses his heart all day."

This regimen improved the patient's condition within days.

"As soon as he was able to walk without aid, I started him on a regular exercise program. Ideally, the aim is to exercise three to four times a week for 20 minutes or more—just walking or, if possible, jogging. Exercise is an important part of a vascular health program because it builds up collateral blood vessels. These are little blood vessels, the size of a hair or two, that enlarge and take over the function of blocked vessels. If those collaterals can be opened, you can save a leg."

Within three weeks, the patient's fat levels dropped from dangerously high to the normal range, without hospitalization. And he showed the difference. "The next time I saw him," says Dr. Lowenberg, "he almost jogged into my office. Without the diet and with his indications, he would have probably succumbed to another stroke or heart attack."

That patient's renewed vitality is characteristic of people on the program. "They become more alert, more interested, because now they are able to be more active," says Dr. Lowenberg. "Many take up old hobbies. They feel that now there's a point to going on and living."

But when it comes to sticking to a special diet, motivation is a problem. Dr. Lowenberg uses an ingenious incentive—a computer readout.

On a desk-top computer, he punches in the patient's data regarding risk factors established through several studies—weight, cholesterol and triglyceride levels, miles walked a day, stress at home and office. The computer then promptly matches that data with the optimal figures and calculates the risk of heart disease.

"The difference between the actual figures and the optimal figures gives the patient a goal to shoot for. There it is in black and white. He can see that he's eating too much beef or that he's 20 pounds overweight and the likelihood of what this might lead to. He can see what he should be doing."

But to persuade patients to actually change their habits, Dr. Lowenberg finds a human touch as essential as a data sheet. "I'm telling my patients that they should change their entire life style—habits of eating, of exercise, even of work and personal relations if they're too stressful. That requires time to put across.

I take several days with each patient, explaining what his disease is, how he got it, and what he can do now to improve his condition and prevent further problems.''

Despite heart attack and bypass, Dr. Lowenberg himself is still active, indeed vigorous, at 65—running a nutritional consultation practice, playing a mean game of doubles tennis and pursuing several hobbies, including poetry. He's a doctor who takes his own medicine and enjoys it.

BOOK V

Vitamin-Rich Foods and Recipes

INTRODUCTION

Hundreds of cookbooks are published in the United States every year. That's a *lot* of recipes. Recipes just for men, artists, athletes, singles—even for specific astrological signs. Recipes for microwaves and barbecue grills. For foods from the pantry, the freezer, the garden.

Yes, you can *find* a recipe for a low-cal, gourmet Italian vegetarian meal that can be cooked in 15 minutes while camping out in Alaska. But it's next to impossible to *know* if that recipe (or any other) supplies lots of thiamine. Or vitamin A. Or B_6.

And that's knowledge you need. What if you're feeling tense and want a meal high in nerve-calming niacin? What if you're trying to shake a cold and want a lunch packed with vitamin C? That's what book 5—Vitamin-Rich Foods and Recipes—is all about. First, you'll find lists for every vitamin that tell you which foods supply extra-big doses of that nutrient. Second, you'll find a recipe section with meals we've singled out for their high vitamin content. (We'll tell you which vitamin the recipes are richest in, of course.) An added benefit is that the recipes are natural—no salt, no sugar, no additives, just healthy foods. By the way, you might want to read this section in the kitchen—the urge for a vitamin-packed meal just may overwhelm you!

126

BEST FOOD SOURCES OF VITAMINS

Best Food Sources of Vitamin A

Food	Portion	Vitamin A (International units)
Liver	3 ounces	45,390
Sweet potato	1 medium	11,940
Carrots, cooked, sliced	½ cup	8,140
Spinach, cooked	½ cup	7,290
Cantaloupe	¼ medium	4,620
Kale, cooked	½ cup	4,565
Broccoli, cooked	1 medium stalk	4,500
Winter squash, mashed	½ cup	4,305
Mustard greens, cooked	½ cup	4,060
Apricots, fresh	3 medium	2,890
Watermelon	1 slice (10-inch diameter, 1 inch thick)	2,510
Endive	1 cup packed	1,650

Best Food Sources of Vitamin A—*Continued*

Food	Portion	Vitamin A (International units)
Leaf lettuce	1 cup packed	1,050
Asparagus	4 medium spears	540
Peas	½ cup	430
Green beans	½ cup	340
Yellow corn	½ cup	330
Parsley, dried	1 tablespoon	303
Egg, hard cooked	1 large	260

Best Food Sources of Thiamine

Food	Portion	Thiamine (milligrams)
Brewer's yeast	1 tablespoon	1.25
Sunflower seeds	¼ cup	0.71
Soybeans, dried	¼ cup	0.58
Wheat germ, toasted	¼ cup	0.44
Beef kidney	3 ounces	0.43
Navy beans, dried	¼ cup	0.33
Soy flour	¼ cup	0.27
Kidney beans, dried	¼ cup	0.24
Beef liver	3 ounces	0.22
Rye flour, dark	¼ cup	0.20
Rolled oats, cooked	1 cup	0.19
Brown rice, raw	¼ cup	0.17
Whole wheat flour	¼ cup	0.17
Chick-peas, dried	¼ cup	0.16
Salmon steak	3 ounces	0.15

Best Food Sources of Thiamine—*Continued*

Food	Portion	Thiamine (milligrams)
Split peas, cooked	½ cup	0.15
Buckwheat flour, dark	¼ cup	0.14
Chicken liver	3 ounces	0.13
Cornmeal	¼ cup	0.12
Collards, without stems, cooked	½ cup	0.11
Asparagus	4 medium spears	0.10

Best Food Sources of Riboflavin

Food	Portion	Riboflavin (milligrams)
Beef kidney	3 ounces	4.1
Beef liver	3 ounces	3.6
Chicken liver	3 ounces	1.5
Calf heart	3 ounces	1.2
Beef heart	3 ounces	1.1
Yogurt, low-fat	1 cup	0.5
Broccoli, cooked	1 medium stalk	0.4
Milk, whole	1 cup	0.4
Almonds	¼ cup	0.3
Brewer's yeast	1 tablespoon	0.3
Brie cheese	2 ounces	0.3
Camembert cheese	2 ounces	0.3
Roquefort cheese	2 ounces	0.3
Wild rice, raw	¼ cup	0.3
Beef, lean	3 ounces	0.2

Best Food Sources of Riboflavin—*Continued*

Food	Portion	Riboflavin (milligrams)
Ricotta cheese, part skim	½ cup	0.2
Soybeans, dried	¼ cup	0.2
Swiss cheese	2 ounces	0.2

Best Food Sources of Niacin

Food	Portion	Niacin (milligrams)
Beef liver	3 ounces	14.0
Tuna, canned in water, undrained	3 ounces	11.3
Chicken, light meat	3 ounces	10.6
Beef kidney	3 ounces	9.1
Swordfish	3 ounces	8.7
Salmon steak	3 ounces	8.4
Halibut	3 ounces	7.2
Peanuts, chopped	¼ cup	6.2
Peanut butter	2 tablespoons	4.8
Beef, lean	3 ounces	3.9
Chicken liver	3 ounces	3.8
Brewer's yeast	1 tablespoon	3.0
Cod	3 ounces	2.7
Brown rice, raw	¼ cup	2.4
Sunflower seeds	¼ cup	2.0
Avocado	½ medium	1.8
Almonds	¼ cup	1.3
Whole wheat flour	¼ cup	1.3

Best Food Sources of Niacin—*Continued*

Food	Portion	Niacin (milligrams)
Navy beans, dried	¼ cup	1.2
Soybeans, dried	¼ cup	1.2
Kidney beans, dried	¼ cup	1.1
Chick-peas, dried	¼ cup	1.0
Dates	¼ cup	1.0

Best Food Sources of Vitamin B_6

Food	Portion	Vitamin B_6 (milligrams)
Banana	1 medium	0.89
Salmon	3 ounces	0.63
Mackerel, Atlantic	3 ounces	0.60
Chicken, light meat	3 ounces	0.51
Beef liver	3 ounces	0.47
Sunflower seeds	¼ cup	0.45
Halibut	3 ounces	0.39
Tuna, canned	3 ounces	0.36
Broccoli, raw	1 medium stalk	0.35
Lentils, dried	¼ cup	0.29
Brown rice, raw	¼ cup	0.28
Beef kidney	3 ounces	0.24
Brewer's yeast	1 tablespoon	0.20
Filberts	¼ cup	0.18
Buckwheat flour, dark	¼ cup	0.14

Best Food Sources of Vitamin B_{12}

Food	Portion	Vitamin B_{12} (micrograms)
Beef liver	3 ounces	93.5
Lamb	3 ounces	2.6
Beef	3 ounces	2.0
Tuna, canned, drained	3 ounces	1.8
Yogurt	1 cup	1.5
Haddock	3 ounces	1.4
Swiss cheese	2 ounces	1.0
Milk, whole	1 cup	0.9
Cottage cheese	½ cup	0.7
Egg	1 large	0.7
Cheddar cheese	2 ounces	0.4
Chicken, light meat	3 ounces	0.4

Best Food Sources of Folate

Food	Portion	Folate (micrograms)
Brewer's yeast	1 tablespoon	313
Orange juice	1 cup	136
Beef liver	3 ounces	123
Black-eyed peas	½ cup	100
Romaine lettuce	1 cup packed	98
Beets	½ cup	67
Cantaloupe	¼ medium	41
Broccoli, cooked	½ cup	38
Brussels sprouts	4 medium	28

Best Food Sources of Pantothenate

Food	Portion	Pantothenate (milligrams)
Beef liver	3 ounces	4.8
Chicken liver	3 ounces	4.6
Beef kidney	3 ounces	2.6
Broccoli, raw	1 medium stalk	1.8
Beef heart	3 ounces	1.4
Turkey, dark meat	3 ounces	1.1
Brewer's yeast	1 tablespoon	1.0
Peanuts	¼ cup	1.0
Peas, dried	¼ cup	1.0
Chicken, dark meat	3 ounces	0.9
Egg, hard cooked	1 large	0.9
Chicken, light meat	3 ounces	0.8
Milk, whole	1 cup	0.8
Mushrooms, raw	½ cup	0.8
Sweet corn	1 medium ear	0.8
Beef, lean	3 ounces	0.7
Sweet potato	1 medium	0.7
Cashews	¼ cup	0.6
Soy flour	¼ cup	0.6
Turkey, light meat	3 ounces	0.6
Brown rice, cooked	¾ cup	0.5
Buckwheat flour, dark	¼ cup	0.4
Rye flour, dark	¼ cup	0.4
Whole wheat flour	¼ cup	0.3

Best Food Sources of Biotin

Food	Portion	Biotin (micrograms)
Chicken liver	3 ounces	146
Calf liver	3 ounces	45
Lamb kidney	3 ounces	36
Rolled oats, uncooked	½ cup	16
Egg, hard cooked	1 large	12
Egg yolk	1 large	10
Haddock	3 ounces	5
Milk	1 cup	5
Halibut	3 ounces	4
Camembert cheese	2 ounces	3
Chicken, dark meat	3 ounces	3
Cod	3 ounces	3
Salmon	3 ounces	3
Tuna, canned in oil	3 ounces	3
Chicken, light meat	3 ounces	2
Lamb, raw lean shoulder	4 ounces	2
Orange	1 medium	2
Tomato, raw	1 medium	2
Turkey, dark meat	3 ounces	2
Whole wheat bread	1 slice	2
Black raspberries	½ cup	1
Cheddar cheese	2 ounces	1
Grapefruit	½ medium	1

Best Food Sources of Choline

Food	Portion	Choline (milligrams)
Soybean lecithin, pure	1 tablespoon	1,450
Beef liver	3 ounces	578
Egg	1 large	412
Fish	3 ounces	100
Soybeans, cooked	½ cup	36

Best Food Sources of Inositol

Food	Portion	Inositol (milligrams)
Grapefruit juice from frozen concentrate	1 cup	912
Orange juice from frozen concentrate	1 cup	490
Great Northern beans	½ cup	440
Cantaloupe	¼ medium	355
Orange	1 medium	307
Whole wheat bread, stone ground	1 slice	288
Kidney beans	½ cup	249
Navy beans, dried	¼ cup	142
Peanut butter, creamy	2 tablespoons	122
Chicken liver	3 ounces	118
Green beans	½ cup	105
Almonds	¼ cup	99
Potato, baked	1 medium	97
Rolled oats, cooked	1 cup	84
Split peas	½ cup	65

Best Food Sources of Inositol—*Continued*

Food	Portion	Inositol (milligrams)
Beef liver	3 ounces	58
Green pepper, cooked	½ cup	57
Tomato, raw	½ cup	54
Zucchini	½ cup	53
Pork chop	3 ounces	38
Onions, raw	¼ cup	22

Best Food Sources of Vitamin C

Food	Portion	Vitamin C (milligrams)
Orange juice, fresh-squeezed	1 cup	124
Green peppers, chopped, raw	½ cup	96
Grapefruit juice	1 cup	93
Papaya	½ medium	85
Brussels sprouts	4 medium	73
Broccoli, chopped, raw	½ cup	70
Orange	1 medium	66
Turnip greens, cooked	½ cup	50
Cantaloupe	¼ medium	45
Cauliflower, chopped, raw	½ cup	45
Strawberries	½ cup	44
Tomato juice	1 cup	39
Grapefruit	½ medium	37
Potato, baked	1 medium	31

Best Food Sources of Vitamin C—*Continued*

Food	Portion	Vitamin C (milligrams)
Tomato, raw	1 medium	28
Cabbage, chopped, raw	½ cup	21
Blackberries	½ cup	15
Spinach, chopped, raw	½ cup	14
Blueberries	½ cup	10
Cherries, sweet	½ cup	8
Mung bean sprouts	¼ cup	5

Best Food Sources of Vitamin D

Food	Portion	Vitamin D (international units)
Halibut liver oil	2 teaspoons	1,120
Herring	3 ounces	840
Cod liver oil	2 teaspoons	800
Mackerel	3 ounces	708
Salmon, Pacific	3 ounces	416
Tuna	3 ounces	168

Best Food Sources of Vitamin E

Food	Portion	Vitamin E (international units)
Wheat germ oil	1 tablespoon	37.2
Sunflower seeds	¼ cup	26.8
Almonds	¼ cup	12.7
Sunflower oil	1 tablespoon	12.7

Best Food Sources of Vitamin E—*Continued*

Food	Portion	Vitamin E (international units)
Pecans, halves	¼ cup	12.5
Hazelnuts	¼ cup	12.0
Safflower oil	1 tablespoon	7.9
Cod liver oil	2 tablespoons	7.8
Wheat germ, raw	¼ cup	6.4
Peanuts	¼ cup	4.9
Corn oil	1 tablespoon	4.8
Peanut butter	2 tablespoons	3.8
Corn oil margarine	1 tablespoon	3.6
Soy oil	1 tablespoon	3.5
Peanut oil	1 tablespoon	3.4
Lobster	3 ounces	2.3
Salmon steak	3 ounces	2.0

Best Food Sources of Vitamin K

Food	Portion	Vitamin K (micrograms)
Turnip greens, cooked	½ cup	471
Broccoli, cooked	1 medium stalk	360
Cabbage, cooked, shredded	½ cup	91
Beef liver	3 ounces	78
Lettuce, chopped	1 cup packed	71
Spinach, chopped, raw	1 cup packed	49
Asparagus	4 medium spears	34

Best Food Sources of Vitamin K—*Continued*

Food	Portion	Vitamin K (micrograms)
Cheese	2 ounces	20
Watercress, finely chopped	¼ cup	18
Peas	½ cup	15
Green beans	½ cup	9
Milk	1 cup	7

Sources for Vitamin Tables

Nutritive Value of American Foods in Common Units, Agriculture Handbook No. 456, by Catherine F. Adams (Washington, D.C.: Agricultural Research Service, U.S. Department of Agriculture, 1975). Vitamin A, Thiamine, Riboflavin, Niacin, Folate, Pantothenate, Biotin, Vitamin C, Vitamin E, Vitamin K.

Composition of Foods: Dairy and Egg Products, Agricultural Handbook No. 8-1, by Consumer and Food Economics Institute (Washington, D.C.: Agricultural Research Service, U.S. Department of Agriculture, 1976). Vitamin A, Riboflavin, Vitamin B_{12}, Pantothenate, Biotin, Vitamin K.

McCance and Widdowson's The Composition of Foods, by A. A. Paul and D. A. T. Southgate (Elsevier North-Holland Biomedical Press, 1978). Biotin, Vitamin D, Vitamin E.

Pantothenic Acid, Vitamin B_6 and Vitamin B_{12}, Home Economics Research Report No. 36, by Martha Louise Orr (Washington, D.C.: Agricultural Research Service, U.S. Department of Agriculture, 1969). Vitamin B_6, Vitamin B_{12}, Pantothenate.

Composition of Foods: Poultry Products, Agriculture Handbook No. 8-5, by Consumer and Food Economics Institute (Washington, D.C.: Science and Education Administration, U.S. Department of Agriculture, 1979). Pantothenate, Biotin.

Introductory Nutrition, by Helen Andrews Guthrie (St. Louis: C. V. Mosby, 1979). Thiamine, Niacin.

Composition of Foods: Spices and Herbs, Agriculture Handbook No. 8-2, by Consumer and Food Economics Institute (Washington, D.C.: Agricultural Research Service, U.S. Department of Agriculture, 1977). Vitamin A.

"Folacin in Selected Foods," by Betty P. Perloff and R. R. Butrum, *Journal of the American Dietetic Association,* February, 1977. Folate.

Human Nutrition, by Benjamin T. Burton, Ph.D. (New York: McGraw-Hill, 1976). Vitamin D.

Modern Nutrition in Health and Disease, by Robert S. Goodhart and Maurice E. Shills (Philadelphia: Lea and Febiger, 1980). Vitamin K.

"Myo-inositol Content of Common Foods: Development of a High-myo-inositol Diet," by Rex S. Clements, Jr., and Betty Darnell, *American Journal of Clinical Nutrition,* September, 1980. Inositol.

"Pantothenic Acid Content of 75 Processed and Cooked Foods," by Joan Howe Walsh, Bonita W. Wyse and R. Gaurth Hansen, *Journal of the American Dietetic Association,* February, 1981. Pantothenate.

U.S. Department of Agriculture and Nutrient Data Research Group, 1981. Choline.

"Vitamin E Content of Foods," by P. J. McLaughlin and John L. Weihrauch, *Journal of the American Dietetic Association,* December, 1979. Vitamin E.

CHAPTER
127

BREAKFASTS

Choo-Choo Granola *(Muesli)*

This tasty breakfast—actually a *muesli*—gets its name from two characteristics: One, it makes you use your jaws, and two, it goes through you like a freight train. To serve it, add milk and top it with several slices of fresh apple, if desired.

vitamin E   **thiamine**

> 2 cups rolled oats
> ⅔ cup wheat germ
> ½ cup sunflower seeds
> ½ cup walnuts, chopped
> ½ cup hulled pumpkin seeds
> ½ cup figs, chopped
> ½ cup dried apricots, chopped

Combine all of the ingredients and store the mixture in a tightly covered glass jar in the refrigerator.

Serves 10.

From *The Natural Healing Cookbook* by Mark Bricklin and Sharon Claessens, Rodale Press, Emmaus, Pa., 1981.

Cottage Cheese Pancakes with Pineapple Yogurt Topping

vitamin B$_{12}$ riboflavin

Topping

> 1 cup crushed pineapple
> 1 tablespoon orange juice
>   concentrate
> ¾ cup yogurt

Pancakes

> 1 cup cottage cheese
> ¾ cup yogurt
> 2 eggs
> ¾ cup whole wheat pastry flour
> ¼ cup wheat germ
> ½ teaspoon baking soda
>   pinch of ground allspice
>   fresh mint leaves (garnish)

To make the topping: In a small bowl, combine the pineapple, orange juice concentrate and yogurt.

To make the pancakes: Combine the cheese, yogurt and eggs in a food processor or blender. Blend them until smooth. Combine the flour, wheat germ, baking soda and allspice and add them to the cheese mixture. Blend the batter just until combined.

Using about ¼ cup per pancake, pour the batter onto a hot oiled or buttered pan or griddle. When it's bubbly, turn it and brown the other side. Serve the pancakes with the topping and garnish with the mint leaves.

Serves 2 to 4.

Breakfast Cereal Mix

Not only can you prepare a custom-made cereal mix in five minutes, but you'll have enough made up to last a week of mornings!

Customize your mix by adding a few tablespoons of seeds, such as sesame or sunflower, or by adding chopped nuts.

thiamine

    2 cups rolled oats
    1 cup bran
    ½ cup wheat germ
    ½ cup soy flakes
    ½ cup raisins
    1 tablespoon brewer's yeast
        (optional)
    2 teaspoons cinnamon (optional)

Combine all of the ingredients in a large bowl. Store the mix in a tightly covered container in the refrigerator.

Makes 4 cups.

From *The Natural Healing Cookbook* by Mark Bricklin and Sharon Claessens, Rodale Press, Emmaus, Pa., 1981.

CHAPTER
128

APPETIZERS AND HORS D'OEUVRES

Fish Pâté

vitamin A

 1 pound sole or flounder fillets
 1 cup firmly packed chopped
   spinach
 1 egg white
 ⅛ teaspoon ground nutmeg
 ½ teaspoon dried basil
 1 cup yogurt
 2 carrots, shredded
 1 cup peas
   parsley sprigs (garnish)

Combine the fish, spinach, egg white, nutmeg and basil in a blender or food processor and puree them. Refrigerate the mixture for 1 hour, then beat in the yogurt, vigorously, until smooth and fluffy.

Boil the carrots and peas for 30 seconds. Drain and fold them into the fish mixture. Pour the mixture into a lightly oiled 8 × 4-inch loaf pan. Smooth the top, then cover the pâté with buttered wax paper and wrap it with foil.

Place the loaf pan into a deep baking dish. Fill the baking dish with water to within 2 inches of the top of the loaf pan. Bake at 375° for 40 minutes, then remove the loaf from the oven, uncover it and let it cool for 10 minutes.

Remove the pâté from the pan by covering it with an inverted platter, then turning it upside down. Blot away any excess liquid before it's served. Garnish with parsley.

Makes 1 loaf.

Sunflower Seed Spread

Use this as a sandwich spread, a filling for stuffed celery or as a dip for raw vegetables.

vitamin E	thiamine	vitamin B_6

    1 cup ground sunflower seeds
    ¼ cup peanut butter
    3 tablespoons vegetable oil

Combine all of the ingredients in a bowl and mix them until smooth.

Makes 1½ cups.

From *The Complete Book of Minerals for Health* by Sharon Faelten, Rodale Press, Emmaus, Pa., 1981.

Chicken Liver Pâté

Perfect in a sandwich, this pâté can double as an appetizer. Formed into a ball and rolled in chopped fresh parsley, it makes a pretty party spread.

vitamin A	riboflavin	pantothenate
niacin	thiamine	vitamin C

    1 onion, diced
    ½ cup diced celery
    ½ green pepper, diced
    2 tablespoons chopped fresh
       parsley
    2 tablespoons vegetable oil or
       butter
    1 pound chicken liver
    1 tablespoon plus 1 teaspoon
       brewer's yeast
    ¼ cup mayonnaise

In a large skillet, sauté the onions, celery, peppers and parsley in the oil or butter until the onions become translucent. Add the chicken liver and continue sautéing for a few minutes. Cover the skillet and cook until the liver is done.

Drain off any excess liquid and reserve it. Puree the liver mixture using a food mill or blender. (If you use a blender, add a little of the reserved liquid to facilitate blending.) Stir in the brewer's yeast. Let the mixture cool, then stir in the mayonnaise. If the pâté is too thick, add a little of the reserved liquid.

Makes 2 cups.

129

SOUPS

Welsh Cock-a-Leekie

vitamin A	riboflavin	niacin
vitamin C		

    1 2½ to 3-pound chicken, cut up
   12 cups chicken stock
    2 pounds veal bones, cut into small pieces
    2 stalks celery with leaves
    2 small carrots
6 to 8 thin leeks, split
    1 bunch parsley
    3 cloves
    2 bay leaves
   ½ cup barley
    1 teaspoon curry powder
    1 teaspoon ground allspice

Place the chicken, stock and veal bones in a soup pot. Bring them to a boil, then lower the heat and skim off the foam. Simmer for 5 minutes. Tie the celery, carrots, 1 leek and the parsley together, and add them to the pot with the cloves and bay leaves. Cover the pot and simmer for 45 minutes.

Remove the chicken and let it cool. Continue cooking the soup for 30 minutes more, then remove the vegetable bouquet and veal bones and discard them. Bring the soup to a boil, slowly add the barley and lower the heat. Trim the leeks, leaving 1 inch of the green part. Cut the leeks into 1-inch lengths and add them to the pot along with the curry and allspice. Simmer, covered, for 40 to 45 minutes, or until the barley is tender.

Meanwhile, remove the skin and bones from the cooled chicken and tear the meat into chunks. Add them to the soup and cook them for 5 minutes, or until heated through. Remove the bay leaves and cloves.

Serves 6 to 8.

From *Creative Cooking with Grains and Pasta* by Sheryl and Mel London, Rodale Press, Emmaus, Pa., 1982.

Fresh Tomato Soup

vitamin C	vitamin A	riboflavin

½ cup minced onion
¼ cup minced celery
¼ cup minced carrot
2 cloves garlic, minced
2 tablespoons butter or vegetable oil
2 pounds tomatoes, peeled, seeded and finely diced
1 bay leaf
¼ cup minced fresh parsley
1 teaspoon minced fresh thyme or ½ teaspoon dried thyme

1 teaspoon minced fresh marjoram
   or ½ teaspoon dried marjoram
1 tablespoon minced fresh basil
4 cups chicken stock or tomato
   juice
   sour cream or yogurt (garnish)
   minced fresh herbs such as
   parsley, chives, basil or
   chervil (garnish)

In a soup pot, sauté the onions, celery, carrots and garlic in the butter or oil until the onions are translucent.

Add the tomatoes, bay leaf, parsley, thyme, marjoram and basil. Cover and cook over low heat for 10 to 15 minutes, or until the mixture is soft and thick.

Gradually stir in the stock or juice. Cover the pot, bring the soup to a boil, reduce the heat and simmer gently for 15 to 20 minutes, or until the vegetables are soft. Remove the bay leaf. If desired, puree the soup, then return it to the heat and warm it thoroughly. Serve it garnished with a little sour cream or yogurt and minced fresh herbs.

Serves 6.

Pennsylvania Dutch Corn Chowder

After a hard day in the fields—or at the office—this traditional chowder and a hunk of whole grain bread make a meal by themselves. Just remember to start it early in the morning or a day in advance.

niacin   **riboflavin**   **vitamin A**

1 3-pound chicken, cut up
1 onion, chopped
1 carrot, sliced

1 stalk celery, sliced
1 sprig fresh thyme or ½ teaspoon
   dried thyme
1 sprig fresh sage or ½ teaspoon
   dried sage
1 sprig fresh rosemary or ½
   teaspoon dried rosemary
6 cups water
2 potatoes, cubed
2 cups corn
¼ cup minced fresh parsley
   (garnish)
2 hard-cooked eggs, sliced
   (garnish)

Place the chicken, onions, carrots, celery, thyme, sage and rosemary in a soup pot. Add the water. Cover the pot and simmer for 1½ hours, or until the chicken is tender. Remove the pot from the heat. Remove the chicken and reserve it. Strain the broth and return it to the soup pot. Remove the chicken skin and bones and discard them. Cut the meat into bite-size pieces and return them to the broth. Refrigerate the broth overnight.

Discard the layer of fat that forms on top. Heat the broth to boiling. Add the potatoes, reduce the heat and cook just until the potatoes are tender, about 15 to 20 minutes. Add the corn and cook for 5 to 7 minutes, or until the corn is tender. Serve the chowder immediately, garnishing each serving with parsley and egg.

Serves 6 to 8.

130

EGGS

Eggs Baked in Leeks

vitamin C

3 or 4 large leeks, split and cut into 1-
inch lengths
2 teaspoons chopped fresh
rosemary or 1 teaspoon dried
rosemary
3 tablespoons butter
4 eggs
¼ cup grated Parmesan cheese
½ cup shredded provolone cheese
1 cup tomato sauce (optional)
2 tablespoons chopped fresh
parsley (garnish)

In a large skillet, sauté the leeks and rosemary in the butter
until tender. Transfer them to a 1½- or 2-quart casserole.

Make four wells in the leeks and carefully break an egg into each. Sprinkle the eggs with the Parmesan and provolone cheese. Bake at 375° until the eggs are set, about 10 minutes. Top the eggs with tomato sauce, if desired, and garnish with parsley.

Serves 2 to 4.

Curried Eggs and Avocados

Serve over rice, bulgur or whole wheat toast.

vitamin E	pantothenate	vitamin B$_{12}$
riboflavin		

```
 3 tablespoons butter
¼ cup minced onion
 3 tablespoons whole wheat flour
 2 teaspoons curry powder (or to
     taste)
 2 cups milk
12 hard-cooked eggs, quartered
 2 avocados, thickly sliced
   chopped fresh parsley (garnish)
```

In a medium-size skillet or saucepan, melt the butter until it is bubbling but not brown. Add the onions and sauté until they are tender and translucent, about 5 minutes.

Add the flour and curry powder and cook, stirring constantly to form a paste. Do not let it brown. Add the milk gradually and continue to stir until the sauce is smooth and medium thick, about 8 minutes. Add the eggs and avocados. Cook, stirring gently, just until they're heated through. Garnish with parsley.

Serves 4 to 6.

Broccoli-Stuffed Eggs

vitamin K   **vitamin C**   **vitamin A**

    2 broccoli stalks (each about 3
        inches long)
    4 hard-cooked eggs, halved
    2 tablespoons water
    1 tablespoon lemon juice
    1 tablespoon cottage cheese
    1 teaspoon French-style mustard
    1 teaspoon minced scallions
    ½ teaspoon tamari or soy sauce
        (preferably reduced sodium)
    ¼ teaspoon paprika

Peel the thin, tough skin from the broccoli stems. Steam the broccoli until tender.

Carefully remove the yolks from the eggs. Place the yolks in a blender with the water, lemon juice, cottage cheese, mustard, scallions, tamari and paprika.

Trim off about ½ inch of the broccoli florets and reserve them for a garnish. Coarsely chop the broccoli and add it to the other ingredients in the blender. Process them on low speed until smooth.

Stuff the egg whites with the yolk mixture, and garnish each half with some of the reserved broccoli florets. Serve them chilled.

Serves 4.

131

MAIN DISHES

Super Chili

vitamin A	vitamin B$_{12}$	riboflavin
vitamin C	pantothenate	niacin
folate		

     2 cups dried kidney beans
     1 pound lean ground beef
    ½ pound calf liver
     1 large onion, quartered
     1 green or sweet red pepper,
          chopped
     3 cloves garlic, crushed
3 to 4 tablespoons chili powder
     2 teaspoons ground cumin
     2 teaspoons dried oregano
    ⅔ cup tomato paste
     1 cup corn
     4 teaspoons tamari or soy sauce
          (preferably reduced sodium)

1 tablespoon blackstrap molasses
dash of cayenne pepper
(optional)

Soak the beans in water overnight. Place the beans in a large saucepan with enough water to cover them, bring them to a boil and simmer them gently until soft, about 1½ hours. Drain them, reserving 1½ cups of the cooking liquid.

Brown the beef in a large, hot, lightly oiled skillet. Place the liver in a blender with a quarter of the onion, and process them on low to medium speed until smooth. Stir the liver into the browning meat. Chop the remaining onion. When the meat is cooked through, add the chopped onions and peppers, garlic, chili powder, cumin and oregano. Cook until the onions become translucent.

Stir in the tomato paste, cooked kidney beans, reserved cooking liquid, corn, tamari, molasses and cayenne, if used. Simmer the chili until the onions and peppers are tender. Serve it hot.

Serves 8.

From *The Natural Healing Cookbook* by Mark Bricklin and Sharon Claessens, Rodale Press, Emmaus, Pa., 1981.

Oxtail, Barley and Braised Cabbage Stew

Here's a hearty one-pot stew from the British Isles that's best eaten on a stormy night in front of a warming wood fire.

vitamin C	**vitamin K**	**vitamin B$_{12}$**
pantothenate	**vitamin E**	**niacin**
riboflavin	**vitamin B$_6$**	

2½ pounds oxtails, cut into 1-inch
pieces

3 tablespoons whole wheat flour
3 tablespoons vegetable oil
2 cloves garlic, minced
4 thin leeks, split and thinly sliced
2 stalks celery with leaves, thinly
   sliced
3 or 4 tomatoes, chopped
2 bay leaves
1 cup barley
¾ teaspoon dried marjoram
2 cups beef stock or water
1½ pounds cabbage, coarsely
   chopped
8 cups boiling water
3 tablespoons butter
1 medium onion, coarsely chopped
2 tablespoons minced fresh dill
sour cream or yogurt (garnish)

Dredge the meat in 2 tablespoons of the flour. Heat the oil in a skillet and brown the meat on all sides. Transfer it to a 3- to 4-quart heavy stew pot. Add the garlic, leeks, celery, tomatoes, bay leaves, barley, marjoram and stock or water. Cover the stew and bring it to boil. Then lower the heat and simmer for 1 hour.

Meanwhile, place the cabbage in a deep bowl and add the boiling water. Let it stand for 5 minutes, then drain it, reserving the liquid.

Heat the butter in a heavy saucepan until it turns brown. Add the onions and remaining tablespoon of flour and cook, stirring constantly, until the mixture is browned. Add the cabbage and stir. Cover the saucepan and simmer for 15 minutes, or until the cabbage turns pinkish in color. (Add a few tablespoons of the reserved liquid if necessary to prevent scorching.)

Add the cabbage mixture to the stew along with 4 cups of the reserved liquid. Cook for 20 minutes or until the meat is tender. Remove the bay leaves. Sprinkle in the dill and serve the stew hot, garnishing each serving with a dollop of sour cream or yogurt.

Serves 6.

Tocana (Romanian Onion Stew with Beef and Peppers)

If you have a penchant for onions, this stew is for you. Serve over cornmeal mush or brown rice.

vitamin C	**thiamine**	**vitamin B$_{12}$**
vitamin B$_6$	**pantothenate**	

- ¾ pound beef chuck, cut into 1-inch cubes
- 1 tablespoon whole wheat flour
- 2 tablespoons butter
- 2 tablespoons olive oil
- 2 pounds Bermuda onions, sliced
- 1 tablespoon cider vinegar
- 2 medium tomatoes, pureed in a blender
- ¼ teaspoon cayenne pepper
- 3 large green peppers, cut into chunks
- 1 cup boiling water

Dredge the meat in the flour. Heat the butter and oil in a heavy 4-quart stew pot and brown the meat on all sides. Lift out the meat with a slotted spoon and set it aside. Add the onions, stir and cover the pot. Cook for 1 to 2 minutes, or until the onions are soft. Uncover the pot and cook over medium heat, stirring occasionally, until the onions are dark brown. Add the vinegar, stir, and return the meat to the pot. Add the pureed tomatoes, cayenne, green peppers and boiling water. Cover the stew and bring it to a boil, then lower the heat to simmer, stir and cook for 45 minutes, or until the meat is tender. Check it during cooking, adding more water if necessary (the stew should be fairly thick).

Serves 4.

Middle Eastern Wheat Kernel, Lamb and Navy Bean Stew

Lime and mint cool this stew.

vitamin B$_{12}$	niacin	vitamin C
thiamine		

      2 tablespoons butter
      2 large onions, sliced
      2 lamb shanks, cut into 2-inch
          pieces
      4 cups water
        pinch of cayenne pepper
    ½ teaspoon turmeric
    ½ cup dried navy beans, soaked in
          water overnight
    ¼ cup wheat kernels, soaked in
          water overnight
      2 tomatoes, cut into chunks
    ¼ teaspoon ground nutmeg
      1 potato, cubed
      1 tablespoon chopped fresh mint
        juice of 1 lime

Heat the butter in large stew pot and sauté the onions until wilted. Add the lamb and cook, stirring frequently, until it's brown. Add the water, cayenne, turmeric and beans. Bring the stew to a boil, lower the heat, cover it and simmer for 1 hour.

Add the wheat kernels, tomatoes and nutmeg and cook for 15 minutes more. Then add the potatoes and simmer for 45 minutes more, or until the wheat kernels and potatoes are tender. Stir in the mint and lime juice. Cook for 5 minutes more.

Serves 4 to 6.

Millet and Parmesan Casserole

Millet is a light, tasty grain that can be used in most dishes that call for rice.

riboflavin   **thiamine**   **niacin**

2	tablespoons butter
1	tablespoon vegetable oil
1	small onion, minced
1	stalk celery, thinly sliced
1	cup millet
2½ to 3	cups chicken stock
1	bay leaf
1	strip lemon rind
¼	cup pine nuts or walnuts
¼	cup currants
10	medium mushrooms, thinly sliced
½	cup grated Parmesan cheese
2	tablespoons grated Parmesan or Romano cheese

Heat the butter and oil in a 2-quart flameproof, ovenproof casserole or ovenproof saucepan, and sauté the onions and celery slowly until they are wilted, about 15 minutes. Add the millet and cook, stirring, for 30 seconds. Add 2½ cups of the chicken stock, the bay leaf, lemon rind, pine nuts or walnuts and currants and bring them slowly to a boil. Cover the casserole and bake at 325° for 20 minutes.

Carefully fold in the mushrooms and ½ cup of Parmesan cheese. If the millet has absorbed all of the stock, add just enough more stock to make the mixture moist. Reduce the heat to 300° and continue cooking for 10 to 15 minutes more. At serving time, remove the bay leaf and lemon rind, and fluff the millet gently with a fork. Sprinkle the top with extra Parmesan or, for a contrasting flavor, grated Romano cheese.

Serves 4.

Stuffed Zucchini

vitamin C

> 4 medium zucchini
> ¼ cup vegetable oil
> 1 medium onion, thinly sliced
> ½ green pepper, finely diced
> 1½ cups cooked brown rice
> 2 cups shredded sharp cheddar
> cheese
> ⅓ cup tomato sauce
> ½ teaspoon minced fresh basil

Cut the zucchini in half, carefully scoop out the pulp and reserve ½ cup. Heat the oil, add the onions and green peppers and sauté. Add the rice. Cook and stir it over high heat until it's lightly browned. Add the zucchini pulp, 1 cup of the shredded cheese, the tomato sauce and basil. (Add a little hot water if the mixture is too dry.)

Stuff the zucchini halves with the mixture. Place the zucchini, stuffed-side up, in a greased baking pan. Bake at 350° for 20 minutes. Top the zucchini with the remaining cheese and return it to the oven for 5 to 10 minutes, or until the cheese melts.

Serves 8.

Hot Vegetable Provençal

vitamin C   vitamin A   vitamin K

```
¼ cup olive oil
2 cups sliced onions
2 cloves garlic, minced
3 green peppers, cut into thin strips
3½ cups cooked tomatoes
1 package (9 ounces) frozen
    artichoke hearts
¼ head cabbage, sliced
¼ teaspoon thyme
1 tablespoon chopped fresh parsley
    (garnish)
```

Heat the oil in a large skillet over medium heat. Sauté the onions, stirring occasionally, until pale yellow and soft. Add the garlic and cook for 1 minute. Add the green peppers, tomatoes, artichoke hearts, cabbage and thyme. Reduce the heat to low. Simmer uncovered for 25 to 30 minutes. Transfer everything to a serving dish and garnish with the parsley.

Serves 6.

Down Home Potato Casserole

thiamine   vitamin C

```
3 pounds potatoes, thinly sliced
2 medium onions, thinly sliced
2½ cups peas
¾ cup shredded Monterey Jack
    cheese
½ cup shredded sharp cheddar
    cheese
```

¼ cup wheat germ
1 teaspoon dried thyme
½ teaspoon cayenne pepper
3 tablespoons butter, softened
2 cups milk

Dry the potato slices. Arrange a third of them in the bottom of a well-buttered 9 × 13-inch baking dish. Top with a third of the onions and sprinkle a third of the peas over the onions.

In a small bowl, combine the Monterey Jack and cheddar cheese, wheat germ, thyme and cayenne. Sprinkle a third of this mixture over the peas. Dot with 1 tablespoon of the butter.

Create two more layers of the ingredients in the same fashion, beginning with potatoes, then onions, peas, cheese mixture and butter. Pour the milk over the top and bake for 30 minutes at 400°. Then reduce the heat to 350° and bake for 20 to 30 minutes more, until the potatoes are tender and the top is golden brown. Let the casserole stand for 15 minutes before it's served.

Serves 6 to 8.

Cheese Soufflé

vitamin B$_{12}$

3 tablespoons butter
3 tablespoons whole wheat flour
1 cup milk
5 eggs, separated
1½ cups grated or crumbled farmer
cheese

Melt the butter in a skillet, stir in the flour until smooth, then remove it from the heat. Slowly stir in the milk until smooth. Return the sauce to the heat and cook until thickened.

Beat the egg yolks until thick, then add the milk sauce to the yolks a little at a time, beating well after each addition. Stir in the cheese.

Beat the egg whites until stiff, then fold them into the cheese mixture, working in plenty of air.

Pour the mixture into a buttered 1½-quart casserole. Bake at 325° for 45 minutes, or until the soufflé is tall and golden brown.

Serves 4.

From *The Complete Dairy Foods Cookbook* by E. Annie Proulx and Lew Nichols, Rodale Press, Emmaus, Pa., 1982.

Stir-Fried Peppers and Tofu

This is a colorful dish and if you can use both red and green peppers, it is even more attractive. It is the perfect centerpiece for a vegetarian dinner.

vitamin A   vitamin C   vitamin B$_6$
vitamin E

2 tablespoons vegetable oil
2 cloves garlic, minced
1 tablespoon grated fresh ginger or
   ½ teaspoon ground ginger
2 carrots, cut diagonally into ¼-
   inch slices
2 green or sweet red peppers, cut
   into 1-inch pieces
5 or 6 scallions, cut into 2-inch pieces
2 tablespoons tamari or soy sauce
   (preferably reduced sodium)
1 tablespoon vinegar
½ pound firm tofu, cubed

Heat the oil in a large skillet or wok. Add the garlic, ginger and carrots and stir-fry for about 2 minutes. Add the peppers and stir-fry for about 3 minutes. Add the scallions and stir-fry for about 1 minute. Add the tamari and vinegar and gently stir in the tofu. Cover and steam the mixture over low heat for about 6 minutes.

Serves 4.

Buck-Corn Burgers

thiamine   niacin

    2 cups buckwheat groats, cooked
    ½ cup corn germ
    1 egg (optional)
    1 small onion, grated
    1 teaspoon poultry seasoning

Puree the cooked groats coarsely in a food processor or with a potato ricer. Combine them with the corn germ, egg (if used), onion and poultry seasoning, then form patties. (If the mixture is too dry to form patties, add a little stock or tomato juice. If it is too soft, refrigerate it for a few hours for easier shaping.) Brown the patties slowly on a well-oiled or buttered griddle or pan until crisp on both sides; or brush them with oil and broil, turning once.

Makes 10.

Lentil Loaf

This lentil dish is good served with broiled tomatoes, a leafy green vegetable, baked winter squash, a big tossed salad—or just about anything else. It's as good cold as it is hot, and it makes delicious sandwiches.

vitamin C

> 1 onion, minced
> 2 cloves garlic, minced
> ¼ pound mushrooms, minced
> 2 tablespoons butter
> 1 cup lentils, ground
> ½ teaspoon dried thyme
>   pinch of ground clove
>   pinch of ground nutmeg
>   pinch of cayenne pepper
> 2 eggs, beaten
> ¾ cup tomato juice
> 2 tablespoons slivered almonds

Cook the onions, garlic and mushrooms in the butter until very soft. Remove them from the heat and stir in the lentils, thyme, clove, nutmeg, cayenne, eggs, tomato juice and almonds. Pour the mixture into a buttered 9 × 5-inch loaf pan and bake at 350° for 30 minutes, or until the top is lightly browned and the loaf is dry.

Serves 6.

Brown Rice, Cheese and Nut Loaf

A delightful medley of tastes and textures, this hearty, crunchy loaf needs only a salad to make a wholesome meal.

thiamine

> 1 tablespoon vegetable oil
> 1 tablespoon butter

   1 onion, chopped
   3 large stalks celery with leaves,
       chopped
   ½ cup chopped cashews
   ½ cup chopped walnuts
   ½ cup sunflower seeds
   1 cup cooked brown rice
   1 cup ricotta cheese
   2 teaspoons chopped fresh chives
   2 tablespoons chopped fresh
       parsley
1½ teaspoons dried thyme
   2 eggs, beaten
   ¼ cup wheat germ
   ¼ cup sesame seeds

In a large skillet, heat the oil and butter, then sauté the onions until limp. Add the celery, cover the skillet and cook for 5 minutes.

In a mixing bowl, combine and mix the cashews, walnuts, sunflower seeds, rice, cheese, chives, parsley, thyme and eggs. Add the onions and celery.

Sprinkle half the wheat germ on the bottom and sides of a greased 9 × 5-inch loaf pan. Turn the mixture into the pan and sprinkle the remaining wheat germ and the sesame seeds on top. Bake at 350° for 1 hour.

Serves 6 to 8.

CHAPTER

132

FISH

Haddock with Ginger Glaze

vitamin B$_{12}$ **niacin**

>   ¼ to ½ cup water
>   ¾ pound haddock fillets
>   1 teaspoon cornstarch
>   ¼ cup cold water
>   1 teaspoon grated fresh ginger
>   1 clove garlic, minced
>   2 teaspoons tamari or soy sauce
>   (preferably reduced sodium)
>   1½ teaspoons cider vinegar
>   1½ teaspoons honey
>   1 scallion, thinly sliced

Bring ¼ cup of water to a boil in a medium skillet. Add the haddock and lower the heat. Poach the fish on one side for 2 to 3 minutes, then turn the fish and poach until it is opaque throughout. Add more water, if necessary.

Dissolve the cornstarch in the cold water. Transfer the fish gently to a warm serving platter. Pour off any water remaining in the skillet. Place the cornstarch mixture, ginger, garlic, tamari, vinegar and honey in the skillet. Over medium heat, stir the sauce until slightly thickened and reduced by almost a third. Pour the ginger sauce over the fish fillets. Top the dish with the scallion, and serve it immediately.

Serves 2.

Peachy Fish Amandine

vitamin E

> ⅓ cup almonds, sliced or chopped
> 3 tablespoons butter
> 1 pound filleted fish
> 3 peaches, sliced

Sauté the almonds briefly in the butter. Remove the almonds when they are golden. Add the fish to the hot butter and sauté for 6 to 8 minutes, or until the fish is just opaque throughout. Transfer it to a serving platter. Top it with the almonds and sliced peaches.

Serves 4.

Salmon Croquettes

vitamin B₁₂   **pantothenate**   **vitamin B₆**
vitamin D

> 1 medium onion, chopped
> 4 scallions, chopped
> 1 tablespoon butter

1 can (15½ or 16 ounces) pink
    salmon, drained and flaked
1 cup cottage cheese
3 eggs
2 egg yolks
2 cups whole wheat bread crumbs
1 tablespoon minced fresh chives
    or 1½ teaspoons dried chives
1 tablespoon minced fresh dill or
    1½ teaspoons dried dill
1 tablespoon minced fresh parsley
    or 1½ teaspoons dried parsley
¼ teaspoon paprika

Sauté the onions and scallions in the butter until the onions are translucent. Transfer them to a large bowl. Add the salmon, cottage cheese, eggs, egg yolks, bread crumbs, chives, dill, parsley and paprika to the bowl and mix well.

Form the mixture, 1 tablespoon at a time, into small croquettes. Place them on a greased cookie sheet and bake at 350° for 20 minutes. The croquettes are done when they're firm to the touch. Or sauté them in butter until browned.

Makes about 35.

Steamed Fish with Spinach and Parmesan Cheese

There's only one word to describe this dish—*sensational!*

| vitamin A | vitamin K | vitamin C |
| vitamin B$_{12}$ | niacin | |

1 pound halibut, haddock or cod
    fillets, cut into four portions

1 pound spinach, chopped and
    cooked
1 egg yolk, beaten
1 small onion, grated
⅛ teaspoon ground nutmeg
¼ cup yogurt
2 teaspoons lemon juice
½ cup grated Parmesan cheese
    mushroom slices (garnish)
    lemon wedges (garnish)

Arrange a piece of cheesecloth along the bottom and up the sides of a perforated or bamboo steamer. Add the fish and steam it over boiling water for 5 to 8 minutes. When the fish is almost done, use the cheesecloth to transfer the fish to a buttered oven-proof casserole.

Drain the spinach. Mix the spinach with the egg yolk, onions, nutmeg, yogurt, lemon juice and half of the Parmesan cheese. Spread the mixture over the steamed fish. Sprinkle it with the remaining cheese and slip it under the broiler until the cheese melts and is lightly browned. Garnish with mushrooms and lemons.

Serves 4.

CHAPTER
133

POULTRY AND LIVER

Turkey Pie

vitamin A   vitamin C   niacin
pantothenate   vitamin B$_6$

         1 green pepper, minced
         4 carrots, thinly sliced
         2 stalks celery, chopped
         2 onions, minced
10 to 12 mushrooms, sliced
         3 tablespoons vegetable oil
         2 cups peas
       ½ teaspoon dried sage
         1 teaspoon dried thyme
         1 teaspoon dried basil
       ¼ cup plus 2 tablespoons butter
       ¼ cup whole wheat flour
         2 cups turkey or chicken stock
         1 cup half-and-half
       ¼ teaspoon ground nutmeg
         pinch of cayenne pepper

4 cups cubed cooked turkey
6 potatoes
½ to ¾ cup milk
¼ cup grated Parmesan cheese

Sauté the green peppers, carrots, celery, onions and mushrooms in the oil until limp. Blanch the peas in simmering water for 3 minutes, then drain them and add them to the other vegetables. Add the sage, thyme and basil.

Melt ¼ cup of the butter in a saucepan and cook until foamy. Stir in the flour and cook for 1 to 2 minutes over low heat. Whisk in the stock and continue cooking, stirring constantly, until the mixture begins to thicken. Stir in the half-and-half and cook until thick enough to coat the back of a spoon. Add the nutmeg and cayenne. In a large bowl, combine the sauce with the cooked vegetables and turkey. Then pour the mixture into a buttered or oiled 9 × 13-inch baking dish.

Cook the potatoes in simmering water until tender. When they're cool enough to handle, peel the potatoes, if desired, and mash them. Beat in the milk, the remaining butter and half of the Parmesan cheese. Spread the potatoes on top of the turkey mixture (or pipe them on with a decorative pastry tube). Sprinkle the top with the remaining cheese. Refrigerate the pie until you're ready to bake it. Bake at 350° until the pie is warm and bubbly and lightly browned on top, about 1 hour.

Serves 6 to 8.

Liver with Mixed Vegetables

vitamin B$_{12}$	vitamin A	riboflavin
vitamin K	pantothenate	vitamin C
niacin	folate	vitamin E
vitamin B$_6$	thiamine	

¾ pound calf liver or baby beef
   liver

3 tablespoons whole wheat flour
2 teaspoons dried basil
2 tablespoons vegetable oil
1 small zucchini
2 scallions, chopped
10 cherry tomatoes, halved
2 teaspoons tamari or soy sauce
(preferably reduced sodium)

Cut the liver into long, thin strips. Combine the flour and basil on wax paper, and dredge the liver slices in the mixture.

Heat 1 tablespoon of the oil in a medium skillet, and sauté the liver over low to medium heat. It should be cooked just until the inside of each strip remains pink. Do not overcook. Transfer the liver to a serving plate and keep it warm.

Cut the zucchini in half crosswise, then lengthwise. Cut each section into long, thin strips. Add the remaining oil to the pan, then add the scallions and stir and cook. When the scallions wilt, add the zucchini. Add a few spoonfuls of water if necessary to keep the vegetables from sticking.

When the scallions and zucchini are slightly softened, add the tomatoes and tamari and stir to combine them. Place a lid on the skillet and allow the vegetables to steam until tender, stirring occasionally, for about 10 minutes. At serving time, arrange the vegetables on two sides of the liver.

Serves 2.

From *The 20-Minute Natural Foods Cookbook* by Sharon Claessens, Rodale Press, Emmaus, Pa., 1982.

Oven-Baked Chicken and Vegetables

vitamin A	niacin	vitamin C
vitamin E	vitamin B$_6$	pantothenate

2 carrots, cut into large pieces
1 large potato, thickly sliced

>   1 sweet potato, thickly sliced
>   1 whole chicken breast, halved and
>   skinned
>   1 onion, thinly sliced
>   ½ cup water

Place the carrots, potatoes and sweet potatoes in a casserole, arranging the chicken breasts on top. Cover them with the onions. Pour the water over all. Cover the casserole and bake at 350° for 1½ hours, or until the chicken and vegetables are tender.

Serves 2.

From *The Natural Healing Cookbook* by Mark Bricklin and Sharon Claessens, Rodale Press, Emmaus, Pa., 1981.

Cashew Chicken with Brown Rice

niacin   pantothenate   vitamin B₆

>   1 cup chopped onion
>   1 clove garlic, minced
>   1 tablespoon vegetable oil
>   1½ cups cottage cheese
>   ¾ cup chicken or turkey stock
>   2 cups cubed cooked chicken
>   breast
>   ½ cup toasted cashews
>   dash of nutmeg
>   2 teaspoons tamari or soy sauce
>   (preferably reduced sodium)
>   1 tablespoon chopped fresh parsley
>   4 cups hot cooked brown rice

In a large skillet, sauté the onions and garlic in the oil until tender. In a blender, combine the cottage cheese and stock. Process them on medium speed until smooth.

Add the blended sauce to the vegetables. Stir in the chicken, cashews, nutmeg, tamari and parsley. Over low heat, stir constantly until the ingredients are hot, but do not let them boil because the cheese sauce may curdle. Serve the mixture over the hot cooked brown rice.

Serves 4.

From *The Natural Healing Cookbook* by Mark Bricklin and Sharon Claessens, Rodale Press, Emmaus, Pa., 1981.

CHAPTER
134

SIDE DISHES

Brussels Sprouts with Sesame Casserole

vitamin C   vitamin E

- 1 small onion, diced
- 1 green pepper, minced
- 1 medium leek, split and chopped
- 1 clove garlic, minced
- 1 tablespoon vegetable oil
- 3 tablespoons sesame seeds
- 1 tablespoon dried oregano
- 1 cup cottage cheese
- 1 tablespoon whole wheat flour
- 2 tablespoons wheat germ
  juice of 1 lemon
- 1 tablespoon tahini (sesame butter)
- 1 teaspoon sesame oil
- ¼ cup stock

3½ cups shredded Brussels sprouts,
     steamed
½ teaspoon paprika

Sauté the onions, peppers, leeks and garlic in the oil over medium-low heat for 10 minutes, or until soft. Stir in the sesame seeds and oregano, and sauté for 3 to 5 minutes more. Remove the vegetables from the heat and set them aside.

In an oiled, deep, 2-quart baking dish, combine the cottage cheese, flour and wheat germ. Mix them well. Fold in the vegetable mixture. In a small bowl, combine the lemon juice, tahini, sesame oil and stock. Blend them well, preferably with a whisk. Alternate folding the tahini mixture and the Brussels sprouts into the cottage cheese mixture. Pat it all down. Cover it tightly. Bake at 300° for 15 minutes, then sprinkle the top with paprika and bake for 15 minutes more.

Serves 4 to 6.

Hawaiian Vegetable Medley

vitamin A   vitamin C

2 tablespoons vegetable oil
1 small onion, chopped
1 green pepper, chopped
1 stalk celery, chopped
2 large carrots, thinly sliced
1 cup green beans, cut into 1-inch
     pieces
¼ cup chicken stock or water
1 cup snow peas
¾ cup crushed pineapple
1 tablespoon tamari or soy sauce
     (preferably reduced sodium)

> 2 teaspoons cornstarch
> 2 tablespoons water
> 1 can (4 ounces) water chestnuts,
>   sliced

Heat the oil in a medium skillet and sauté the onions, green peppers and celery for 3 to 5 minutes. Do not let them brown. Add the carrots, green beans and stock. Simmer, covered, until the vegetables are tender, about 10 to 12 minutes. Add the snow peas, pineapple and tamari, and simmer for 2 minutes more. Dissolve the cornstarch in the water. Add the water chestnuts and cornstarch mixture to the skillet. Cook, stirring constantly, until the liquid is thickened.

Serves 4.

From *Rodale's Basic Natural Foods Cookbook* edited by Charles Gerras, Rodale Press, Emmaus, Pa., 1984.

Orange Rice Pilaf

This is a grand production. It takes a little longer, but the delight with which it is always received justifies the extra effort. Make it for a special occasion, or just make it—and dinner will be special.

vitamin C

> 1 tablespoon vegetable oil
> 2 tablespoon butter
> 1 onion, minced
> 2 cups brown rice
> 2 cups orange juice
> 2 cups boiling water
> 12 cloves
> 1 small piece cinnamon stick

¼ teaspoon ground ginger
3 tangerines or oranges, peeled and
sectioned
½ cup raisins
¼ cup sliced almonds
1 tablespoon honey

In a large saucepan, heat the oil and 1 tablespoon of the butter and sauté the onions until soft. Add the rice and continue cooking for 5 minutes, stirring constantly. Add the orange juice to the boiling water. Pour that over the rice. Add the cloves, cinnamon and ginger. Cover the saucepan and simmer for 40 minutes, or until the liquid is absorbed. Remove the cloves and cinnamon stick.

Reserve 6 tangerine or orange sections. Stir in the remaining sections and the raisins. In a small skillet, heat the remaining tablespoon of butter and sauté the almonds until golden. Place the rice in a serving dish and top it with the reserved fruit and the sautéed almonds. Drizzle the top with the honey.

Serves 6 to 8.

Asparagus Amandine

vitamin K   **vitamin E**   **vitamin C**

1 tablespoon butter
⅓ cup sliced or slivered almonds
1 cup sliced mushrooms
¼ cup minced fresh parsley
2 teaspoons grated lemon rind
1 pound asparagus

In a large frying pan, melt the butter. Add the almonds and mushrooms. Cook over low heat, stirring often, until the almonds are golden and the mushrooms are tender. Stir in the parsley and lemon rind.

Using white kitchen string, tie the asparagus spears into small bundles about 2 to 3 inches in diameter. (Make sure all of the spears in each bundle are about the same thickness.)

Bring a very large pot of water to a boil. Carefully lower the bundles into the water. Cook at a boil just until the asparagus is tender, about 5 minutes.

Remove the asparagus from the water. Remove the string and place the asparagus on a serving platter. Cover it with the almonds and mushrooms.

Serves 4.

From *Cooking with the Healthful Herbs* by Jean Rogers, Rodale Press, Emmaus, Pa., 1983.

Applesauce-Filled Squash

vitamin A   vitamin C

2 acorn squashes
1 cup applesauce
2 teaspoons lemon juice
¼ cup raisins
2 tablespoons molasses
2 tablespoons chopped walnuts
1 tablespoon butter
¼ teaspoon cinnamon

Cut the squashes in half and remove the seeds. Combine the applesauce, lemon juice, raisins, molasses and walnuts. Fill the squashes with this mixture. Dot the tops with the butter and sprinkle them with the cinnamon. Place the squashes, filled-side up, in a baking dish. Pour hot water into the dish to a depth of about ½ inch. Cover the dish and bake at 375° for 30 minutes. Then uncover the dish and bake for another 30 minutes.

Serves 4.

Carrots, Cauliflower and Pumpkin Seeds

vitamin A

> 1 tablespoon vegetable oil
> 1 medium onion, sliced into thin
>   rings
> 2 cups cauliflower florets
> 2 medium carrots, sliced diagonally
> 1 tablespoon minced fresh parsley
> ¼ cup hulled pumpkin seeds

In a large skillet, heat the oil, then add the onions. Sauté them over medium heat for 1 to 2 minutes. Stir in the cauliflower florets and carrots. Add a few spoonfuls of water and steam the vegetables until tender, about 15 minutes, stirring occasionally. (Add a little more water if necessary.) Toss the vegetables with the parsley and pumpkin seeds. Serve them hot.

Serves 4.

Gingered Apples and Sweet Potatoes

vitamin A   vitamin E   vitamin C

> 2 medium sweet potatoes
> 2 tart apples
> ½ cup apple cider or chicken stock
> ½ teaspoon grated fresh ginger
>   dash of cinnamon

Cut the sweet potatoes in half lengthwise, then cut them crosswise into thin slices. Quarter the apples and cut them into thin slices.

Place the sweet potatoes and apples in layers in an 8 × 8-inch baking dish. Pour on the cider or stock, sprinkle the top with the ginger, and dust it with the cinnamon.

Bake at 350° for 45 minutes or until the sweet potatoes are tender.

Serves 4.

Spinach with Wheat Germ, Nuts and Raisins

Even those who profess to hate spinach will love this supernutritious version.

vitamin A	vitamin E	vitamin K
vitamin C	thiamine	

    1 pound spinach
    2 tablespoons butter or margarine
    1 clove garlic, minced
      pinch of cayenne pepper
    ¼ cup raisins
    ¼ cup sunflower seeds or chopped
        walnuts
    ¼ cup toasted wheat germ
    ¼ cup grated Parmesan cheese

Immerse the spinach in boiling water, then drain it immediately. Chop it coarsely and reserve it.

Heat the butter or margarine in a large skillet. Add the garlic and cayenne and sauté for 2 minutes. Stir in the raisins and sunflower seeds or walnuts. Mix the skillet contents until well blended. Place the mixture in a 1-quart ovenproof casserole. Combine the wheat germ and cheese. Sprinkle them over the top of the casserole, and broil until the cheese is lightly browned, about 2 minutes.

Serves 4.

Creamy Potato Salad, Utah Style

vitamin C   pantothenate

    4 large boiled potatoes, cut into 1-
      inch cubes
    4 hard-cooked eggs, diced
    ⅓ cup grated mild onions
    1 teaspoon dry mustard
    2 tablespoons honey
    2 eggs, beaten
    3 tablespoons butter, melted
    ½ cup hot cider vinegar
    1 cup heavy cream, whipped

Toss the potatoes, hard-cooked eggs and onions in a large bowl until well mixed. Chill them.

Blend the mustard and honey in the top of a double boiler, then stir in the beaten eggs. Stir in the butter and vinegar. The mixture should be smooth. Cook it over simmering water until it's thick enough to coat a spoon. Cool it to room temperature.

Fold in the whipped cream. Stir the vinegar mixture into the salad and chill it all thoroughly before it's served.

Serves 4 to 6.

From *The Complete Dairy Foods Cookbook* by E. Annie Proulx and Lew Nichols, Rodale Press, Emmaus, Pa., 1982.

Green Beans with Dill and Walnut Sauce

Give green beans a gourmet touch.

vitamin C

    1 pound green beans
    ½ cup walnuts

   3 tablespoons mild vinegar
1½ tablespoons chopped fresh dill
   ¼ teaspoon French-style mustard
   1 tablespoon minced sweet red
        pepper

Steam the green beans just until crisp-tender. While the beans are steaming, place the walnuts, vinegar, dill and mustard in a blender. Process them on low to medium speed until they make a relatively smooth sauce. When the green beans are done, toss them with the sauce and the minced pepper. Serve them hot or chilled.

Serves 6.

CHAPTER

135

SALADS

Brown Rice Tabbouleh

vitamin C   riboflavin

   2 cups cooked brown rice
1½ cups chopped fresh parsley
  ½ cup chopped scallions
  ½ cup chopped fresh mint
  ¾ cup chopped tomatoes
  ¼ teaspoon cinnamon
  ¼ cup lemon juice
  ¼ cup olive oil

In a medium-size mixing bowl, combine the brown rice, parsley, scallions, mint, tomatoes and cinnamon. Combine the lemon juice and oil. Pour them over the tabbouleh and toss it to coat it evenly.

Serves 4 to 6.

Cauliflower and Pine Nut Tomato Salad

vitamin C   vitamin E   vitamin A

    2 pounds tomatoes, peeled, seeded
        and minced
    2 cloves garlic, minced
    2 tablespoons lemon juice
    ½ cup olive oil
    ⅛ teaspoon cayenne pepper
   10 fresh basil leaves, minced
    ¼ cup minced fresh parsley
    ½ cup pine nuts
    1 large head cauliflower, broken
        into florets

Place the tomatoes in a ceramic or glass bowl. Mix in the garlic, lemon juice, oil, cayenne, basil and parsley. Cover the bowl and let it stand at room temperature for 2 hours. Stir the mixture occasionally. Then chill it for 1 hour.

Spread the pine nuts on a baking sheet and toast them at 300° for 10 to 15 minutes, stirring occasionally. Bake just until golden, being careful not to overbrown the nuts. Set them aside and let them cool.

Steam the cauliflower just until tender, about 7 minutes. Cool, cover and chill it.

To serve the salad, arrange the cauliflower on a serving dish, pour the tomato mixture over it and sprinkle the top with the pine nuts.

Serves 6.

From *Rodale's Soups and Salads Cookbook and Kitchen Album* edited by Charles Gerras, Rodale Press, Emmaus, Pa., 1981.

California Chicken and Almond Salad

niacin   vitamin E

   3 cups cubed cooked chicken
1½ cups coarsely chopped celery
   2 scallions, minced
  ½ cup almonds, coarsely chopped
  ½ cup mayonnaise
  ½ cup yogurt
   1 tablespoon lemon juice
   1 avocado, mashed
   2 tablespoons minced fresh dill
   6 lettuce leaves

In a large mixing bowl, combine the chicken, celery, scallions and almonds. Cover and chill them.

In a small mixing bowl, whisk together the mayonnaise, yogurt, lemon juice, avocado and dill. Beat the dressing until creamy. Cover and chill it.

Just before serving time, arrange a lettuce leaf on each plate. Toss the dressing and salad together and place a mound on each leaf.

Serves 6.

From *Rodale's Soups and Salads Cookbook and Kitchen Album* edited by Charles Gerras, Rodale Press, Emmaus, Pa., 1981.

CHAPTER

136

BEVERAGES

Icy Melon Delight

vitamin C

> ½ cup chopped cantaloupe
> ½ cup chopped pineapple
> 2 tablespoons yogurt or buttermilk
> 3 ice cubes
> ¼ teaspoon vanilla extract
> dash of nutmeg
> fresh mint sprigs (garnish)

Place the cantaloupe, pineapple, yogurt or buttermilk, ice cubes, vanilla and nutmeg in a blender and process them on high speed until smooth. Serve the drink over ice in two tall chilled glasses. Garnish with mint.

Serves 2.

Bananaberry Shake

This shake is thick, creamy and better than a milk shake. And you can use whichever fruits are in season.

vitamin C

1 cup yogurt
½ cup milk
1 cup fresh or frozen strawberries, raspberries, chopped peaches or other fruit
1 banana
1 apple
1 tablespoon plus 1 teaspoon chopped nuts
1 tablespoon plus 1 teaspoon honey
1 tablespoon plus 1 teaspoon brewer's yeast
1 teaspoon vanilla extract

Combine all of the ingredients in a blender and process them until fairly smooth. If necessary, thin the shake with a little more milk.

Makes 4 cups.

CHAPTER
137

DESSERTS AND SNACKS

Sunflower Sesame Treats

vitamin B₆   **pantothenate**

¾ cup ground sunflower seeds
¼ cup tahini (sesame butter)
½ cup shredded coconut
¼ cup honey
⅓ cup toasted wheat germ
1 cup minced dates or raisins

In a medium-size mixing bowl, combine the sunflower seeds and tahini. One at a time, mix in the coconut, then the honey, wheat germ and dates or raisins. Mix everything together thoroughly. Separate the mixture into two portions. Place each portion on a separate piece of wax paper. Form each into a roll about 4 inches long. Wrap it securely in wax paper and chill it thoroughly. For serving, unwrap the rolls and cut them into ½-inch slices. Store them in the refrigerator.

Makes about 16.

Lemon Walnut Frozen Yogurt

This keeps well in a 0° freezer for two or three days.

vitamin B$_{12}$

> 2 teaspoons unflavored gelatin
> 2 tablespoons boiling water
> 2 cups yogurt
> ½ cup nonfat dry milk
> ⅓ cup honey
>   grated rind of 2 lemons
> ¼ cup lemon juice
> 1 egg white
> ¼ cup chopped walnuts

Dissolve the gelatin in the boiling water. In a mixing bowl, combine the yogurt, dry milk, honey, lemon rind, lemon juice and dissolved gelatin and mix them well with a whisk. Chill the mixture for 45 minutes. Transfer it to the drum of an ice cream maker and process it until it's half-frozen. Beat the egg white until soft peaks form, fold it into the half-frozen yogurt mixture along with the walnuts, and continue processing until the mixture is firm. Transfer it to a freezer container and store it at 0° in the freezer. Before it's served, let it soften a little.

Serves 4.

From *Cooking with Fruit* by Marion Gorman, Rodale Press, Emmaus, Pa., 1983.

Apple Crepes with Raspberry Syrup

vitamin C

Crepes

> 3 eggs
> ⅔ cup whole wheat pastry flour

½ teaspoon honey
1 cup water

Syrup

2 cups fresh or frozen raspberries
2 tablespoons honey
½ teaspoon vanilla
2 teaspoons arrowroot or
    cornstarch
¼ cup water

Filling

5 tart apples, thinly sliced
2 tablespoons butter
1 tablespoon honey
3 tablespoons raisins
½ teaspoon cinnamon

fresh or frozen raspberries
(garnish)

To make the crepes: In a large mixing bowl, beat the eggs. Add the flour and mix well. Add the honey and water and mix to a smooth batter with the consistency of light cream. Pour the batter into a pitcher and let it stand for 30 minutes.

To make the syrup: In a small saucepan, combine the raspberries, honey and vanilla. Stir them over low heat until just below boiling. Mix the arrowroot or cornstarch and water and add them to the raspberry mixture. Cook the syrup over low heat until thickened, about 5 minutes. Strain it through a coarse sieve.

To make the filling: Sauté the apples in the butter until slightly soft. Stir in the honey, raisins and cinnamon. Remove the filling from the heat and cover it to keep it warm.

Pour ¼ cup of the batter into a lightly buttered 8-inch skillet or crepe pan and tilt it to spread the batter evenly. Cook the crepe for 1 minute on each side. Remove it from the pan and place it on a towel. Repeat the procedure with the remaining batter. Do not stack the crepes.

Using about 3 tablespoons per crepe, spoon the filling down the center of each crepe and fold both sides over. Garnish with raspberries.

Serves 4.

Banana Wheat Germ Pudding

A delicious dessert that's great for breakfast!

vitamin E

> 2 cups milk
> 1 cup mashed bananas
> 2 eggs, beaten
> 2 tablespoons honey
> ½ cup raisins
> 1 teaspoon grated lemon rind
> ½ cup wheat germ

Scald the milk in a large saucepan. Mix in the bananas, eggs, honey, raisins, lemon rind and wheat germ. Turn the mixture into a buttered 1-quart casserole and bake at 350° for 50 minutes, or until a knife inserted into the pudding comes out clean. Let it stand for 15 minutes before it's served.

Serves 6.

Almond Cheesecake

The flavor is so extraordinary, you won't believe this is a "health" dish—with about one-half the calories and one-third the fat of ordinary cheesecake.

vitamin E

Crust

    ¼ cup sunflower seeds
    ½ cup wheat germ
    1 tablespoon vegetable oil
    1 teaspoon honey

Filling

    2 cups ricotta cheese
    1 cup low-fat cottage cheese
    3 eggs
    2 egg whites
    ½ cup honey
 1½ teaspoons vanilla extract
    ¼ cup blanched almonds, chopped
    1 teaspoon grated lemon rind
    1 tablespoon whole wheat flour

To make the crust: Grind the sunflower seeds in a blender with short bursts on high speed. In a small bowl, combine the ground sunflower seeds and wheat germ. Add the oil and honey and stir the mixture with a fork until combined. Press it into a lightly oiled 9-inch springform pan, covering the bottom and halfway up the sides.

To make the filling: Remove any lumps from the ricotta and cottage cheese by mashing them with a wooden spoon against the sides of a large mixing bowl. (The cottage cheese can also be pressed through a sieve for smoothness.)

Beat the eggs and egg whites together in a medium-size bowl until light. Add them to the cheese mixture along with the honey, vanilla, almonds, lemon rind and flour. Stir the mixture until it's combined. For a light-textured cheesecake, beat the mixture for 5 to 10 minutes on high speed with an electric mixer.

Pour the cheese mixture into the prepared crust and bake at 350° for 45 to 60 minutes. Turn off the heat and let the cheesecake cool in the oven with the door ajar for about an hour. Remove it from the oven and let it cool to room temperature before chilling it. Chill the cheesecake for at least 6 hours before it's served.

Serves 12.

From *The Natural Healing Cookbook* by Mark Bricklin and Sharon Claessens, Rodale Press, Emmaus, Pa., 1981.

Butter Almond Cookies

Delicate and delightful.

vitamin E

> ½ cup butter, at room temperature
> ½ cup honey
> 1 egg, beaten
> ½ cup blanched almonds
> 1 teaspoon vanilla extract
> 1 cup whole wheat flour

Beat together the butter and honey. Beat in the egg. Place the almonds in a blender and grind them with short bursts on high speed. Stir them into the batter with the vanilla. Add the flour and stir just until the batter is smooth.

Drop the batter by the tablespoon onto two lightly oiled

baking sheets. Bake at 375° for 8 to 10 minutes, or until the edges of the cookies are brown.

Makes 2 dozen.

From *The 20-Minute Natural Foods Cookbook* by Sharon Claessens, Rodale Press, Emmaus, Pa., 1982.

CHAPTER
138

BREADS AND MUFFINS

Super Squash Muffins

Moist and delicious, these muffins are best piping hot from the oven. Any leftovers can be reheated for later enjoyment.

thiamine   **folate**

¼ cup brewer's yeast
1½ cups whole wheat pastry flour
1 teaspoon baking soda
1 cup mashed cooked squash
⅓ cup honey
⅓ cup melted butter or vegetable oil
1 egg
¼ cup chopped nuts
¼ cup raisins

Mix the brewer's yeast, flour and baking soda in a large bowl. Combine the squash, honey, butter or oil and egg in a small bowl. Pour the liquid ingredients into the flour mixture.

Stir in the nuts and raisins. Spoon the batter into greased muffin cups, filling each about two-thirds full. Bake at 350° for 20 minutes.

Makes about 16.

Whole Wheat Hamburger Buns

thiamine   **niacin**

¼ teaspoon plus 2 tablespoons
   honey
   pinch of ginger
½ cup warm water
1 tablespoon dry yeast
5 to 5½ cups whole wheat flour
¼ cup nonfat dry milk
1 egg
¼ cup vegetable oil
1⅓ cups milk
3 tablespoons butter, melted
   sesame seeds (garnish)

In a small bowl, stir ¼ teaspoon honey and the ginger into the warm water until they're dissolved. Add the yeast but do not stir it in. Set the bowl aside until the yeast is foamy, about 10 minutes.

In a large mixing bowl, combine two cups of the flour with the dry milk. Add the yeast mixture, egg, oil, 2 tablespoons of honey and the milk. Blend the mixture thoroughly. Begin adding more flour, 1 cup at a time, until the dough is too stiff to beat with a spoon or electric beater. Then mix the dough with a dough hook, or knead it by hand for about 5 minutes. The dough should be somewhat sticky, neither runny nor dry. Cover it and let it rise until doubled, about 45 to 60 minutes.

Divide the dough into 15 equal pieces and shape them into balls. Place them on a well-oiled baking sheet. Flatten them slightly, brush the tops with the melted butter, and garnish them with sesame seeds. Allow them to rise until puffed, about 30 minutes. Bake at 350° for 15 to 20 minutes.

Makes 15.

From *Bread Winners* by Mel London, Rodale Press, Emmaus, Pa., 1979.

Whole Wheat Biscuits

thiamine   niacin

2 cups whole wheat flour
2 teaspoons baking powder
¼ cup butter
⅔ to ¾ cup buttermilk

In a medium-size mixing bowl, sift together the flour and baking powder. Cut in the butter until the mixture is the consistency of coarse cornmeal. Make a well in the center of the mixture, and mix in just enough buttermilk for the dough to hold together. With lightly floured hands, knead the dough lightly. Press or roll out the dough until it's ¾ inch thick, then cut it into 8 pieces with a floured biscuit cutter. (If you don't have a cutter, roll the dough into 8 balls and flatten them slightly.) Place the biscuits touching one another in a well-buttered 8 × 8-inch baking dish. Bake at 400° for 20 to 25 minutes. Eat them as soon as possible, since they do not keep well.

Makes 8.

Double-Barreled Oatmeal Bread

We call this loaf double-barreled because it's loaded with lots of fiber from the oats, in addition to lots of yeast. Yet, for all its hardware, it's an amazingly light bread.

thiamine   folate   pantothenate
niacin

```
          1  tablespoon dry yeast
         ½  cup warm water
         ¾  cup buttermilk or milk
         ¼  cup honey
          2  tablespoons butter
2½ to 2¾  cups whole wheat flour
         ¾  cup rolled oats
          1  egg, beaten
         ¼  cup plus 2 tablespoons brewer's
               yeast
```

Sprinkle the tablespoon of yeast over the warm water. Set it aside until the yeast bubbles. In a small saucepan, combine the buttermilk or milk, honey and butter. Heat them until the butter melts. Cool the mixture to lukewarm, then stir in the bubbling yeast.

Combine 1½ cups of the flour and the oats in a large bowl. Stir in the yeast mixture and the egg. Beat vigorously to combine them. Stir in the brewer's yeast and enough additional flour to make a stiff dough. (Go easy; too much flour will make the bread heavy.) Work the dough together well, but do not knead it. (It will be too sticky to knead.)

Transfer the dough to a well-oiled bowl. Brush the top with oil. Cover the bowl and let the dough rise in a warm place until doubled in size, about 1 hour. Punch it down, then transfer it to a well-greased 9 × 5-inch loaf pan. Let it rise until doubled again, about 45 minutes. Bake at 375° for about 35 minutes. If the top browns too fast, cover it with foil.

Makes 1 loaf.

Bravo Banana Bread

thiamine   folate

1½ cups whole wheat pastry flour
¼ cup brewer's yeast
1 teaspoon baking soda
1 cup mashed bananas
⅓ cup vegetable oil or melted butter
⅓ cup honey
⅓ cup orange juice
1 egg
2 teaspoons vanilla

Butter a 9 × 5-inch loaf pan. Line the pan with a piece of parchment paper cut to cover the bottom and extend up the 9-inch sides to about ½ inch above the edges. Butter the paper.

In a large bowl, combine the flour, brewer's yeast and baking soda. In another bowl, combine the bananas, oil or butter, honey, orange juice, egg and vanilla. Mix the liquid ingredients into the dry ones. Pour the mixture into the prepared pan. Bake at 325° for 50 minutes, or until a wooden pick inserted into the center comes out clean. Remove the bread from the pan and immediately peel off the paper.

Makes 1 loaf.

INDEX

A

Abruptio placentae, 246
Absorption of nutrients, factors
  affecting, 23–28
Acetaldehyde, in cigarette smoke,
  46, 64–65
Acetylcholine, 233
Acne, 557
  vitamin A in, 390–93, 569, 708
  zinc in, 391–92, 708
Addiction to heroin, and
  detoxification with vitamin C,
  299–302
Additives in food
  affecting absorption of
    nutrients, 27
  eye problems from, 562
  Yellow No. 5, 163
Adolescence
  delinquency in, 449–54
  folate deficiency in, 461
  weight problems in, 676–77
Adrenal glands, 502
Adriamycin side effects,
  prevention with vitamin E,
  50–51
Advertisements, misleading
  statements in, 14
Aflatoxins, 539–40
Aging, 401–14
  absorption of nutrients in,
    27–28
  · antioxidants affecting, 394–400
  biotin deficiency in, 229
  capillary problems in, 305
  folate deficiency in, 212–13
  malnutrition in, 434
  nutrient needs in, 33–39

osteoporosis in, 318
pyridoxine levels in, 177, 466
shingles in, 550, 551
thiamine requirements in, 126
vitamin B_{12} deficiency in, 188
vitamin D metabolism in,
  324–26
vitamin E needs in, 373,
  397–400
Alcohol intake, 44–46
  folate deficiency from, 213
  in pregnancy, 676
  protective effects of vitamin C
    in, 541
  sperm count affected by, 508
  thiamine loss from, 127
  vision affected by, 87–88
  vitamin C absorption after, 252
Aldose reductase, inhibitors of,
  306–7, 428
Allergies, 633
  bioflavonoids in, 314
  to food, 451–52, 697
  hay fever in, 483–87, 633
  pantothenate in, 219
Amblyopia, nutritional, 561
p-Aminobenzoic acid, 222–24
  interaction with sulfa drugs, 69
Anaphylaxis, vitamin C in, 486
Anemia
  in folate deficiency, 460
  megaloblastic, 204
  pernicious, 67–68, 184, 214
  in riboflavin deficiency, 144–45
  sickle cell, vitamin E in,
    361–62
Angina pectoris. *See* Heart disease
Antacids, effects of, 44, 414